T0382689

Neuromonitoring in Neonatal and Pediatric Critical Care

Drs. Hahn and Wusthoff have masterfully organized and edited this stunning monograph on neuromonitoring in neonatal and pediatric critical care. There is excellent coverage of general and practical considerations with sections devoted individually to neonatal, pediatric, and cardiac intensive care monitoring, *and* 30+ illustrative cases that are concise, instructive, and integrated into the earlier chapters as exemplars. Strong coverage of quantitative EEG, with side-by-side comparisons to conventional EEG, is especially helpful. This book is a welcome addition of immense value to both trainees and experienced practitioners of clinical neurophysiology and pediatric epilepsy.

Phillip L. Pearl MD, Boston Children's Hospital, Harvard Medical School, USA

This is an outstanding, comprehensive, accessible, and well-illustrated book that will be of use to nurses and physicians at different levels of training and from any background, including neurology, critical care, and neonatology, interested in ICU EEG neuromonitoring and the uses and potential of quantitative EEG. Each chapter combines detailed and critical assessments of the literature with liberal use of informative figures that have examples of EEG and quantitative EEG patterns or effective summaries of treatment or diagnostic pathways. One of the book's many strengths is the way the authors treat ICU EEG monitoring as part of a neuromonitoring program and provide a comprehensive overview of the many operational issues required to justify and create such a program. An entire chapter is devoted specifically to nursing, again with a comprehensive scope addressing both interpretation of EEG signals and practical applications of performing EEGs. Developmental issues are addressed across multiple chapters and special populations and pathophysiologies including, for example, ECMO, cardiac arrest, and infants with congenital heart disease. Readers should be aware that the focus is almost exclusively on EEG. With that caveat, this book will be an essential clinical reference and teaching resource for practitioners from multiple specialties who care for neonates and children in intensive care units.

Mark S. Wainwright MD PhD, Pediatric Neurocritical Care Program, University of Washington, Seattle, USA

This book, edited by Cecil Hahn and Courtney Wusthoff and written by many experts in the field, was urgently needed. The last book on investigating the neonatal brain was published more than a decade ago and many advances have been made since. We find extensive information on aEEG, EEG, EEG trends, and a bit on NIRS and evoked potentials in the chapter on neuromonitoring after cardiac arrest. This book does not only address the neonatal brain, but also takes you to the paediatric intensive care unit and the cardiac intensive care unit. The final part provides more than 30 cases, which are referred to at the beginning of each chapter and which I found very interesting and useful.

Linda de Vries, University of Utrecht, Netherlands

The chapters of this excellent textbook run the gamut of practical and logistical aspects of setting up monitoring, to interpreting results and using EEG monitoring for prediction of cardiac arrest and ischemia. The chapters are to the point and the writing crisp. Part 4 was instructive to me, and I've spent my professional life in the CICU. This should be required reading for ICU fellows (PICU, NICU, and CICU), as well as neurology residents.

Daniel J. Licht MD, Professor of Neurology, Department of Pediatrics Distinguished Endowed Chair, Director of the J. and S. Wolfson Family Laboratory for Clinical and Biomedical Optics, Children's Hospital of Philadelphia, USA

Neuromonitoring in Neonatal and Pediatric Critical Care

Edited by

Cecil D. Hahn
The Hospital for Sick Children, University of Toronto

Courtney J. Wusthoff
Lucile Packard Children's Hospital Stanford, Stanford University

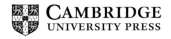
CAMBRIDGE
UNIVERSITY PRESS

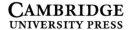

CAMBRIDGE
UNIVERSITY PRESS

University Printing House, Cambridge CB2 8BS, United Kingdom

One Liberty Plaza, 20th Floor, New York, NY 10006, USA

477 Williamstown Road, Port Melbourne, VIC 3207, Australia

314–321, 3rd Floor, Plot 3, Splendor Forum, Jasola District Centre, New Delhi – 110025, India

103 Penang Road, #05–06/07, Visioncrest Commercial, Singapore 238467

Cambridge University Press is part of the University of Cambridge.

It furthers the University's mission by disseminating knowledge in the pursuit of education, learning, and research at the highest international levels of excellence.

www.cambridge.org
Information on this title: www.cambridge.org/9781107145696
DOI: 10.1017/9781316536001

First published 2022

Printed in the United Kingdom by TJ Books Limited, Padstow Cornwall

A catalogue record for this publication is available from the British Library.

Library of Congress Cataloging-in-Publication Data
Names: Hahn, Cecil, editor. | Wusthoff, Courtney, editor.
Title: Neuromonitoring in neonatal and pediatric critical care / edited by Cecil Hahn, Courtney Wusthoff.
Description: Cambridge ; New York, NY : Cambridge University Press, 2022. | Includes bibliographical references and index.
Identifiers: LCCN 2022011257 | ISBN 9781107145696 (hardback) | ISBN 9781316536001 (ebook)
Subjects: MESH: Electroencephalography – methods | Infant | Child | Neurophysiological Monitoring – methods | Seizures – diagnosis | Central Nervous System Diseases – diagnosis | Heart Diseases – diagnosis
Classification: LCC RJ488.5.E44 | NLM WL 150 | DDC 618.92/8047547–dc23/eng/20220404
LC record available at https://lccn.loc.gov/2022011257

ISBN 978-1-107-14569-6 Hardback

....

Contents

Contents

Contributors

Nicholas S. Abend
Departments of Neurology and Pediatrics, The Perelman School of Medicine at the University of Pennsylvania, and The Children's Hospital of Philadelphia, Philadelphia, Pennsylvania

Shefali Aggarwal
Department of Pediatrics, Texas Tech University Health Sciences Center, El Paso, Texas

Daad Alsowat
King Faisal Specialist Hospital and Research Centre, Riyadh, Saudi Arabia

Saadet Mercimek-Andrews
Department of Medical Genetics, Faculty of Medicine and Dentistry, University of Alberta, Edmonton, Alberta

Brian Appavu
University of Arizona College of Medicine – Phoenix, Departments of Child Health and Neurology, Phoenix Children's Hospital, Phoenix, Arizona

Emilie Bourel-Ponchel
INSERM UMR 1105, University of Picardie Jules Verne, Amiens, France

Geraldine B. Boylan
INFANT Research Centre & Department of Paediatrics and Child Health, University College Cork, Cork, Ireland

Ersida Buraniqi
Division of Epilepsy and Clinical Neurophysiology, Department of Neurology, Boston Children's Hospital, Harvard Medical School, Boston, Massachusetts

Jessica L. Carpenter
Division of Pediatric Neurology, University of Mississippi Medical Centre, Jackson, Mississippi

Robert R. Clancy
Departments of Neurology and Pediatrics, The Perelman School of Medicine, at the University of Pennsylvania, and The Children's Hospital of Philadelphia, Philadelphia, Pennsylvania

Genevieve Du Pont-Thibodeau
Sainte-Justine University Hospital, University of Montréal, Montréal, Québec

Erin M. Fedak Romanowski
Division of Pediatric Neurology, C.S. Mott Children's Hospital, University of Michigan, Ann Arbor, Michigan

Marina Gaínza-Lein
Instituto de Pediatría, Facultad de Medicina, Universidad Austral de Chile, Valdivia, Chile

William Gallentine
Department of Neurology and Pediatrics, Lucile Packard Children's Hospital, Palo Alto, California

Cristina Go
Division of Neurology, Department of Paediatrics, British Columbia Children's Hospital, Vancouver, British Columbia

Cecil D. Hahn
Division of Neurology, The Hospital for Sick Children and Department of Paediatrics, University of Toronto, Toronto, Ontario

Puneet Jain
Division of Neurology, The Hospital for Sick Children and Department of Paediatrics, University of Toronto, Toronto, Ontario

Crystal M. Keller
Department of Neurology, Duke University, Durham, North Carolina

Saptharishi Lalgudi Ganesan
Paediatric Critical Care, Children's Hospital – London Health Sciences Center; Department of Paediatrics, Schulich School of Medicine & Dentistry, Western University; Western Institute for Neuroscience, Western University, London, Ontario

Chusak Limotai
Chulalongkorn Comprehensive Epilepsy Center of Excellence, King Chulalongkorn Memorial Hospital, The Thai Red Cross Society; Division of Neurology, Department of Medicine, Faculty of Medicine, Chulalongkorn University, Bangkok, Thailand

Jainn-Jim Lin
Division of Pediatric Critical Care and Pediatric Neurocritical Care, Chang Gung Children's Hospital and Chang Gung Memorial Hospital, Chang Gung University College of Medicine; Graduate Institute of Clinical Medical Sciences, College of Medicine, Chang Gung University, Taoyuan, Taiwan

Brian Livingstone
Duke University Health System, Durham, North Carolina

Tobias Loddenkemper
Division of Epilepsy and Clinical Neurophysiology, Department of Neurology, Boston Children's Hospital, Harvard Medical School, Boston, Massachusetts

Shavonne Massey
Departments of Neurology and Pediatrics, The Perelman School of Medicine at the University of Pennsylvania, The Children's Hospital of Philadelphia, Philadelphia, Pennsylvania

Bláthnaid McCoy
Blackrock Clinic, County Dublin, Ireland

Deirdre M. Murray
Department of Paediatrics and Child Health, University College Cork, Cork, Ireland

Sylvie Nguyen The Tich
Service de Neurologie Pédiatrique, Hôpital Roger Salengro, CHRU de Lille, France

Iris Noyman
Pediatric Neurology Unit, Pediatric Division, Soroka Medical Center and The Faculty of Health Sciences, Ben- Gurion University of the Negev, Beer-Sheva, Israel

Ayako Ochi
Division of Neurology, The Hospital for Sick Children, and Department of Paediatrics, University of Toronto, Toronto, Ontario

Akihisa Okumura
Department of Pediatrics, Aichi Medical University, Nagakute, Japan

Andreea M. Pavel
INFANT Centre, University College Cork, Cork, Ireland and Department of Paediatrics and Child Health, University College Cork, Cork, Ireland.

Elena Pavlidis
Child Neurology and Neurorehabilitation Unit, Department of Pediatrics, Bolzano Regional Hospital, Bolzano, Italy

Eric T. Payne
Section of Pediatric Neurology, Alberta Children's Hospital, and Department of Pediatrics, University of Calgary, Calgary, Alberta

Elana F. Pinchefsky
Division of Neurology, Department of Paediatrics, Sainte-Justine University Hospital Center, University of Montréal; CHU Sainte Justine Research Center, Department of Neurosciences, Montréal, Québec

Ronit Pressler
Department of Clinical Neurophysiology, Great Ormond Street Hospital; Developmental Neurosciences Department, University College London, Great Ormond Street Institute of Child Health, London, UK

Kathi S. Randall
Synapse Care Solutions

Carlos I. Salazar
Division of Neurology, The Hospital for Sick Children, and Department of Paediatrics, University of Toronto, Toronto, Ontario

Iván Sánchez Fernández
Department of Neurology, Boston Medical Centre, Boston, Massachusetts

Jonathan Santoro
Division of Neurology, Department of Pediatrics, Children's Hospital Los Angeles; Department of Neurology, Keck School of Medicine, University of Southern California, Los Angeles, California

Shatha Shafi
Paediatric Neurologist, Epileptologist and Clinical Neurophysiologist, Prince Sultan Military Medical City, Riyadh, Saudi Arabia

Renée A. Shellhaas
Division of Pediatric Neurology, C.S. Mott Children's Hospital and University of Michigan, Ann Arbor, Michigan

Emily W. Y. Tam
Division of Neurology, The Hospital for Sick Children, and Department of Paediatrics, University of Toronto, Toronto, Ontario

Alexis A. Topjian
Department of Anesthesiology and Critical Care Medicine, The Children's Hospital of Philadelphia and the Perelman School of Medicine at the University of Pennsylvania, Philadelphia, Pennsylvania

Tammy Tsuchida
Departments of Neurology and Pediatrics, Children's National Health System, George Washington University School of Medicine, Washington, District of Columbia

Adam Wallace
Division of Pediatric Neurology, Department of Neurology, University of Wisconsin School of Medicine and Public Health, Madison, Wisconsin

Sarah S. Welsh
Department of Anesthesiology and Critical Care Medicine, The Children's Hospital of Philadelphia and the Perelman School of Medicine at the University of Pennsylvania, Philadelphia, Pennsylvania

Robyn Whitney
Division of Pediatric Neurology, Department of Pediatrics, McMaster Children's Hospital, McMaster University, Hamilton, Ontario

Diane Wilson
Division of Neonatology, Department of Paediatrics, The Hospital for Sick Children; Faculty of Nursing, University of Toronto, Toronto, Ontario

Rudolph Wong
Phoenix Children's Hospital, University of Arizona College of Medicine, Tucson, Arizona

Courtney J. Wusthoff
Division of Child Neurology, Department of Neurology, Neurological Sciences & Pediatrics, Stanford University; Lucile Packard Children's Hospital Stanford, California

Elissa Yozawitz
Division of Child Neurology, Department of Neurology and Department of Pediatrics, Albert Einstein College of Medicine and Montefiore Medical Center, Bronx, New York

Acknowledgements

We are indebted to the efforts and support of many individuals who made this book possible.

First, we gratefully acknowledge the contributors, each of whom gave their time to share their remarkable expertise while patiently accommodating our editorial requests over several years. We are grateful to the editorial staff at Cambridge University Press for their guidance and support in this project from its conception to publication.

Dr. Hahn thanks all of the neurodiagnostic technologists at The Hospital for Sick Children for their tireless front-line support in the care of critically ill neonates and children: Roy Sharma, Amrita Viljoen, Ann Richards, Chantal O'Neill, Justine Staley, Lee Robles, Paula Melendres, Sherida Somaru and Ying Wu. Dr. Hahn would like to thank O. Carter Snead III for his visionary leadership which enabled the creation of the SickKids critical care EEG monitoring program, and the many epilepsy fellows, neurophysiologists and epileptologists whose extraordinary teamwork and dedication have sustained the program's growth.

Dr. Wusthoff thanks all of the neurodiagnostic technologists at Lucile Packard Children's Hospital Stanford, whose talents in EEG have allowed us to help children in even the most challenging circumstances: Betty Cobb, Lisa Elliott, Mauricio Rodriguez, Noel Amezquita, Zachary Fuchs, Melanie Lemke, Rose Morlock, Jillian Mazloum, Shahla Young, Jenna Hayes, Borak Phang, and Patty Romero. Many thanks to those clinical neurophysiology and pediatric epilepsy fellows who aided in identifying cases and examples for this text, including Harsheen Kaur and Kavya Rao. Dr. Wusthoff offers her ongoing gratitude to Robert Clancy, whose mentorship has been a cornerstone over many years.

We are grateful to our families for their support and patience: Freya and Alorani; Felix, Javier, and Daniel. Your patience and understanding of the many nights and weekends spent writing and revising have been immensely generous.

Finally, we wish to thank the families and children who have allowed for us to care for them in the most difficult times, and to learn from you so we may better care for others.

Overview of Continuous EEG Monitoring in Critically Ill Neonates and Children

Shavonne L. Massey and Nicholas S. Abend

Key Points

- Seizures are common in critically ill children with acute encephalopathy. Most seizures have no accompanying clinical signs, and therefore detection requires continuous EEG monitoring.
- Guidelines recommend at least 24 hours of continuous EEG monitoring in critically ill neonates and children with clinical and EEG risk factors for seizures.
- Seizures have been associated with worse short- and long-term outcomes in neonates and children, even after adjusting for acute encephalopathy etiology and markers of brain injury severity.
- Although EEG-guided anti-seizure therapy has been shown to reduce seizure burden, it remains to be proven that the resulting reductions in seizure burden improve outcomes.

Introduction

Continuous EEG (cEEG) monitoring offers bedside, noninvasive, diffuse, and continuous information about brain function. These characteristics allow clinicians to assess brain function, evaluate for changes in brain function over time, and identify electrographic seizures that are often not clinically observable (Figure 1.1). These advantages have led to widespread and increasing use of cEEG in critically ill patients across the age spectrum. This chapter introduces cEEG in critically ill neonates and children including seizure epidemiology (incidence and risk factors), the relationship between electrographic seizures and outcome, available consensus statements and guidelines, and role of quantitative EEG.

Electrographic Seizures in Critically Ill Neonates

Incidence

Seizures are a common manifestation of neurological injury and dysfunction in the neonatal period. Across childhood, the occurrence of seizures is highest during the neonatal period [1], with an estimated incidence of 1–3.5 per 1000 live births in term neonates, greater than 25 per 1000 live births in preterm neonates, and 58 per 1000 live births for very low birth weight neonates [1, 2]. A 1998–2002 population-based study from the California Office of Statewide Planning and Development identified the seizure incidence as 0.95 per 1000 live births in term neonates. Risk factors for neonatal seizures were categorized as intrinsic to the neonate, mother, and birthing process

[1, 3]. Intrinsic neonatal risk factors were male sex and low birth weight. Maternal risk factors included nulliparity, age greater than 40 years, race (with a decreased risk in Asian and Hispanic mothers compared to Caucasian mothers), and the presence of diabetes independent of macrosomia. The most significant intrapartum risk factor was maternal fever (as a marker for maternal infection). Additional risk factors included prolonged second stage of labor, fetal distress, cesarean section or surgically assisted vaginal delivery, and "catastrophic" delivery involving placental abruption, uterine rupture, or cord prolapse. Additional risk factors have been less consistent and include an increased risk for African American mothers, young maternal age (18–24 years), preeclampsia, heavy smoking, obesity, and asthma [1].

Risk Factors

There are many etiologic precipitants for neonatal seizures. Hypoxic-ischemic encephalopathy, stroke, intracranial hemorrhage, intracranial infection, and cerebral malformations are reported to cause up to 85% of neonatal seizures [4]. The Neonatal Seizure Registry consortium of seven tertiary care pediatric centers in the United States prospectively studied a cohort of 426 neonates with seizures who underwent cEEG. The most common seizure etiologies were hypoxic-ischemic encephalopathy in 38%, ischemic stroke in 18%, neonatal onset epilepsy in 13%, intracranial hemorrhage in 11%, neonatal genetic epilepsy syndrome in 6%, congenital cerebral malformation in 4%, and benign familial neonatal epilepsy in 3% [5]. In term neonates, hypoxic-ischemic encephalopathy is the most common precipitant, accounting for about 40–50% of cases [1, 2, 5]. Hypoxic-ischemic encephalopathy occurs in 1–2.5 per 1000 live births, is a clinical syndrome characterized by neonatal depression with laboratory evidence of systemic acidosis [6], and is associated with increased rates of acute mortality, seizures, prolonged hospitalizations, and subsequent neurodevelopmental problems, particularly in neonates with moderate and severe hypoxic-ischemic encephalopathy [7–9]. Therapeutic hypothermia is often used as a neuroprotective strategy [10], and it may reduce acute seizure exposure in neonates with moderate hypoxic-ischemic encephalopathy [11–14]. Less common etiologies include metabolic derangements, mitochondrial or metabolic disorders, inborn errors of metabolism, and neonatal epilepsy syndromes. Fewer studies in the preterm population indicate intraventricular hemorrhage is the most common seizure precipitant [12–14].

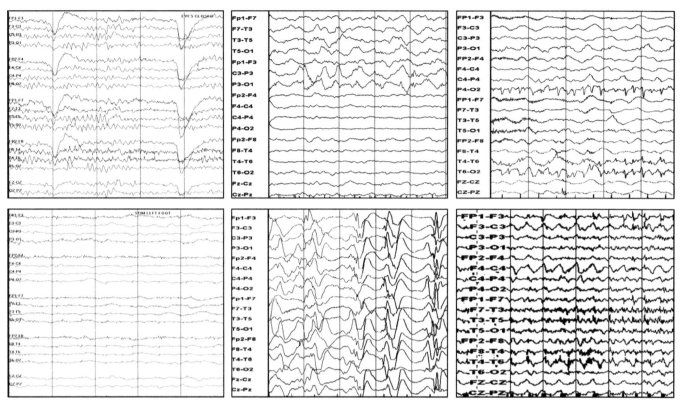

Figure 1.1 Five-second conventional EEG images from critically ill children who all appeared similarly encephalopathic to clinicians. Left top shows a normal EEG pattern, bottom left shows attenuation, middle top shows hemispheric asymmetry, middle bottom shows periodic epileptiform discharges, and the right top and bottom show electrographic seizures.

The EEG background may also help identify neonates at risk for electrographic seizures [15]. A cohort of 51 neonates, including 8 premature neonates, was monitored with cEEG, and the EEG background was graded in five categories: normal, immature for gestational age, mild abnormalities, moderate abnormalities, and severe abnormalities. Seizures occurred in 45% of the cohort, and 96% of the neonates with seizures had an abnormal EEG background. A severely abnormal EEG background predicted the highest risk for seizures while neonates with normal or immature backgrounds had a low risk for seizures. All premature neonates with seizures had mild to severely abnormal background while premature neonates without seizures all had normal or immature EEG backgrounds. The EEG backgrounds remained relatively consistent over the course of the recording (ranging 16–119 hours), with nearly 70% maintaining identical grading from onset to the end of the recording [16].

Diagnosis

There are three broad neonatal seizures types: (1) "clinical-only," which is a sudden paroxysm of abnormal clinical change that does not correlate with a simultaneous EEG seizure; (2) "electroclinical," which is a clinical seizure coupled with an EEG seizure; and (3) "EEG-only," which is an EEG seizure that is not associated with any outwardly visible clinical signs [17]. EEG-only seizures are also called subclinical or nonconvulsive seizures. An electrographic neonatal seizure is defined as

a sudden, abnormal EEG event defined by a repetitive and evolving pattern with a minimum 2 microvolt voltage and duration of at least 10 seconds (Figure 1.2) [17].

Neonatal seizure diagnosis has evolved from a clinical diagnosis to a frequently EEG-based diagnosis for two main reasons. First, paroxysmal abnormal movements or events are common, and it can be very difficult to determine which represent seizures. In a study that included 415 clinically diagnosed neonatal seizures, the suspected seizures were categorized by the four semiology categories: clonic, tonic, myoclonic, and subtle [4]. All clinically diagnosed seizures classified as focal clonic or focal tonic had an EEG correlate. Alternatively, none of the clinically diagnosed seizures classified as generalized tonic or subtle had an EEG correlate. About one-third of clinically diagnosed myoclonic seizures had an EEG correlate. Interestingly, the seizures that had a consistent electrographic correlate (focal clonic and tonic) only comprised about 16% of the clinically diagnosed seizures, while the suspected seizures that more often had no electrographic correlate (generalized tonic and subtle) comprised 55% of the clinically diagnosed seizures. Myoclonic seizures that inconsistently had an electrographic correlate were also common, comprising 25% of the clinically diagnosed seizures. Focal EEG seizures had a high correlation with focal brain lesion and favorable short-term outcome, while clinical seizures without electrographic correlate were associated with diffuse processes, such as hypoxic-ischemic encephalopathy, and unfavorable short-term

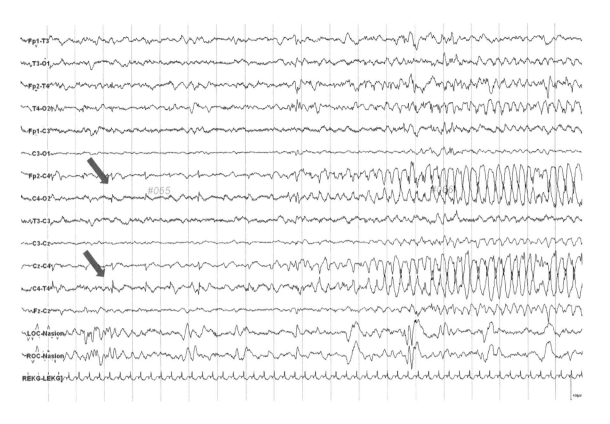

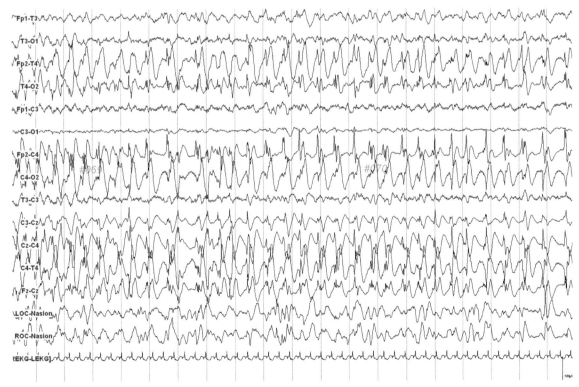

Figure 1.2 Electroclinical seizure in a full-term neonate. (a) The seizure begins with rhythmic 1 Hz sharp waves in the right central region (C4). (b) The sharp waves evolve in amplitude and frequency in the right central region (C4) and spreads to the right temporal region (T4). Thirty seconds after electrographic onset of the seizure, the infant exhibited a left arm clonic seizure.

outcomes [18]. Similarly, a retrospective audit of 43 neonates with 160 electrographic seizures found 56% of the neonates had clinical signs with the electrographic seizure, and, of those, 89% had multiple clinical features. The most common clinical features seen were subtle seizures: ocular movements (70%), oro-lingual movements (56%), and autonomic changes (56%). In contrast, clonic movements and tonic movements were seen at any point during seizure in only 23% and 25% of neonates, respectively [19]. These studies indicate that although focal tonic and clonic movements are often associated with electrographic seizure, they occur less commonly than subtle clinical movements, which are inconsistently associated with electrographic seizures.

Considering the aforementioned studies, it is understandable that a solely clinical diagnosis of neonatal seizures is difficult for clinicians. A study of 51 neonates undergoing video EEG demonstrated the difficulties that practitioners face. Nine neonates had electrographic seizures and three neonates had clinical seizures. On video review, only one-third of the electrographic seizures had a clinical correlate while two-thirds of the seizures were EEG-only. In total, clinical staff correctly identified only 9% of the seizures based on clinical observation. Simultaneously, clinical staff identified numerous movements that were clinically concerning for seizures, and only 27% had an electrographic correlate [20]. Similarly, a study showed video clips from 20 neonates with abnormal movements to 137 healthcare professionals, including nurses and doctors with varying degrees of experience, each of whom opined on the nature of the movements. Overall, 50% of the abnormal movements were correctly identified as seizures, with clonic movements more often correctly identified than subtle movements. Inter-observer agreement was poor [21]. These data indicate that clinical seizure diagnosis is problematic since clinicians underdiagnose seizures without an identifiable clinical correlate and incorrectly classify paroxysmal neonatal movements as seizures, potentially leading to unnecessary anti-seizure medication administration.

The second reason clinical seizure diagnosis is difficult is that electroclinical seizures represent a minority of the true neonatal seizure burden in most neonates experiencing seizures. EEG-only seizures are very common in neonates. Across neonatal cohorts, rates of EEG-only seizures identified by both cEEG and amplitude-integrated EEG (aEEG) range from 10% to 79% [22–25]. EEG-only seizures may occur before any treatment, and they are even more common after anti-seizure medication administration. Further, about 50% of neonates experience electroclinical dissociation in which there is an uncoupling of electrographic seizure activity and clinical signs following treatment with an anti-seizure medication [26]. Thus, administration of an anti-seizure medication terminates clinically evident seizures, but EEG-only seizures persist.

For these reasons, it is now recognized that clinical diagnosis alone is insufficient to optimally quantify neonatal seizures. Clinical seizure diagnosis both overestimates that non-ictal events are seizures (leading to unnecessary exposure to anti-

seizure medications with potential adverse effects) and underestimates the true incidence of seizure in neonates (potentially missing treatment and yielding seizure-induced secondary brain injury). As a result, there is increasing use of cEEG in neonatal intensive care units [27, 28–30].

Among neonates with seizures, the seizure exposure is often high. Neonatal status epilepticus has been defined as present when the summed duration of seizures comprising $\geq$50% of an arbitrarily defined 1 hour epoch [17]. Across critically ill neonates, the incidence of status epilepticus has been reported as 10%–60% [24, 25, 31, 32].

Prognostication Using Neonatal EEG

While seizure identification and the differential diagnosis of paroxysmal events are the primary reasons to perform cEEG monitoring in neonates, another important indication is assessment of the EEG background (Figure 1.3) [15]. EEG background assessment may help to predict neurodevelopmental outcomes, particularly in neonates with hypoxic-ischemic encephalopathy, in whom clinical variables are not reliable predictors of outcomes [31, 33]. However, EEG background, while more objective than some clinical features or examination signs, also only imperfectly predicts outcomes [34–37]. A 2016 systematic review included EEG and aEEG studies from 1960 to 2014 assessing EEG background features in neonates with hypoxic-ischemic encephalopathy. A total of 31 studies were identified with 1948 term neonates ($\geq$36 weeks gestational age) with hypoxic-ischemic encephalopathy who had neurodevelopmental outcome information available at 12 months of age or older. Given the time span of the studies, therapeutic hypothermia was only used in 23% of neonates. The review found that burst suppression, low voltage, and flat EEG tracings were the most accurate predictors of unfavorable neurodevelopmental outcomes, having both high sensitivity and specificity. Individual studies used a mixture of structured and unique measures to determine outcomes. For the meta-analysis, neurodevelopmental outcomes were recorded in a binary fashion with normal outcome defined as any normal, minor, or mildly abnormal outcomes in individual testing and abnormal outcome defined as a moderate or severely abnormal or death outcome. Burst suppression had a pooled sensitivity of 0.87 and pooled specificity of 0.82, low voltage had a pooled sensitivity of 0.92 and pooled specificity of 0.99, and flat tracing had a pooled sensitivity of 0.78 and pooled specificity of 0.99. Though three predictive background features were found, the authors noted a lack of standardized definitions used for neonatal EEG background terms across the studies. EEG type was also not standardized across studies, with 45% using cEEG, 45% using aEEG, and 10% using a combination [38].

Serial EEGs, particularly when background abnormalities persist, have stronger predictive value for outcomes than single EEG assessments. A retrospective study reviewed a heterogeneous group of 58 newborns with neonatal seizures who had at least two EEG recordings during the neonatal period and follow-up at 30–40 months. The persistence of abnormal background activity on sequential EEGs was more significantly

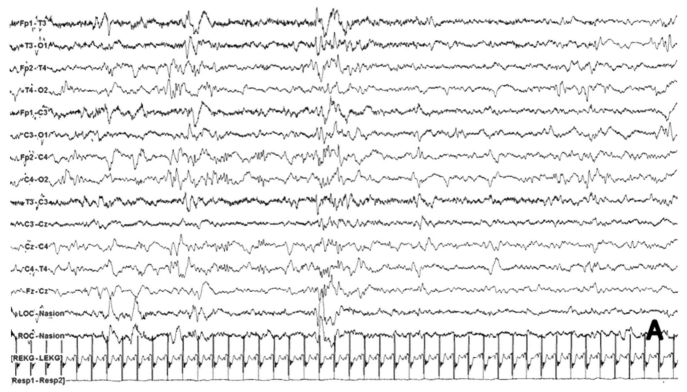

Figure 1.3 Neonatal EEG background patterns. (A) Normal EEG background of an awake term neonate consisting of continuous, low-moderate voltage (25–50 microvolts peak-to-peak) delta and theta activity with overriding beta activity. This pattern is also referred to as "activité moyenne." (B) Excessively discontinuous EEG of a term neonate in quiet sleep. The EEG is considered discontinuous because of prolonged (greater than 6 seconds) inter-burst intervals [arrow denotes onset] that are composed of low-voltage (less than 25 microvolts) mixed-frequency activity. (C) Burst suppression EEG of a term neonate, defined as invariant EEG bursts separated by prolonged and attenuated (less than 5 microvolts) inter-burst intervals. Bursts [denoted by stars] are characterized by sharply contoured, high-voltage (often greater than 200 microvolts) mixed-frequency activity with imbedded spike wave discharges. (D) Electrocerebral inactivity on EEG with the absence of all discernable cerebral activity, defined by lack of any EEG activity greater than 2 microvolts. This is also referred to as "electrocerebral silence" or "isoelectric EEG."

associated with neurodevelopmental delays (relative risk 2.20; p=0.006), as well as the development of postnatal epilepsy (relative risk 1.8; p=0.041). The development of an abnormal EEG background between the first and second EEG (first EEG is normal, second EEG is abnormal) increased the risk of neurodevelopmental delays (relative risk 2.20). Regarding specific background abnormalities, the presence of burst suppression on any EEG was associated with postnatal epilepsy (p=0.013) and postnatal death (p=0.034) [39]. Continuous EEG monitoring carries the benefit of assessing EEG background across multiple time points, like the benefit of serial EEGs.

Electrographic Seizures in Critically Ill Children

Incidence

Observational studies of interdisciplinary neurological critical care services at large pediatric institutions describe seizures and status epilepticus as the most commonly managed conditions [40, 41]. A study in a quaternary care children's hospital described that among 373 pediatric neurocritical care consultations over one year, 18% of consults related to an admission diagnosis of status epilepticus, 35% of consultations related to evaluation of seizures or possible seizures, and cEEG

monitoring was performed in 19% of patients [40]. A second study from a quaternary care children's hospital described that among 615 pediatric neurocritical care consultations over a 32-month period, 48% of diagnoses related to epilepsy, seizures, or status epilepticus. EEG was often used, including cEEG monitoring in 28% [41].

Studies of critically ill children undergoing clinically indicated cEEG monitoring report electrographic seizures occur in 10%–50% of patients (Figure 1.4). Further, about one-third of critically ill children with electrographic seizures have a sufficiently high seizure burden to be categorized as electrographic status epilepticus [42–63]. Studies have used varying definitions for electrographic status epilepticus, but a common criterion has been 50% of any 1-hour epoch containing seizure activity. For example, this could constitute a single 30-minute seizure or five 6-minute seizures. The largest epidemiological study of cEEG monitoring in the pediatric intensive care unit was a retrospective study in which 11 tertiary care pediatric institutions each enrolled 50 consecutive subjects, thereby yielding 550 subjects. Electrographic seizures occurred in 30% of subjects. Among subjects with electrographic seizures, electrographic status epilepticus occurred in 33% of subjects and exclusively EEG-only seizures occurred in 35% of subjects [54]. These data are consistent with other single center studies [44, 47, 49–51, 53, 55–57, 59, 61–63]. The indications for cEEG

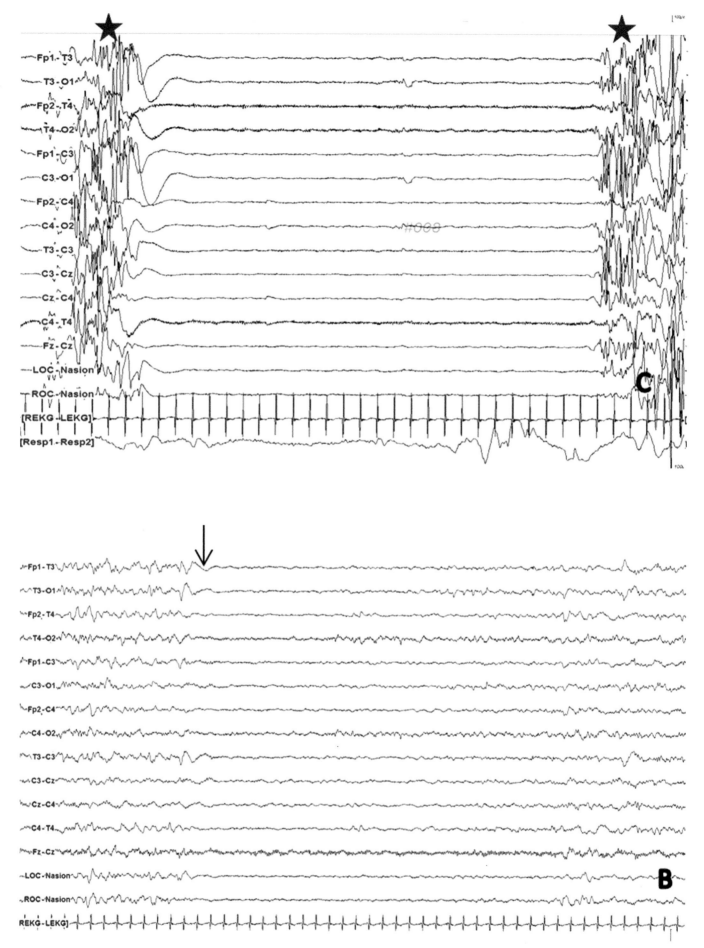

Figure 1.3 (Cont.)

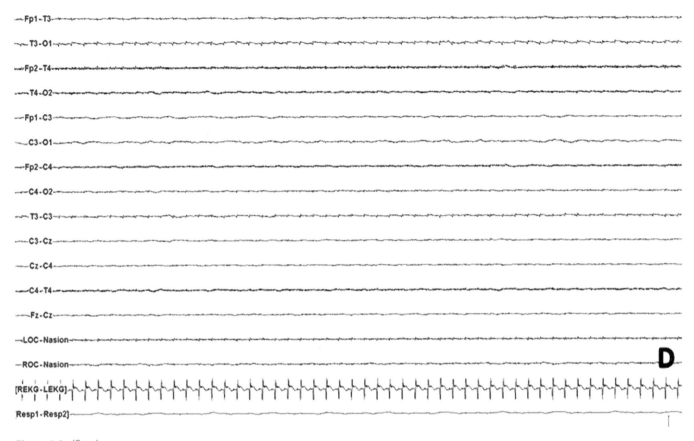

Figure 1.3 (Cont.)

monitoring varied across these studies. Some studies included only patients with known acute structural neurological disorders (e.g., hypoxic-ischemic brain injury, encephalitis, or traumatic brain injury), while other studies included patients with encephalopathy due to broader and more heterogeneous diagnoses (e.g., both primary neurological and primary medical conditions). Inclusion criteria variability may explain the broad reported electrographic seizure incidences since lower electrographic seizure incidences are reported by studies with broader inclusion criteria. Additionally, many of the studies were small as reflected in the wide 95% confidence intervals in Figure 1.4. When individual subjects from these studies are combined, the overall electrographic seizure diagnosis rate is 34% and the electrographic status epilepticus diagnosis rate is 14% [64].

Risk Factors

Continuous EEG monitoring is resource-intensive, and seemingly small utilization and workflow changes have substantial impacts on equipment and personnel needs [65, 66]. Thus, identifying children at higher risk for experiencing electrographic seizures may be beneficial in optimally directing limited cEEG monitoring resources. Several risk factors for electrographic seizures have been reported: (1) younger age (infants as compared to older children) [49, 52, 54, 57, 59]; (2) the occurrence of convulsive seizures [50, 54, 55] or convulsive

status epilepticus [49] prior to initiation of cEEG monitoring; (3) the presence of acute structural brain injury [48–50, 52, 53, 55, 57, 61]; and (4) the presence of interictal epileptiform discharges [49, 53–55] or periodic epileptiform discharges [44]. Importantly, EEG-only seizures occur in children who have not received paralytics recently or ever during their intensive care unit stay [56, 59]. This indicates that clinically evident changes are not simply masked by paralytic administration, but that there is an electromechanical uncoupling (or electromechanical dissociation) between the electrographic seizures and observable seizure manifestations.

Unfortunately, these risk factors may have limited clinical utility in selecting patients to undergo cEEG monitoring. Although statistically significant, the absolute difference in the proportion of children with and without electrographic seizures based on the presence or absence of a risk factor is often only 10%–20%. Seizure prediction models combining multiple risk factors might allow better targeting of cEEG monitoring within the resource limitations of an individual medical center. A recent study derived and validated an electrographic seizure prediction model with fair to good discrimination, indicating that most, but not all, patients were appropriately classified. If a center implemented the broadest cEEG monitoring use recommended by the model, 58% of patients without electrographic seizures would be identified as not needing cEEG monitoring, thereby reducing cEEG monitoring utilization. However, 14% of patients with

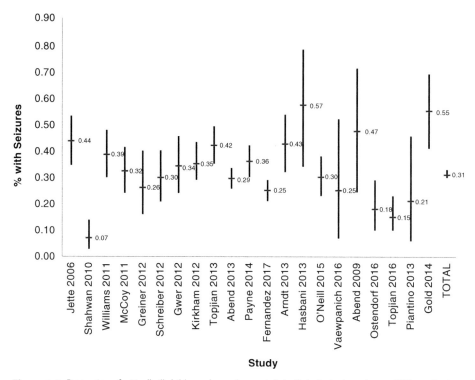

Figure 1.4 Proportion of critically ill children who underwent clinically indicated continuous EEG monitoring with electrographic seizures and electrographic status epilepticus. Each individual study is listed on the x-axis, with vertical lines representing the 95% confidence interval for each. Adapted to add additional publications from original image reprinted from *Epilepsy and Behavior*, 49, Abend NS, Electrographic status epilepticus in children with critical illness: Epidemiology and outcome. 223–7, 2015, with permission from Elsevier.

electrographic seizures would not undergo cEEG monitoring, so their seizures would not be identified and managed [67]. Further development of seizure prediction models in more homogeneous cohorts using additional variables might yield improved performance characteristics.

Timing

Decisions regarding the duration of cEEG monitoring must balance the goal of identifying electrographic seizures against practical concerns regarding resources required to perform cEEG monitoring. Observational studies of critically ill children undergoing clinically indicated cEEG monitoring have reported that about 50% of patients with electrographic seizures are identified with 1 hour of cEEG monitoring and 90% of patients with electrographic seizures are identified with 24–48 hours of cEEG monitoring (Figure 1.5) [44, 47, 49, 50, 53, 55, 56, 59]. However, there are limitations to these data. Most of the studies calculated timing based on cEEG monitoring initiation, which is generally not the same as the onset of the acute brain insult. Additionally, patients generally underwent 1–3 days of clinically indicated cEEG monitoring, so some patients may have had electrographic seizures after cEEG monitoring was discontinued. Based on these data, the Neurocritical Care Society's Guideline for the Evaluation and Management of Status Epilepticus strongly recommends performing cEEG monitoring for 48 hours to identify electrographic status epilepticus in comatose children following an

acute brain insult [68]. Similarly, the American Clinical Neurophysiology Society's Consensus Statement on CEEG monitoring in Critically Ill Children and Adults recommends performing cEEG monitoring for at least 24 hours in children at risk for electrographic seizures [69]. A survey of neurologists regarding cEEG monitoring utilization described that most perform 24–48 hours of cEEG monitoring when screening for electrographic seizures [70].

Determining whether to monitor for 24 or 48 hours has a substantial impact on resource utilization. Monitoring for 48 hours identifies slightly more patients with electrographic seizures than monitoring for 24 hours, but since all patients including those who don't experience electrographic seizures must be monitored for an extra day, there is substantial additional resource utilization [65, 66]. A cost-effectiveness analysis used estimated variable costs directly related to cEEG monitoring and estimates of electrographic seizure occurrence from a literature review; this found that the cost-effectiveness of 24 hours of cEEG monitoring per patient identified experiencing seizures was relatively stable across seizure probabilities. However, for 48 hours of cEEG monitoring, as the probability of electrographic seizures decreased the incremental cost-effectiveness ratio increased substantially [66]. Optimized value-based cEEG monitoring approaches might use broad inclusion criteria for 24 hours of cEEG monitoring but select only high-risk patients using a seizure prediction model to determine which patients need additional monitoring to 48 hours or longer.

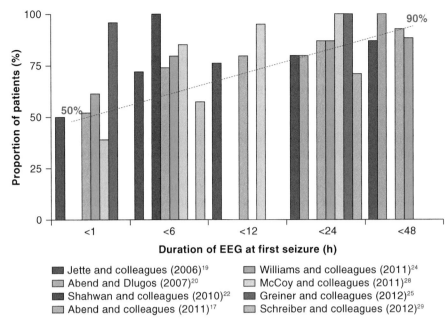

Figure 1.5 Duration of EEG monitoring at onset of the first electrographic seizure in critically ill children. Reprinted from *Lancet Neurology*, 12(12), Abend NS, Wusthoff CJ, Goldberg EM, Dlugos DJ. Electrographic seizures and status epilepticus in critically ill children and neonates with encephalopathy. 1170–9, 2013, with permission from Elsevier.

Relationship between Seizures and Outcomes

Greater electrographic seizure exposures are associated with worse outcomes in critically ill neonates and children. However, the extent to which electrographic seizures produce secondary brain injury versus serve as biomarkers of more severe acute brain injury remains uncertain. Further, the extent to which electrographic seizures produce secondary brain injury is likely dependent on a complex interplay between acute brain injury etiology, seizure exposure, and seizure management strategies. Even seizure exposure may be complex and related to multiple seizure characteristics including duration, anatomical extent, morphology, frequency, and voltage. Despite these complexities, many studies have identified associations between seizures, particularly high seizure exposures, and unfavorable outcomes. This holds true even after adjusting for variables reflecting acute brain injury etiology, acute brain injury severity, and critical illness severity. These data indicate that in at least some patients, electrographic seizures may cause secondary brain injury and subsequently worse neurobehavioral outcomes.

Observational Studies in Neonates

Neonates with seizures have increased short-term and long-term risks of mortality and morbidity. While the underlying seizure etiology substantially determines outcome, there is some evidence that seizures independently worsen outcomes.

Retrospective studies have assessed the relationship between seizures and neurodevelopmental outcomes. A study evaluated 56 neonates with hypoxic-ischemic encephalopathy who underwent therapeutic hypothermia, cEEG monitoring, and subsequent magnetic resonance imaging (MRI). Seizures

occurred in 30% of the cohort. The presence of seizures conferred an increased risk of moderate to severe injury on MRI (relative risk 2.3, p=0.02). Neonates with seizures were more likely to display cortical or near total brain injury on MRI [71]. Similarly, in a heterogeneous cohort of 68 neonates at risk for seizures who underwent cEEG monitoring, the presence of seizures was associated with increased risk of death due to neurological causes in the first year of life (relative risk 7, p<0.02) and of cerebral palsy (relative risk 2, p<0.05). Seizure burden was associated with microcephaly (p=0.04), severe cerebral palsy (p=0.03), and failure to thrive (p=0.03) [72]. In a study of 311 full-term neonates with seizures monitored with aEEG, 65 neonates (18%) had clinical or electrographic status epilepticus. Among the subgroup of neonates with hypoxic-ischemic encephalopathy, longer duration of status epilepticus was associated with worse outcome (215 minutes of seizures in poor outcome versus 85 minutes of seizures in good outcome, p<0.05) [73].

Two studies have evaluated the response to anti-seizure medications to assess the relationship between neonatal seizures and outcomes. A retrospective study of 52 neonates monitored with EEG for seizures graded both seizure severity (mild, moderate, severe) and change in severity over time. Neonates were stratified by their response to anti-seizure medications in the neonatal period. There was no association between anti-seizure medication response and later developmental outcomes. However, seizure severity did predict outcomes, with mild- and moderate-severity seizures associated with normal (p=0.002) or moderate (p=0.007) outcomes [74]. Seizure refractoriness may also confer worsened outcomes. A retrospective study of 46 term neonates with refractory neonatal seizures due to heterogeneous etiologies used the number of anti-seizure medications administered as a surrogate measure of seizure severity. Among neonates who received ≤2 anti-seizure medications versus ≥3 anti-seizure medications, normal development occurred in 50% versus 5%, moderate disability occurred in 20% versus 27%, and severe disability occurred in 30% versus 68% (p<0.01) [75].

Although the above studies demonstrate a consistent association between seizure burden, refractoriness to treatment, and outcome, their univariate analyses did not adjust for the severity of the underlying brain injury, an important potential confounder. Several studies have performed multivariate analyses adjusting for variables reflecting brain injury severity [76–79]. A multicenter prospective study of 85 neonates ≥36 weeks gestational age with moderate-severe hypoxic-ischemic encephalopathy treated with therapeutic hypothermia and undergoing aEEG identified seizures in 52%, including 35% with high seizure burden (>15 minutes per hour) or status epilepticus. In multivariate analyses accounting for severity of underlying injury as reflected by aEEG background and Apgar scores, high seizure burden remained associated with a severe pattern of MRI injury (odds ratio 5, 95% confidence interval 1.47–17.05, p=0.01) [76]. Similarly, a prospective study of 77 neonates with hypoxic-ischemic encephalopathy of at least 36 weeks gestational age evaluated for largely clinical seizure occurrence and seizure severity. Even after adjustment for MRI severity of hypoxic-ischemic brain injury, every 1-point increase in the seizure severity scale was associated with a 4.7-point reduction in intelligence quotient (IQ). The median IQ for neonates with no seizures, mild/moderate seizures, and severe seizure burdens were 97, 83, and 67, respectively. After adjustment for MRI severity, the seizure severity score was also associated with an increased odds of an abnormal neuro-motor score (odds ratio 20, 95% confidence interval 3–140) [77]. A multicenter prospective cohort of 49 neonates of at least 36 weeks gestational age with moderate to severe hypoxic-ischemic encephalopathy treated with therapeutic hypothermia was monitored with aEEG for occurrence of seizure. Seizures occurred in 59% of neonates and seizure burden was scored as low (no seizures or <15 minutes of seizure per 1 hour) or high (>15 minutes of seizure per 1 hour). A multivariate analysis that included seizure burden and aEEG discontinuity demonstrated an association between high seizure burden and severe MRI brain injury with an odds ratio of 4.2 for severe MRI injury with high seizure burden (95% confidence interval 1.01–17.5, p=0.05). Although severe MRI injury was associated with unfavorable neurodevelopmental outcomes (Pearson's R 0.62, p<0.001), the direct relationship between seizure burden and neurodevelopmental outcome was not assessed [78]. Together, these studies using multivariate analyses indicate that even after adjusting for variables reflecting hypoxic-ischemic injury severity, seizures are associated with worse MRI injury and worse neurobehavioral outcomes.

Randomized Controlled Trials in Neonates

Two randomized controlled trials exploring the effects of treating subclinical seizures in neonates with hypoxic-ischemic encephalopathy have demonstrated that EEG-guided therapy

can reduce seizure burden and that higher seizure burden is associated with worse neurodevelopmental and neuroimaging outcomes [80, 81]. A multicenter study of 63 infants with hypoxic-ischemic encephalopathy monitored all neonates ≥37 weeks gestational age with aEEG. At the time of the first seizure on aEEG, 33 neonates who experienced seizures were randomized to treatment of all seizures (clinical and aEEG) or treatment of only the clinically evident seizures. However, all neonates underwent aEEG, so the true seizure burden was available for all. There was a non-significant trend toward lower seizure burden on aEEG in the group with treatment of all seizures (195 versus 503 minutes). Further, neonates who died had experienced a higher seizure burden than survivors (428 minutes versus 164 minutes). Additionally, MRI injury severity correlated with seizure burden among the entire cohort (p<0.001) and among the neonates treated for only clinical seizures (p=0.001). However, there was no significant difference in MRI injury severity between the two treatment groups (p=0.292) [80].

A second randomized controlled trial enrolled neonates ≥36 weeks gestational age with moderate to severe hypoxic-ischemic encephalopathy or neonates with clinical seizures. All underwent continuous EEG to assess seizure burden, but neonates were randomized to treatment of all seizures (clinical and cEEG) or only the clinically evident seizures. Thirty-five neonates who had been randomized experienced seizures and thus provided the analyzed study cohort with 15 in the EEG-guided treatment group and 20 in the group treating only clinical seizures. Neonates with status epilepticus were excluded from analysis. The median duration of seizures was significantly lower in the EEG than clinical group (449 versus 2226 seconds, p=0.02). There were also a lower number of seizures in the electrographic seizure group than the clinical seizure group (median of 7 versus 12, [p=0.04]), and the time to treatment completion was lower in the electrographic seizure group than the clinical seizure group (mean of 79 minutes versus 170 minutes, [p=0.04]). When combining both treatment groups, higher seizure burden was associated with worse MRI injury scores (p<0.03) and lower performance on Bayley neurodevelopmental testing (cognitive composite R=0.502 p=0.03; motor composite R=0.497 p=0.01; language composite R=0.444 p=0.03). However, there were no significant differences in MRI injury score or neurodevelopmental outcome between the two treatment groups, likely due to the small sample size [81].

Observational Studies in Children

Several studies in critically ill children have identified an association between electrographic seizures, particularly with high seizure exposures, and worse outcomes. This association holds even after adjustment for potential confounders related to acute encephalopathy etiology, acute encephalopathy severity, and critical illness severity. A prospective observational study of EEG in 204 critically ill neonates and children found occurrence of electrographic seizures was associated with a higher risk of unfavorable neurological outcome (odds ratio 15.4) in a multivariate analysis that included age, etiology, pediatric index of mortality score, Adelaide coma score, and EEG background categories [51].

Several other studies aimed to evaluate the effect of seizure burden and categorically classified children as having no seizures, electrographic seizures, or electrographic status epilepticus. A single-center study of 200 children in the pediatric intensive care unit with outcome assessed at discharge identified an association between electrographic status epilepticus and higher mortality (odds ratio 5.1) and worsening Pediatric Cerebral Performance Category scores (odds ratio 17.3) in multivariate analyses including seizure category, age, acute neurological disorder, prior neurodevelopmental status, and EEG background categories. Electrographic seizures less than electrographic status epilepticus were not associated with worse outcomes [82]. A multicenter study of 550 children in the pediatric intensive care unit reported an association between electrographic status epilepticus and mortality (odds ratio 2.4) in a multivariate analysis that included seizure category, acute encephalopathy etiology, and EEG background categories. Electrographic seizures not classified as electrographic status epilepticus were not associated with mortality [54].

A single-center prospective study evaluated 259 critically ill infants and children who underwent cEEG monitoring. There were electrographic seizures in 36% of subjects, and 9% of those with seizures had electrographic status epilepticus. The mean maximum hourly seizure burden (proportion of each hour containing seizures) was 16% in subjects with neurological decline versus 2% in subjects without neurological decline. In a multivariate analysis that adjusted for diagnosis and illness severity, for every 1% increase in the maximum hourly seizure burden, the odds of neurological decline increased by 1.13. Maximum hourly seizure burdens of 10%, 20%, and 30% were associated with odds ratios for neurological decline as measured using the Pediatric Cerebral Performance Category scores of 3.3, 10.8, and 35.7, respectively. [58].

A study addressing long-term outcome obtained follow-up data at a median of 2.7 years following admission to the pediatric intensive care unit in 60 encephalopathic children who were neurodevelopmentally normal prior to admission to the pediatric intensive care unit and underwent clinically indicated cEEG monitoring. Multivariate analysis including acute neurological diagnosis category, EEG background category, age, and several other clinical variables identified an association between electrographic status epilepticus and unfavorable Glasgow Outcome Scale (Extended Pediatric Version) category (odds ratio 6.36), lower Pediatric Quality of Life Inventory scores (median of 23.07 points lower), and an increased risk of subsequently diagnosed epilepsy (odds ratio 13.3). Children with electrographic seizures not classified as electrographic status epilepticus did not have worse outcomes in this study [83].

Summary

Taken together, these studies indicate that at least in some critically ill neonates and children, there may be a dose-dependent or threshold effect of electrographic seizures upon outcomes, with high seizure exposures having clinically relevant adverse impacts. This threshold may vary based on age, brain injury etiology, and seizure characteristics such as the extent of brain involved and electroencephalographic morphology. However, an important caveat to these data is that most of these were observational studies in which clinicians did identify and manage electrographic seizures, yet despite this management, electrographic seizures remained associated with worse outcomes. It is possible that seizure identification and management did partially improve outcomes that would have been worse if the seizures had not been identified and managed. Thus, optimized seizure identification and management approaches might yield improved outcomes. Further study is needed to develop optimal management strategies and assess their impact on outcomes.

Clinical Practice Guidelines and Consensus Statements

Neonates

There are three guidelines and consensus statements related to EEG in neonates: those published by the American Clinical Neurophysiology Society [15, the World Health Organization [84], and the American Academy of Pediatrics [10].

In 2011 the American Clinical Neurophysiology Society published a guideline on cEEG monitoring in the neonate created by a panel of expert neurophysiologists based on extensive literature review [15]. The guideline describes two main purposes of cEEG monitoring in the neonate: (1) electrographic seizure identification, and (2) encephalopathy assessment. There are several indications related to electrographic seizure identification (Table 1.1). First, cEEG monitoring may be used to determine whether paroxysmal clinical events are seizures. The likelihood that such events are electroclinical seizures is increased in high-risk populations, including those with acute encephalopathy, cardiac or pulmonary conditions that increase the risk for acute brain injury, central nervous system infection, brain trauma, inborn errors of metabolism, perinatal stroke, prematurity with intraventricular hemorrhage, and genetic syndromes. Second, cEEG monitoring may be used to identify EEG-only seizures that have no identifiable clinical correlate and can only be identified using cEEG monitoring. Third, cEEG monitoring may be used during weaning of anti-seizure medications to evaluate for recurrent seizures. Fourth, cEEG monitoring can be used to characterize burst suppression. Regarding encephalopathy assessment, cEEG provides a marker of brain function. Tracking changes in the EEG background over time may identify changes in an encephalopathic infant whose neurological status may not be assessed by clinical examination. Some EEG background features are predictive of long-term outcomes [15] and a normal EEG background has been associated with a low risk of acute seizures [85]. All high-risk neonates should be monitored for at least 24 hours to screen for electrographic seizures,

Table 1.1 Neonatal populations at high risk for seizures, adapted from the American Clinical Neurophysiology Society's Guideline on Continuous Electroencephalography Monitoring in Neonates, *J Clinical Neurophysiology* 2011.

Category	Examples
Acute neonatal encephalopathy	HIE, postnatal collapse
Cardiac or pulmonary risk for brain injury	ECMO, congenital heart defects perioperatively
CNS infection	Meningitis, encephalitis
CNS trauma	Subarachnoid bleeding, nonaccidental trauma
Inborn errors of metabolism	Organic and amino acidurias, urea cycle defects
Stroke	Arterial stroke, venous thrombosis
At-risk preterm infants	Acute IVH
Genetic/syndromic disease	Cerebral dysgenesis, multiple anomalies with encephalopathy
Use of paralytic medications	As indicated by postoperative or ventilatory management

even if clinically concerning movements have not occurred. Multiple studies in high-risk groups show that most acute seizures occur within 24–72 hours of the acute brain insult [24, 76, 86–89]. If seizures are identified, then the guideline recommends continuing cEEG monitoring for an additional 24 hours after the last electrographic seizure to ensure full resolution. If cEEG monitoring is used for differential diagnosis of abnormal paroxysmal events, then it is recommended that cEEG monitoring continue until all events have been captured adequately on EEG and the presence or absence of an electrographic correlate can be assessed. Technical standards for EEG recording and reporting are further detailed in the American Clinical Neurophysiology Society's Standardized EEG Terminology and Categorization for the Description of CEEG monitoring in Neonates (see Chapter 2) [17].

In 2011 the World Health Organization published a guideline on neonatal seizures that was a multidisciplinary effort based on a formal literature review published with the guideline [84]. While neonatal seizure treatment recommendations were considered weak with low evidence, all recommendations regarding cEEG monitoring were considered strong, with the expert panel finding that desirable effects of cEEG monitoring outweigh any undesirable effects. More specifically, the guideline strongly recommended that in specialized facilities where cEEG monitoring is available, all clinical seizures should be confirmed by EEG and all electrical seizures should be treated, including those without clinical correlate only identifiable using cEEG.

In 2014 a clinical report from the American Academy of Pediatrics reviewing neonatal encephalopathy and the use of therapeutic hypothermia recognized that there was variation in the neuromonitoring capabilities of centers performing therapeutic hypothermia [10]. The committee concluded that centers offering therapeutic hypothermia should be capable of providing comprehensive care for affected neonates, which includes seizure detection and monitoring with some form of EEG (conventional EEG or amplitude-integrated EEG).

Children

There are two guidelines and consensus statements related to cEEG monitoring in critically ill children: those published by the Neurocritical Care Society [68] and the American Clinical Neurophysiology Society [69, 90].

The Neurocritical Care Society's Guidelines for the Evaluation and Management of Status Epilepticus recommends 48 hours of cEEG monitoring to identify electrographic seizures in at-risk patients including (1) patients with persisting altered mental status for more than 10 minutes after convulsive seizures or status epilepticus, and (2) encephalopathic children after resuscitation from cardiac arrest, with traumatic brain injury, with intracranial hemorrhage, or with unexplained encephalopathy. If status epilepticus occurs (including electrographic status epilepticus), then the guideline recommends that management should continue until both clinical and electrographic seizures are halted [68].

The American Clinical Neurophysiology Society's Consensus Statement on Continuous EEG monitoring in Critically Ill Children and Adults recommends cEEG monitoring for 24–48 hours in children at risk for seizures. EEG monitoring indications include: (1) recent convulsive seizures or convulsive status epilepticus with altered mental status, (2) cardiac arrest resuscitation or with other forms of hypoxic-ischemic encephalopathy, (3) stroke (intracerebral hemorrhage, ischemic stroke, and subarachnoid hemorrhage), and (4) encephalitis and altered mental status with related medical conditions. The consensus statement provides additional detailed recommendations regarding personnel, technical specifications, and overall workflow [69, 90].

Summary

Multiple guidelines regarding cEEG monitoring in neonates and children provide a wide range of indications focused on identification of electrographic seizures that may be difficult or impossible to diagnose by clinical observation alone. These guidelines call for relatively wide use of cEEG monitoring based on the presumption that seizure identification and management reduce secondary brain injury and improve outcomes. While seizures are certainly common in many of the cohorts recommended for monitoring making cEEG monitoring reasonable, few data are available to guide management when seizures are identified. Further study of both specific anti-seizure medications and overall seizure management approaches is needed, since to serve as a neuroprotective strategy, seizure identification using cEEG monitoring must be followed by evidence-based optimized seizure management.

Quantitative EEG for Electrographic Seizure Identification

There are two key problems with expanding cEEG monitoring in critically ill neonates and children. First, cEEG monitoring among critically ill patients is resource-intensive and requires substantial electroencephalographer time to review the full tracing. Second, since cEEG monitoring is generally only reviewed intermittently by electroencephalographers and EEG technologists, delays may occur between electrographic seizure onset and management initiation. Quantitative EEG techniques may improve cEEG monitoring review efficiency by electroencephalographers and allow more involvement by bedside clinicians, which could improve the speed of electrographic seizure identification.

Quantitative EEG techniques separate the complex EEG signal into components (such as amplitude and frequency) and compress time in the display, thereby permitting display of several hours of EEG data on a single image that may be interpreted more easily and rapidly than conventional EEG [91]. The most commonly utilized quantitative EEG techniques are amplitude-integrated EEG (aEEG), which is based on amplitude, and color density spectral array (CDSA), which is based on both amplitude and frequency.

Neonates

The most commonly used form of quantitative EEG monitoring for neonates is aEEG (Figure 1.6). This is a bedside EEG monitoring tool that employs 2–4 electrodes that yield either a single- or dual-channel EEG recording. Often, electrodes are placed in the bilateral central regions for maximal seizure detection [92]. Alternative strategies involve placing electrodes over bilateral frontal or bilateral parietal regions or an averaged hemispheric or regional recording, though this may decrease sensitivity. Compared to cEEG, aEEG allows more rapid electrode application and interpretation of aEEG data by neonatologists and neonatal nurses at bedside. A survey of perinatal practitioners in the United States found that 55% of respondents reported aEEG use in their neonatal intensive care units, with higher rates in academic centers. The most common reasons for aEEG use were decisions regarding seizure treatment (~80%), decisions regarding therapeutic hypothermia initiation (~50%), to guide counseling and prognosis (~50%), and to aid decisions surrounding medication dosages and treatment durations (~35%) [30].

The aEEG has an established role in encephalopathy assessment despite variable concordance between aEEG background features and clinical outcomes [93, 94]. The role of aEEG for seizure identification is more nuanced since although seizure identification with aEEG is imperfect, it is readily available and superior to clinical seizure identification. A study in neonates with hypoxic-ischemic encephalopathy performed aEEG in all neonates but randomized neonates to have management based on clinical observation alone or clinical observation plus use of aEEG data. Neonates in whom clinicians could use aEEG data had shorter total duration of seizures [95]. These data indicate that while imperfect, aEEG may have a meaningful clinical

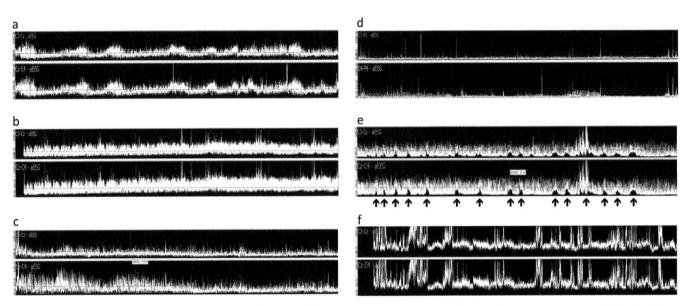

Figure 1.6 Amplitude-integrated EEG (aEEG) examples. (a) Normal aEEG with 6-hour compressed time scale using bilateral central channels (C3-Cz, Cz-C4). Minimum amplitudes are consistently between greater than 5 microvolts and maximum amplitudes are greater than 10 microvolts. There is evidence of variability with sleep–wake cycling. (b) Improving aEEG with 24-hour compressed time scale and bilateral central channels (C3-Cz, Cz-C4). Initially, minimum amplitudes are low (≤5 microvolts) with maximum amplitudes of 5 microvolts and greater. During the 24-hour recording, amplitudes gradually improve with minimum amplitudes greater than 5 microvolts and maximum amplitudes greater than 10 microvolts. (c) Abnormal aEEG with 6-hour compressed time scale and bilateral central channels (C3-Cz, Cz-C4). Amplitudes are persistently diminished with minimum amplitudes of ≤5 microvolts and the majority of maximum amplitudes ≤10 microvolts. (d) Severely abnormal aEEG with 6-hour compressed time scale and bilateral central channels (C3-Cz, Cz-C4). Amplitudes are persistently attenuated with all minimum and maximum amplitudes less than 10 microvolts. (e) Seizures on aEEG with 6-hour compressed time scale and bilateral central channels (C3-Cz, Cz-C4). Seizures are characterized by a sudden change in amplitude in a notch-like or bell-shaped morphology. There are numerous seizures in this 6-hour recording, denoted by arrows. (f) Electrode artifact on aEEG with 6-hour compressed time scale and bilateral central channels (C3-Cz, Cz-C4). Note the abrupt and extremely high voltage (100 microvolts) of the nature of the tracing.

impact in reducing seizure exposure. While aEEG may answer the binary question of whether an EEG record contains any seizures with relatively high accuracy, individual seizure discrimination is lower than with cEEG, potentially resulting in an under-estimate of seizure burden, including underdiagnosis of status epilepticus [96, 97].

The discordance in seizure identification between cEEG and aEEG is due to both modifiable and non-modifiable factors. An aEEG is less accurate in identifying seizures that are brief in duration, slow in frequency, or low in amplitude, or originate from cerebral locations that are distant from the recording electrodes [98]. These factors are innate to the seizure and generally not influenced by aEEG display characteristics or user training, though once seizure location is established a limited electrode scheme could be placed to maximize specific regional seizure identification. One modifiable factor affecting aEEG interpretation is the experience of the aEEG interpreter; non-experienced users have been shown to miss at least 50% of seizures using aEEG alone [99]. Though users with more experience theoretically have improved seizure identification, some studies show that individual seizure detection by this experienced group remains low, with aEEG readers with at least one year of experience identifying only 12–38% of individual seizures [97]. In addition to the false negatives associated with aEEG, false positives may occur. Given the lack of additional EMG, EKG, respiratory, and ocular channels that often aid the electroencephalographer in distinguishing between cerebral and artifactual changes on the EEG, artifact can be misinterpreted as seizure [96]. Finally, the majority of aEEG is interpreted by neonatology staff rather than electroencephalographers, and neonatologists self-report low confidence in their ability to perform aEEG interpretation. Survey data of neonatologists describe that only 7% of neonatologists report feeling very confident about aEEG interpretation while 31% feel not confident about aEEG interpretation [27].

Given the above limitations of aEEG, the American Clinical Neurophysiology Society's guideline on EEG monitoring in neonates recommended that cEEG monitoring remain the gold standard for seizure identification in neonates and that cEEG should be used whenever available. The guideline described that aEEG can act as a complementary tool to aid in rapid bedside diagnosis of seizures followed by confirmation with cEEG. When cEEG is not available, aEEG can be used for seizure screening, but if a seizure is suspected on aEEG, then it should be confirmed on cEEG when cEEG is available [15].

Children

Quantitative EEG test characteristics are still being established in critically ill children, and use of quantitative EEG is not as widespread as aEEG in neonates (Figure 1.7). In one study, 27 color density spectral array and aEEG tracings were reviewed by 3 electroencephalographers. The median sensitivity for seizure identification was 83% using CDSA and 82% using aEEG. However, for individual tracings the sensitivity varied from 0 to 100%, indicating excellent performance for some patients and poor performance for other patients, likely related to individual seizure characteristics. A false positive (event identified as a seizure that was not a seizure based on conventional EEG review) occurred

about every 17–20 hours [100]. In a second study, 84 CDSA images were reviewed by 8 electroencephalographers. Sensitivity for seizure identification was 65%, which indicated that some electrographic seizures were not identified. Only about half of seizures were identified by 6 or more of the raters, indicating problems with inter-rater agreement. Specificity was 95%, which indicated that some non-ictal events were misdiagnosed as seizures [101]. A study of CDSA and envelope trend EEG review by electroencephalographers found that seizure identification was impacted by both modifiable factors (interpreter experience, display size, and quantitative EEG method) and non-modifiable factors inherent to the EEG pattern (maximum spike amplitude, seizure duration, seizure frequency, and seizure duration) (Figure 1.7) [102].

Critical care providers are generally continually in the pediatric intensive care unit and have expertise using other screening modalities. Involving these providers might allow more rapid electrographic seizure identification. A study provided 20 critical care physicians (attending physicians and fellows) and 19 critical care nurses with a brief training session regarding color density spectral array and then asked participants to determine whether each of 200 CDSA images contained electrographic seizures. The images were created from conventional EEG derived from critically ill children resuscitated from cardiac arrest, and the true seizure incidence was 30% based on electroencephalographer review of the conventional EEG tracings. Among critical care providers reviewing CDSA images, the sensitivity was 70% (indicating that some electrographic seizures were not identified) and the specificity was 68% (indicating that some images categorized as containing EEG seizures did not contain seizures based on conventional EEG review). Given the 30% seizure incidence used in the study, the positive predictive value was 46% and the negative predictive value was 86% [103].

Summary

Data in neonates and children indicate that commercially available quantitative EEG techniques permit identification of many but not all seizures, and sometimes non-ictal events might be misidentified as seizures based on isolated quantitative EEG review. While imperfect, these techniques may be valuable when conventional cEEG is not available and may improve the efficiency of cEEG monitoring review by electroencephalographers. Since quantitative EEG techniques lead to misclassification of some non-ictal events as seizures, potentially leading to unnecessary anti-seizure medication administration, confirmation by conventional EEG review is indicated when quantitative EEG techniques suggest seizures are present. Such confirmation is particularly important for patients with refractory events to confirm that these events represent seizures prior to escalating to management with high-dose or multiple anti-seizure medications.

Further development of quantitative techniques, display optimization (including specific quantitative EEG trends and the duration of EEG displayed on a screen), and improved quantitative EEG training methods may allow these techniques to become even more valuable adjuvants to cEEG data. Additionally, synergistic methods could make use of the efficiency and bedside availability of quantitative EEG methods and the accuracy of

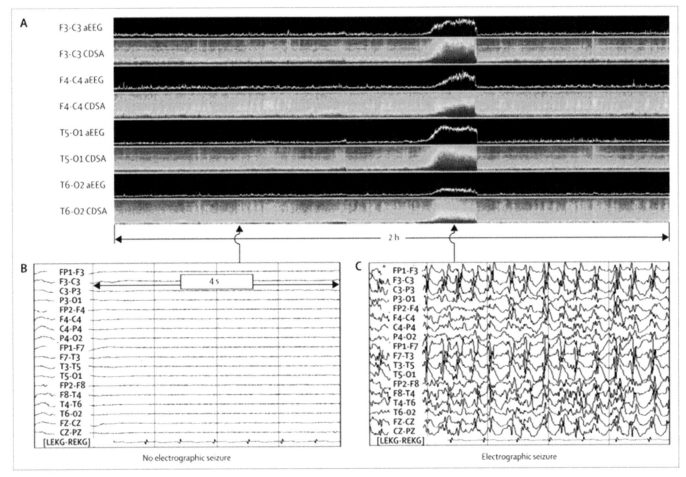

Figure 1.7 Amplitude-integrated EEG (aEEG) and color density spectral array (CDSA) image showing an electrographic seizure in a critically ill child. The electrographic seizures are characterized by increases in amplitude (displayed as increases on the y-axis) on the aEEG and CDSA tracings, and also by an increase in power (displayed as warmer colors) on the CDSA tracing. Reprinted from *Lancet Neurology*, 12(12), Abend NS, Wusthoff CJ, Goldberg EM, Dlugos DJ. Electrographic seizures and status epilepticus in critically ill children and neonates with encephalopathy. 1170–9, 2013, with permission from Elsevier.

conventional cEEG tracings. Quantitative EEG might be used at bedside to allow for rapid and frequent screening with confirmation of ongoing seizures by conventional EEG review prior to treatment initiation. Additionally, review of the initial portion of conventional EEG might be used to fine-tune the optimal quantitative EEG display at bedside for individual patients. This type of strategy was utilized by a randomized controlled trial of electrographic versus clinical seizure treatment in neonates that found that the combined strategy resulted in decreased acute seizure burden [81].

Conclusions

Continuous EEG monitoring of critically ill neonates and children offers an opportunity to assess and monitor cerebral function to guide overall therapy and identify electrographic seizures which are associated with unfavorable outcomes. Further research is needed to optimally target cEEG monitoring resources to the highest risk patients, develop management strategies that synergistically utilize quantitative EEG and conventional EEG, better understand the impact of electrographic seizures on patient outcomes, and develop optimized evidence-based seizure management strategies.

References

1. Glass HC, Wu YW. Epidemiology of neonatal seizures. *J Pediatr Neurol.* 2009;7:13–17.

2. Lawrence R, Inder T. Neonatal status epilepticus. *Semin Pediatr Neurol.* 2010;17(3):163–8.

3. Glass HC, Pham TN, Danielsen B, et al. Antenatal and intrapartum risk factors for seizures in term newborns: a population-based study, California 1998–2002. *J Pediatr.* 2009;154(1):24–8 e1.

4. Volpe JJ. Neonatal seizures. In Volpe JJ, editor. *Neurology of the Newborn.* Philadelphia: WB Saunders Elsevier; 2008, pp. 203–7.

5. Glass HC, Shellhaas RA, Wusthoff CJ, et al. Contemporary profile of seizures in neonates: a prospective cohort study. *J Pediatr.* 2016;174:98–103.e1.

6. Allen KA, Brandon DH. Hypoxic ischemic encephalopathy: pathophysiology and experimental treatments. *Newborn Infant Nurs Rev.* 2011;11(3):125–33.

7. Robertson CM, Perlman M. Follow-up of the term infant after hypoxic-ischemic encephalopathy. *Paediatr Child Health.* 2006;11(5):278–82.

8. Massaro AN, Murthy K, Zaniletti I, et al. Short-term outcomes after perinatal hypoxic ischemic encephalopathy: a report from the Children's Hospitals Neonatal Consortium HIE focus group. *J Perinatol.* 2015;**35**(4):290–6.

9. Simbruner G, Mittal RA, Rohlmann F, et al. Systemic hypothermia after neonatal encephalopathy: outcomes of neo.nEURO.network RCT. *Pediatrics.* 2010;**126**(4): e771–8.

10. Committee on Fetus and Newborn; Papile, L-A, Baley JE, Benitz I, et al. Hypothermia and neonatal encephalopathy. *Pediatrics.* 2014;**133**(6):1146–50.

11. Low E, Boylan GB, Mathieson SR, et al. Cooling and seizure burden in term neonates: an observational study. *Arch Dis Child Fetal Neonatal Ed.* 2012;**97**(4):F267–72.

12. Vasudevan C, Levene M. Epidemiology and aetiology of neonatal seizures. *Semin Fetal Neonatal Med.* 2013;**18**(4):185–91.

13. Pisani F, Facini C, Pelosi A, et al. Neonatal seizures in preterm newborns: a predictive model for outcome. *Eur J Paediatr Neurol.* 2016;**20**(2):243–51.

14. Sheth RD, Hobbs GR, Mullett M. Neonatal seizures: incidence, onset, and etiology by gestational age. *J Perinatol.* 1999;**19**(1):40–3.

15. Shellhaas RA, Chang T, Tsuchida T, et al. The American Clinical Neurophysiology Society's guideline on continuous electroencephalography monitoring in neonates. *J Clin Neurophysiol.* 2011;**28**(6):611–17.

16. Laroia N, Guillet R, Burchfiel J, McBride MC. EEG background as predictor of electrographic seizures in high-risk neonates. *Epilepsia.* 1998;**39**(5):545–51.

17. Tsuchida TN, Wusthoff CJ, Shellhaas R, et al. American clinical neurophysiology society standardized EEG terminology and categorization for the description of continuous EEG monitoring in neonates: report of the American Clinical Neurophysiology Society Critical Care Monitoring Committee. *J Clin Neurophysiol.* 2013;**30**(2):161–73.

18. Mizrahi EM, Kellaway P. Characterization and classification of neonatal seizures. *Neurology.* 1987;**37**(12):1837–44.

19. Nagarajan L, Palumbo L, Ghosh S. Classification of clinical semiology in epileptic seizures in neonates. *Eur J Paediatr Neurol.* 2012;**16**(2):118–25.

20. Murray DM, Boylan GB, Ali I, et al. Defining the gap between electrographic seizure burden, clinical expression and staff recognition of neonatal seizures. *Arch Dis Child Fetal Neonatal Ed.* 2008;**93**(3):F187–91.

21. Malone A, Anthony Ryan C, Fitzgerald A, et al. Interobserver agreement in neonatal seizure identification. *Epilepsia.* 2009;**50**(9):2097–101.

22. Clancy RR, Legido A, Lewis D. Occult neonatal seizures. *Epilepsia.* 1988;**29**(3):256–61.

23. Connell J, Oozeer R, de Vries L, Dubowitz LM, Dubowitz V. Continuous EEG monitoring of neonatal seizures: diagnostic and prognostic considerations. *Arch Dis Child.* 1989;**64**(4 Spec No):452–8.

24. Naim MY, Gaynor JW, Chen J, et al. Subclinical seizures identified by postoperative electroencephalographic monitoring are common after neonatal cardiac surgery. *J Thorac Cardiovasc Surg.* 2015;**150**(1):169–78.

25. Hahn JS, Vaucher Y, Bejar R, Coen RW. Electroencephalographic and neuroimaging findings in neonates undergoing extracorporeal membrane oxygenation. *Neuropediatrics.* 1993;**24**(1):19–24.

26. Scher MS, Alvin J, Gaus L, Minnigh B, Painter MJ. Uncoupling of EEG-clinical neonatal seizures after antiepileptic drug use. *Pediatr Neurol.* 2003;**28**(4):277–80.

27. Boylan GB, Burgoyne L, Moore C, O'Flaherty B, Renni JM. An international survey of EEG use in the neonatal intensive care unit. *Acta Paediatr.* 2010;**99**(8):1150–5.

28. Glass HC, Kan J, Bonifacio SL Ferriero DM. Neonatal seizures: treatment practices among term and preterm infants. *Pediatr Neurol.* 2012;**46**(2):111–15.

29. Filan PM, Inder TE, Anderson PJ, Doyle LW, Hunt RW. Monitoring the neonatal brain: a survey of current practice among Australian and New Zealand neonatologists. *J Paediatr Child Health.* 2007;**43**(7–8):557–9.

30. Shah NA, Van Meurs KP, Davis AS. Amplitude-integrated electroencephalography: a survey of practices in the United States. *Am J Perinatol.* 2015;**32**(8):755–60.

31. Glass HC, Wusthoff CJ, Shellhaas RA, et al. Risk factors for EEG seizures in neonates treated with hypothermia: a multicenter cohort study. *Neurology.* 2014;**82**(14):1239–44.

32. Nash KB, Bonifacio SL, Glass HC, et al. Video-EEG monitoring in newborns with hypoxic-ischemic encephalopathy treated with hypothermia. *Neurology.* 2011;**76**(6):556–62.

33. Murray DM, Ryan CA, Boylan GB, et al. Prediction of seizures in asphyxiated neonates: correlation with continuous video-electroencephalographic monitoring. *Pediatrics.* 2006;**118**(1):41–6.

34. Monod N, Pajot N, Guidasci S. The neonatal EEG: statistical studies and prognostic value in full-term and pre-term babies. *Electroencephalogr Clin Neurophysiol.* 1972;**32**(5):529–44.

35. Rowe JC, Holmes GL, Hafford J, et al. Prognostic value of the electroencephalogram in term and preterm infants following neonatal seizures. *Electroencephalogr Clin Neurophysiol.* 1985;**60**(3):183–96.

36. Murray DM, Boylan GB, Ryan CA, Connolly S. Early EEG findings in hypoxic-ischemic encephalopathy predict outcomes at 2 years. *Pediatrics.* 2009;**124**(3):e459–67.

37. Takeuchi T, Watanabe K. The EEG evolution and neurological prognosis of neonates with perinatal hypoxia [corrected]. *Brain Dev.* 1989;**11**(2):115–20.

38. Awal MA, Lai MM, Azemi G, et al. EEG background features that predict outcome in term neonates with hypoxic ischaemic encephalopathy: A structured review. *Clin Neurophysiol.* 2016;**127**(2):285–96.

39. Khan RL, Nunes ML, Garcias da Silva LF, Costa da Costa J. Predictive value of sequential electroencephalogram (EEG) in neonates with seizures and its relation to neurological outcome. *J Child Neurol.* 2008;**23**(2):144–50.

40. Bell MJ, Carpenter J, Au AK, et al. Development of a pediatric neurocritical care service. *Neurocrit Care.* 2009;**10**(1):4–10.

41. LaRovere KL, Graham RJ, Tasker RC, Pediatric Critical Nervous System Program (pCNSp) Pediatric neurocritical care: a neurology consultation model and implication for education and training. *Pediatr Neurol.* 2013;**48**(3):206–11.

42. Abend, NS, Wusthoff CJ, Goldberg EM, Dlugos DJ. Electrographic seizures and status epilepticus in critically ill children and neonates with encephalopathy. *Lancet Neurol.* 2013;**12** (12):1170–9.

43. Hosain SA, Solomon GE, Kobylarz EJ. Electroencephalographic patterns in unresponsive pediatric patients. *Pediatr Neurol.* 2005;**32**(3):162–5.

44. Jette N, Claasen J, Emerson RG, et al. Frequency and predictors of nonconvulsive seizures during continuous electroencephalographic monitoring in critically ill children. *Arch Neurol.* 2006;**63**(12):1750–5.

45. Abend NS, Dlugos DJ. Nonconvulsive status epilepticus in a pediatric intensive care unit. *Pediatr Neurol.* 2007;**37**(3):165–70.

46. Tay SK, Hirsch LJ, Leary L, et al. Nonconvulsive status epilepticus in children: clinical and EEG characteristics. *Epilepsia.* 2006;**47** (9):1504–9.

47. Shahwan A, Bailey C, Shekerdemian L, Harvey AS. The prevalence of seizures in comatose children in the pediatric intensive care unit: a prospective video-EEG study. *Epilepsia.* 2010;**51** (7):1198–1204.

48. Abend NS, Topjian A, Ichord R, et al. Electroencephalographic monitoring during hypothermia after pediatric cardiac arrest. *Neurology.* 2009;**72** (22):1931–40.

49. Williams K, Jarrar R, Buchhalter J. Continuous video-EEG monitoring in pediatric intensive care units. *Epilepsia.* 2011;**52**(6):1130–6.

50. Greiner HM, Holland K, Leach JL, et al. Nonconvulsive status epilepticus: the encephalopathic pediatric patient. *Pediatrics.* 2012;**129**(3):e748–55.

51. Kirkham FJ, Wade AW, McElduff F, et al. Seizures in 204 comatose children: incidence and outcome. *Intensive Care Med.* 2012;**38**(5):853–62.

52. Arango JI, et al. Posttraumatic seizures in children with severe traumatic brain injury. *Childs Nerv Syst.* 2012;**28** (11):1925–9.

53. Piantino JA, Wainwright MS, Grimason M, et al. Nonconvulsive seizures are common in children treated with extracorporeal cardiac life support. *Pediatr Crit Care Med.* 2013;**14** (6):601–609.

54. Abend NS, Arndt DH, Carpenter JL, et al. Electrographic seizures in pediatric ICU patients: cohort study of risk factors and mortality. *Neurology.* 2013;**81**(4):383–91.

55. McCoy B, Sharma R, Ochi A, et al. Predictors of nonconvulsive seizures among critically ill children. *Epilepsia.* 2011;**52**(11):1973–8.

56. Schreiber JM, Zelleke T, Gaillard WD, et al. Continuous video EEG for patients with acute encephalopathy in a pediatric intensive care unit. *Neurocrit Care.* 2012;**17** (1):31–8.

57. Arndt DH, Lerner JT, Matsumoto JH, et al. Subclinical early posttraumatic seizures detected by continuous EEG monitoring in a consecutive pediatric cohort. *Epilepsia.* 2013;**54** (10):1780–8.

58. Payne ET, Yan Zhao X, Frndova H, et al. Seizure burden is independently associated with short term outcome in critically ill children. *Brain.* 2014;**137** (Pt 5):1429–38.

59. Abend NS, Gutierrez-Collina AM, Topjian AA, et al. Nonconvulsive seizures are common in critically ill children. *Neurology.* 2011;**76**(12):1071–7.

60. Gold JJ, Crawford JR, Glaser C, et al. The role of continuous electroencephalography in childhood encephalitis. *Pediatr Neurol.* 2014;**50** (4):318–23.

61. Greiner MV, Greiner HM, Caré MM, et al. Adding insult to injury: nonconvulsive seizures in abusive head trauma. *J Child Neurol.* 2015; **30** (13):1778–84.

62. Gwer S, Idro R, Fegan G, et al. Continuous EEG monitoring in Kenyan children with non-traumatic coma. *Arch Dis Child.* 2012;**97**(4): 343–9.

63. Hasbani DM, Topjian AA, Friess SH, et al. Nonconvulsive electrographic seizures are common in children with abusive head trauma. *Pediatr Crit Care Med.* 2013;**14**(7):709–15.

64. Abend NS. Electrographic status epilepticus in children with critical illness: Epidemiology and outcome. *Epilepsy Behav.* 2015;**49**:223–7.

65. Gutierrez-Colina AM, Topjian AA, Dlugos DJ, Abend NS. EEG monitoring in critically ill children: indications and strategies. *Pediatric Neurology.* 2012;**46**:158–161.

66. Abend NS, Topjian AA, Williams S. How much does it cost to identify a critically ill child experiencing electrographic seizures? *J Clin Neurophysiol.* 2015;**32**(3):257–64.

67. Yang A, Arndt DH, Berg RA, et al. Development and validation of a seizure prediction model in critically ill children. *Seizure.* 2015;**25**:104–11.

68. Broph GM, Bell R, Claassen J, et al. Guidelines for the evaluation and management of status epilepticus. *Neurocrit Care.* 2012;**17**(1):3–23.

69. Herman ST, Abend NS, Bleck TP, et al. Consensus statement on continuous EEG in critically ill adults and children, part I: indications. *J Clin Neurophysiol.* 2015;**32**(2):87–95.

70. Abend NS, Dlugos DJ, Hahn CD, et al. Use of EEG monitoring and management of non-convulsive seizures in critically ill patients: a survey of neurologists. *Neurocrit Care.* 2010;**12** (3):382–9.

71. Glass HC, Nash KB, Bonifacio SL, et al. Seizures and magnetic resonance imaging-detected brain injury in newborns cooled for hypoxic-ischemic encephalopathy. *J Pediatr.* 2011;**159** (5):731–735 e1.

72. McBride MC, Laroia N, Guillet R. Electrographic seizures in neonates correlate with poor neurodevelopmental outcome. *Neurology.* 2000;**55**(4):506–13.

73. van Rooij LG, de Vries LS, Handryastuti S, et al. Neurodevelopmental outcome in term infants with status epilepticus detected with amplitude-integrated electroencephalography. *Pediatrics.* 2007;**120**(2):e354–63.

74. Painter MJ, Sun Q, Scher MS, Janosky J, Alvin J. Neonates with seizures: what predicts development? *J Child Neurol.* 2012;**27**(8):1022–6.

75. Maartens IA, Wassenberg T, Buijs J, et al. Neurodevelopmental outcome in full-term newborns with refractory neonatal seizures. *Acta Paediatr.* 2012;**101**(4):e173–8.

76. Shah DK, Wusthoff CJ, Clarke P, et al. Electrographic seizures are associated with brain injury in newborns undergoing therapeutic hypothermia. *Arch Dis Child Fetal Neonatal Ed.* 2014;**99**(3):F219–24.

77. Glass HC, Glidden D, Jeremy RJ, et al. Clinical neonatal seizures are independently associated with outcome in infants at risk for hypoxic-ischemic brain injury. *J Pediatr.* 2009;**155** (3):318–23.

78. Dunne JM, Wertheim D, Clarke P, et al. Automated electroencephalographic discontinuity in cooled newborns predicts cerebral MRI and neurodevelopmental outcome. *Arch Dis Child Fetal Neonatal Ed.* 2017;**102**(1): F58–64.

79. Meyn DF, Jr., Ness J, Ambalavanan N, Carlo WA. Prophylactic phenobarbital and whole-body cooling for neonatal hypoxic-ischemic encephalopathy. *J Pediatr.* 2010;**157**(2):334–6.

80. van Rooij LG, Toet MC, van Huffelen AC, et al. Effect of treatment of subclinical neonatal seizures detected with aEEG: randomized, controlled trial. *Pediatrics.* 2010;**125**(2):e358–66.

81. Srinivasakumar P, Zempel J, Trivedi S, et al. Treating EEG seizures in hypoxic ischemic encephalopathy: a randomized controlled trial. *Pediatrics.* 2015;**136**(5):e1302–9.

82. Topjian AA, Gutierrez-Colina AM, Sanchez SM, et al. Electrographic status epilepticus is associated with mortality and worse short-term outcome in critically ill children. *Crit Care Med.* 2013;**41**(1):215–23.

83. Wagenman KL, Blake TP, Sanchez SM, et al. Electrographic status epilepticus and long-term outcome in critically ill children. *Neurology.* 2014;**82**(5):396–404.

84. WHO, *Guidelines on Neonatal Seizures.* World Health Organization; 2011.

85. Glauser TA, Clancy RR. Adequacy of routine EEG examinations in neonates with clinically suspected seizures. *J Child Neurol.* 1992;**7**(2):215–20.

86. Wusthoff CJ, Dlugos DJ, Gutierrez-Colina A, et al. Electrographic seizures during therapeutic hypothermia for neonatal encephalopathy. *J Child Neurol.* 2011;**26**(6):724–728.

87. Lynch NE, Stevenson NJ, Livingstone V, et al. The temporal evolution of electrographic seizure burden in neonatal hypoxic ischemic encephalopathy. *Epilepsia.* 2012;**53**(3):549–57.

88. Clancy RR, Sharif U, Ichord R, et al. Electrographic neonatal seizures after infant heart surgery. *Epilepsia.* 2005;**46**(1):84–90.

89. Shah DK, Zempel J, Barton T, Lukas K, Inder TE. Electrographic seizures in preterm infants during the first week of life are associated with cerebral injury. *Pediatr Res.* 2010;**67**(1):102–6.

90. Herman ST, Abend NS, Bleck TP, et al. Consensus statement on continuous EEG in critically ill adults and children, part II: personnel, technical specifications, and clinical practice. *J Clin Neurophysiol.* 2015;**32**(2):96–108.

91. Scheuer ML, Wilson SB. Data analysis for continuous EEG monitoring in the ICU: seeing the forest and the trees. *J Clin Neurophysiol.* 2004;**21**(5):353–78.

92. Wusthoff CJ, Shellhaas RA, Clancy RR. Limitations of single-channel EEG on the forehead for neonatal seizure detection. *J Perinatol.* 2009;**29**(3):237–42.

93. de Vries, LS, Hellstrom-Westas L. Role of cerebral function monitoring in the newborn. *Arch Dis Child Fetal Neonatal Ed.* 2005;**90**(3):F201–7.

94. Clancy RR, Dicker L, Cho S, et al. Agreement between long-term neonatal background classification by conventional and amplitude-integrated EEG. *J Clin Neurophysiol.* 2011;**28**(1):1–9.

95. van Rooij LG, de Vries LS, van Huffelen AC, Toet MC. Additional value of two-channel amplitude integrated EEG recording in full-term infants with unilateral brain injury.

Arch Dis Child Fetal Neonatal Ed. 2010;**95**(3):F160–8.

96. Shah DK, Mackay MT, Lavery S, et al. Accuracy of bedside electroencephalographic monitoring in comparison with simultaneous continuous conventional electroencephalography for seizure detection in term infants. *Pediatrics.* 2008;**121**(6):1146–54.

97. Shellhaas RA, Soaita AI, Clancy RR. Sensitivity of amplitude-integrated electroencephalography for neonatal seizure detection. *Pediatrics.* 2007;**120**(4):770–7.

98. Shellhaas RA, Clancy RR. Characterization of neonatal seizures by conventional EEG and single-channel EEG. *Clin Neurophysiol.* 2007;**118**(10):2156–61.

99. Rennie JM, Chorley G, Boylan GB, et al. Non-expert use of the cerebral function monitor for neonatal seizure detection. *Arch Dis Child Fetal Neonatal Ed.* 2004;**89**(1):F37–40.

100. Stewart CP, Otsubo H, Ochi A, et al. Seizure identification in the ICU using quantitative EEG displays. *Neurology.* 2010;**75**(17):1501–8.

101. Pensirikul AD, Beslow LA, Kessler SK, et al. Density spectral array for seizure identification in critically ill children. *J Clin Neurophysiol.* 2013;**30**(4):371–5.

102. Akman CI, Micic V, Thompson A, Riviello JJ, Jr. Seizure detection using digital trend analysis: Factors affecting utility. *Epilepsy Res.* 2011;**93**(1):66–72.

103. Topjian AA, Fry M, Jawad AF, et al. Detection of electrographic seizures by critical care providers using color density spectral array after cardiac arrest is feasible. *Pediatr Crit Care Med.* 2015;**16**(5):461–7.

Technical Aspects of Neurophysiological Monitoring

Erin M. Fedak Romanowski and Renée A. Shellhaas

Illustrative Case

Case 1 Pitfalls in aEEG Interpretation

Key Points

- An electroencephalogram (EEG) reflects the summation of electrical activity arising from excitatory and inhibitory post synaptic potentials of pyramidal neurons.
- EEG electrodes are traditionally placed on the scalp according to the International 10–20 system of electrode placement.
- There are a number of different montages that may be used to best analyze an EEG and allow for interpretation of the spatial distribution and localization of the EEG activity across the cortex. Neonates may require a reduced montage.
- Full EEG data remain the gold standard of neurophysiological monitoring; however, reduced montage and quantitative EEG techniques have allowed providers, particularly in the neonatal and pediatric intensive care units, to have supplementary data to interpret, in real time, at the patient's bedside or via remote access.

Physiology

An electroencephalogram (EEG) reflects the summation of electrical activity arising from excitatory and inhibitory post synaptic potentials of pyramidal neurons [1]. The release of a neurotransmitter onto a post-synaptic membrane creates post-synaptic potentials. Certain neurotransmitters are excitatory, such as glutamate and acetylcholine, while others, such as gamma-aminobutyric acid (GABA), are inhibitory. When an excitatory neurotransmitter depolarizes a post-synaptic membrane, this opens sodium and/or calcium channels, and creates an excitatory post-synaptic potential (EPSP). When an inhibitory neurotransmitter acts on a post-synaptic membrane, potassium and/or chloride channels open, and therefore inhibit the membrane potential so that sodium channels are not opened and depolarization cannot occur. This produces an inhibitory post-synaptic potential (IPSP). The sum of these potentials creates the surface scalp EEG activity. EEG essentially displays the difference in electrical voltage between two different recording locations (y-axis) over time (x-axis) [2]. Approximately 6 cm^2 of cortex must be activated to create enough electrical activity to be visible on a scalp EEG [1, 2].

Electrodes

Electrode Placement

EEG electrodes are traditionally placed on the scalp according to the International 10–20 system of electrode placement

(Figure 2.1), based on the recommendations of the General Assembly of the International Federation of Clinical Neurophysiology (IFCN) [3] and the American Clinical Neurophysiology Society (ACNS) [4]. Electrodes are placed based on bony landmarks: nasion, inion, and preauricular, and then at specific proportional intervals to create standard distances between electrodes.

The ACNS recommends a minimum of 21 electrodes for the 10–20 placement system, with each electrode labeled based on its anatomic location [4]. The letter "C" is used for the central head locations, "F" for frontal, "P" for parietal, "O" for occipital, and "T" for temporal. Numbers are then also used to indicate placement, with odd numbers located over the left hemisphere and even numbers over the right hemisphere. Lower numbers indicate electrodes closer to the midline, and the letter "z" (for zero) is used to indicate midline electrodes [5].

Under certain circumstances, additional electrodes may be needed for more detailed localization. In this case, the 10–10 system is used, with electrodes placed in closer proximity to each other. The additional electrodes are located at points halfway between the traditional 10–20 positions [6]. Temporal electrodes in the 10–20 system are labeled differently in the 10–10 system, with T3 and T4 instead labeled as T7 and T8, respectively. T5 and T6 in the 10–20 system are instead labeled as P7 and P8 respectively in the 10–10 system [3, 4, 5] (Figure 2.1).

For neonates (any infant less than 44–48 weeks postmenstrual age), a reduced number of electrodes is commonly used due to small head size, lack of EEG activity in the frontopolar head regions, or restrictive environments such as the neonatal ICU, where a full electrode array may not be possible. In these situations, the ACNS has recommended use of a 10–20 system modified for neonates that includes the following 11 electrodes: Fp1, Fp2, C3, Cz, C4, T7 (T3), T8 (T4), O1, O2, A1, and A2. Alternatively, using Fp3 and Fp4 in place of Fp1 and Fp2 is acceptable for frontal electrode coverage [4] (Figure 2.1). The addition of extracerebral channels (ECG, EMG, respiratory leads and pulse oximetry) is also recommended, both to assist with differentiating sleep–wake stages and to enable the EEG reader to distinguish artifacts from cerebral activity (see below).

Electrode Types

EEG electrodes are applied to the scalp to permit the direct recording of electrical current. In a standard EEG recording, the electrodes are cup-shaped and 1 cm in diameter. Most cup

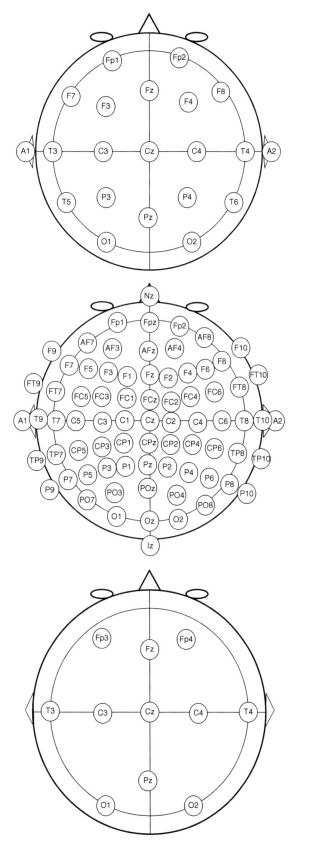

Figure 2.1 (a) Standard International 10–20 electrode positions; (b) modified 10–10 electrode positions; (c) 10–20 electrode placement, modified for neonates.

electrodes have a flat rim to maximize skin contact and a hole in the center to facilitate the addition of conductive paste or gel. Electrodes can be made from platinum, tin, or gold, but the most common type is made from silver oxidized with chloride, which allows for adequate ion exchange with the conducting gel [5, 7]. For patients requiring prolonged EEG monitoring, it is helpful to use electrodes that are compatible with magnetic resonance imaging (MRI) and computed tomography (CT) scanning to prevent the need for frequent removal and reapplication. Removal and reapplication of EEG electrodes may exacerbate scalp breakdown and increases the chance of missing seizures or other important information during the longer time intervals during which the EEG is disconnected. A gold-plated silver electrode system has been shown to be safe and cause minimal artifact during MRI, and a conductive plastic electrode system has been shown to be safe and cause minimal artifact during both CT and MRI [8, 9].

An alternative to cup electrodes is needle electrodes, placed subdermally in the scalp. These have the advantage of being less easily dislodged and often recording with superior impedance. While commonly used in Europe, these are less often used in North America due to concerns for needlestick injuries and infection risk.

Methods of Affixing EEG Electrodes

Prior to attaching electrodes, the EEG technologist prepares the patient's scalp with a skin preparation solution, which removes excess oil and debris in order to decrease impedance. Impedance should typically be less than 5 kΩ and is tested after electrode application by an ohmmeter, typically on the EEG machine [5]. For patients with delicate skin (e.g., newborns) for whom aggressive scalp preparation could be harmful, a higher impedance (10 kΩ) is usually acceptable. Electrode cups are filled with a conductive paste or gel and held in place with adhesives, and/or pressure from head caps or wraps. If a prolonged EEG study is anticipated, the use of collodion or other adhesive pastes is preferable because the prolonged use of head wraps can predispose to pressure sores, particularly under forehead electrodes. Collodion is an adhesive substance formulated from pyroxylin, a nitrated cellulose that is typically dissolved in diethyl ether and ethyl alcohol. When collodion is drying, the vapors of the diethyl ether solvent emit a strong odor that can be unpleasant; however, routine use of collodion has been shown to meet occupational health and safety standards when adequate ventilation is maintained. Nevertheless, because of this unpleasant odor, alternative adhesive pastes are favored by many EEG laboratories [5, 10–12].

Polarity

Each EEG channel has two inputs (commonly referred to as G1 and G2) that measure the voltage difference between two electrodes. Pairs of input electrodes can be rearranged to create a variety of different montages (described below). By convention, an upward deflection on the EEG indicates negative polarity, meaning that the voltage at input 1 is more negative than input 2 ("negative to positive = up"). Conversely,

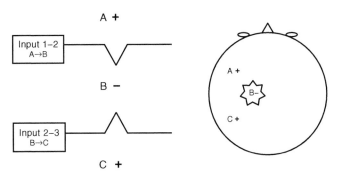

Figure 2.2 Input 1 (A) is more positive than input 2 (B), creating a downward deflection. Input 2 (B) is more negative than input 3 (C), creating an upward deflection. The most negative point between the two channels is B. This creates a phase reversal in a bipolar montage.

a downward EEG deflection indicates positive polarity, with more positive voltage at input 1 as compared to input 2 ("positive to negative = down") [1, 5] (Figure 2.2).

Montages

An EEG montage is a specific arrangement of EEG electrode channels and is designed to permit comparisons of the electrical voltage between the channels. There are a number of different montages that may be used to best analyze an EEG, and allow for interpretation of the spatial distribution and localization of the EEG activity across the cortex. The ACNS has proposed a guideline for the standard montages that are to be used in clinical EEG laboratories, paraphrased as follows: A minimum of 16 channels should be recorded simultaneously; however, a larger number of channels is encouraged. It is recommended that all 21 electrodes of the 10–20 system be used. A minimum of longitudinal bipolar, transverse bipolar and referential montages should be used in every recording. Electrode connections should be clearly indicated at the beginning of each montage, the pattern of electrode connections should be simple, and montages easy to comprehend. The tracings from the more anterior electrodes should be displayed above the more posterior electrodes, and at least some of the montages should be comparable across all EEG laboratories [4].

Bipolar Montages

A bipolar montage refers to the comparison of two electrodes compared at inputs 1 and 2, respectively. Active electrodes are connected to both inputs, without one common electrode. The montage is formed by a chain of these electrodes, typically linked either in a longitudinal (anterior to posterior) or transverse (left to right) orientation across the scalp (Figure 2.3). As an example, such a chain of channels could appear as follows: Fp1-F3, F3-C3, C3-P3, P3-O1. In this example, the first channel in the chain is Fp1-F3. Input 1 of channel 1 is Fp1, and input 2 of channel 1 is F3. The second channel is F3-C3, with F3 as input 1 and C3 as input 2. In a bipolar montage, the aim is to identify the electrode registering the maximum voltage. Bipolar montages are most helpful to analyze localization in signals that are rapidly changing across space. They are less

useful for the assessment of differences in amplitude, or signals with a broad field.

A longitudinal bipolar montage, as mentioned, sequentially links electrode pairs to be analyzed anteriorly to posteriorly in a sagittal plane (commonly referred to as the "double banana" montage). A transverse bipolar montage allows for electrical activity to be analyzed left to right, in a coronal plane. The circumferential bipolar montage allows for analysis in an axial plane [1, 2, 5].

Referential Montages

A referential montage refers to the comparison of one active electrode at input 1 to a presumably neutral reference electrode at input 2. The same common reference electrode is used as input 2 for every channel in the montage (Figure 2.3). An example of such a montage is: Fp1-Cz, F3-Cz, C3-Cz, P3-Cz, O1-Cz. In this example, the first channel in the chain is Fp1-Cz, and input 1 is Fp1, while the common reference electrode, Cz, is input 2. The ideal neutral reference electrode is inactive to the activity of interest, although this is not always possible. To some degree, the neutral reference electrode is always somewhat active.

Many times an *average reference* is used. This is obtained by electronically averaging the voltage in all of the scalp electrodes together and using this information as the "average reference" (note: the frontopolar electrodes may be omitted from the average due to predictable extracerebral artifact). An example of a chain using an average reference is: Fp1-Avg, F3-Avg, C3-Avg, P3-Avg, O1-Avg.

Referential montages are helpful for analyzing waveform morphology, amplitude, and signals with a broad field. They are less useful for localizing rapidly changing signals, and caution must be used in determining the correct, least active electrode as the reference electrode. For example, a Cz reference electrode may be helpful for analyzing activity presumed to be far from the vertex, but could distort a trace recorded in sleep, since the typical sleep EEG is most active at the central vertex. A montage using the auricular electrodes as a reference ("ipsilateral ears" for example) may be helpful for activity presumed to be maximal far from the ears or temporal head regions, but could distort the record of a person with seizures or epileptiform discharges that arise from the temporal lobe [1, 2, 5].

Neonatal Montages

For children older than 48 weeks postmenstrual age, the conventional International 10–20 system described above should be applied [13]. Pediatric, adolescent, and adult patients' EEGs are recorded using the same system. Neonates require a modified montage, due to small head size. As described above, the suggested minimum reduced array consists of electrodes placed at these positions: Fp3, Fp4, C3, Cz, C4, T7 (T3), T8 (T4), O1, O2, A1, and A2 (bilateral auricular electrodes). The Fp3 and Fp4 electrode positions are recommended because of the newborn's natural paucity of EEG activity in the frontopolar head regions. Fp3 is located midway between the typical Fp1 and F3 electrode positions. There are several montages that are used commonly in neonatal EEG monitoring, and these commonly combine single- and double-distance electrodes [5, 13, 14]. Unlike EEG for older infants and children, a single montage is typically adequate for neonatal EEG records (Table 2.1).

Neonatal EEGs are subject to misinterpretation due to rhythmic artifact from respirations, pulse, EKG, patting, sucking, and a variety of limb, eye, and head movements. It is, therefore, recommended that a minimum of two channels devoted to extra-cerebral variables, such as EKG and respiratory leads, be included in the neonatal EEG montage. Ideally, electromyography (EMG) channels representing chin, limb, and bilateral eye movements are also included [15].

Since the native EEG frequencies of a newborn are in the low delta range, it is typical practice to review a neonatal EEG display at 15 mm/second, instead of the standard 30 mm/second used for children and adults. This allows for better appreciation of slower frequencies, as well as discontinuity, interhemispheric synchrony, and state changes [16] (Figure 2.4).

Filters

Filters are used in digital EEG recording to either reduce or emphasize particular frequencies of electrical activity, and to help compensate for artifact related to electrical power. Scalp EEG reading software frequently has standard settings that include frequencies between a band of 0.5 and 70 Hz. This allows for the emphasis to be placed on medium frequency range activity, when appropriate [2]. Common high frequencies that may distort an EEG recording include myogenic artifact, while sweat artifact (e.g., salt bridges) and movement

artifact are the most common low frequencies that may distort a recording. While filters can be extremely helpful, they must be used deliberately and sparingly, lest desired activity be masked and important abnormalities rendered undetectable.

Table 2.1 Commonly used sample montages for neonates. Extracerebral channels should also be included (e.g., respiratory, EKG, EMG)

Channel	1	2*
1	Fp1-C3	Fp1-F3
2	C3-O1	F3-C3
3	Fp1-T3	C3-P3
4	T3-O1	Fp2-F4
5	Fp2-C4	F4-C4
6	C4-O2	C4-P4
7	Fp2-T4	F7-T3
8	T4-O2	T3-T5
9	T3-C3	T5-O1
10	C3-CZ	F8-T4
11	CZ-C4	T4-T6
12	C4-T4	T6-O2

*Not all of these electrode positions are used in the International 10–20 system modified for neonates.

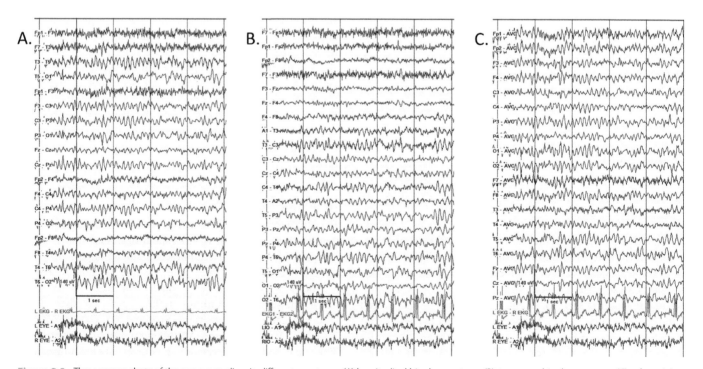

Figure 2.3 Three screen-shots of the same recording, in different montages: (A) longitudinal bipolar montage; (B) transverse bipolar montage; (C) referential (average) montage.

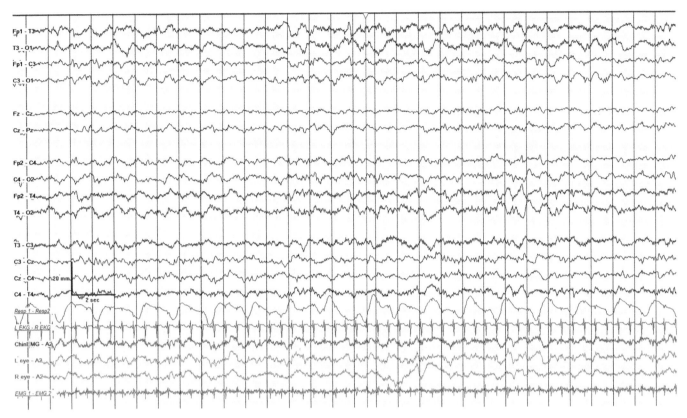

Figure 2.4 This is a neonatal EEG with the limited montage, including extracerebral channels at the bottom of the recording: respiratory (blue), EKG (red), chin EMG (purple), eye movements (green), and limb EMG (pink).

High-Frequency Filters

A high-frequency filter (HFF), also referred to as a "low-pass filter," is used to reduce or attenuate unwanted fast frequencies. The commonly used default setting is 70 Hz. Application of a 70 Hz low-pass filter dampens frequencies higher than 70 Hz and allows lower frequencies to be appreciated more easily. This filter can be adjusted as necessary. For example, reducing the low-pass filter (e.g., to 30 Hz or to 15 Hz) can allow for more detailed evaluation of slower frequencies that are obscured by myogenic artifact (e.g., during a seizure) [5].

Low-Frequency Filters

A low-frequency filter (LFF) is also referred to as a "high-pass filter," as it filters lower frequencies and allows high frequencies to be displayed. The default setting for a low-frequency filter is typically 0.5 Hz. When this filter is applied, the EEG will not display frequencies less than 0.5 Hz [5]. The high-pass filter frequency can be adjusted to reduce the impact of low-frequency extracerebral artifact.

Notch Filter

The notch filter aids in eliminating the most common type of electrical artifact. This is typically set at 60 Hz in North America and 50 Hz in Europe, corresponding to electrical frequencies used regionally. Electrical artifact arises from other nearby machines, medical equipment or electronics, as these devices are most often powered with alternating current [2, 5]. In most EEG labs, the filter is not required as standard laboratories are electrically protected. Electrical artifact is most commonly seen in the inpatient setting, particularly in the ICU (Figure 2.5).

Extracerebral Channels

Extracerebral electrodes include EKG, EMG (submental, extremities), respiratory leads, and/or pulse oximetry. Channels such as EKG, respiratory, or pulse oximetry allow for examination of extracerebral causes for the patient's clinical event, such as primary cardiac arrhythmia, apnea, or desaturation events. This information may provide further clinical clues regarding the underlying etiology of the patient's index events.

Extracerebral channels also allow for examination of potential artifacts. Respiratory or pulse artifact can create rhythmic delta activity on the EEG, which may be perceived and treated as a seizure if the EEG reader does not have access to the extracerebral channel. Repetitive movements can be seen on the EMG channel, and correlating this with myogenic artifact on EEG can be extremely helpful when determining whether a movement is due to a seizure or to a nonseizure paroxysmal event.

Time-locked video recording is also essential, both for neonatal and pediatric EEG monitoring. Review of the video can assist with detecting artifact (e.g., from patting an infant), description of event semiology, and determining if an electrographic seizure has any clinical correlate. To be most useful,

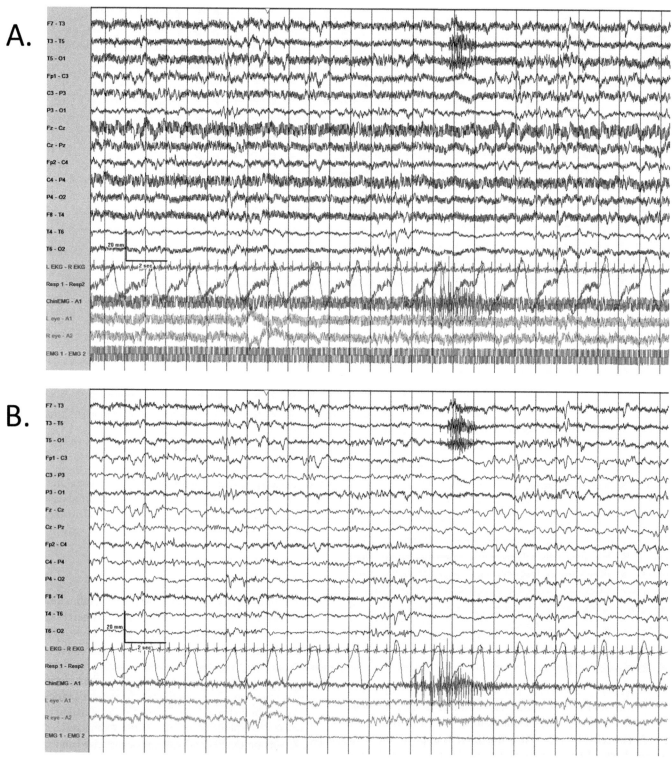

Figure 2.5 This neonatal EEG illustrates the same record with notch filter off (A) versus on (B).

Activation Procedures

a bedside observer who can press a patient event button and document any events of concern is essential.

Activation procedures are typically performed when obtaining a baseline routine EEG, or at the start of a non-urgent long-term EEG monitoring study. These procedures are performed in order to elicit specific epileptiform abnormalities or to provoke focal slowing. They also produce characteristic, normal physiological responses. These tests are not performed on neonates, patients who are unable to cooperate, or those who are critically ill.

24

Hyperventilation

Hyperventilation is performed by having a patient breathe quickly and deeply for 3–5 minutes. It is normal for patients to exhibit diffuse slowing during hyperventilation. In particular, children's hyperventilation response can be quite robust and rhythmic. This activation technique can be especially useful for patients with suspected genetic generalized epilepsy (particularly childhood or juvenile absence epilepsy), because hyperventilation activates generalized spike-wave discharges and can provoke absence seizures. In patients with focal cortical dysfunction, hyperventilation may elicit focal EEG slowing over the affected region. Hyperventilation is contra-indicated for patients with severe pulmonary or cardiac disease, acute or recent stroke, or significant cerebrovascular disease, due to the risk of vasoconstriction and reduced cerebral perfusion [1, 13, 17].

Photic Stimulation

Photic stimulation is also a routinely performed activating procedure, during which the patient is exposed to a brief series of flashing lights at specific frequencies ranging from 1 to 30 Hz. It is normal to see a "photic driving response" on EEG, which is characterized by symmetric bi-occipitally predominant surface negative deflections occurring at the same time and frequency as the flashes of light. Sometimes, these driving responses can occur at harmonic or subharmonic frequencies, relative to the light flashes. Photic stimulation can induce a photoparoxysmal response for some patients. This typically consists of a generalized epileptiform discharge (spike-wave or polyspike-wave) occurring in response to the photic stimulation. In order to confirm the association of the discharge with the photic stimulus, the EEG technologist will typically repeat the same flash frequency that initially induced the photoparoxysmal response. If the discharges occur again, the response is said to be reproducible and photic stimulation should be terminated in order to avoid provocation of a photoparoxysmal convulsion. If the photoparoxysmal response persists after the photic stimulation ends, the patient may have a photosensitive epilepsy syndrome [17].

Quantitative EEG

Full array EEG data remain the gold standard of neurophysiological monitoring. In recent years, the volume of EEG studies has increased substantially, and many centers do not have the capabilities or personnel to individually interpret real-time full EEG data 24 hours per day, 7 days of the week. Reduced montage and quantitative EEG techniques have allowed providers, particularly in the neonatal and pediatric intensive care units, to have supplementary data to interpret, in real time, at the patient's bedside or via remote access. Although these tools are not equivalent to full EEG, the information they provide can be extremely helpful in centers where EEG technologists and/or neurophysiologists are not continuously available or ICU monitoring volumes are high. These techniques are also interesting and exciting research tools.

Amplitude-Integrated EEG

Conventional long-term monitoring EEG is the gold standard for monitoring neonates at risk for seizures [14]. In many neonatal nurseries or ICUs, however, long-term monitoring EEGs and clinical neurophysiologists are not consistently available; amplitude-integrated EEG (aEEG) can be a useful tool. In most cases, the aEEG electrodes can be applied by bedside nurses or other NICU staff, and the aEEG can be interpreted without the assistance of a neurophysiologist if necessary [18, 19]. Both hydrogel and needle electrodes are commonly employed for aEEG recordings. Hydrogel electrodes have the advantage of not breaking the skin, but can be easily dislodged and may provide higher impedance values. Needle electrodes provide better, and more consistent, impedance, but require subdermal insertion.

Amplitude-integrated EEG records activity from one or two channels, using electrodes typically placed over the biparietal head regions (P3 → P4) or bilateral central-parietal positions (C3 → P3; C4 →P4). The biparietal derivation was chosen for single channel recording in neonates as this is the over the cerebrovascular watershed regions – areas that are most susceptible to ischemia and to seizures [20]. In the international 10–20 system, modified for neonates, P3 and P4 electrodes are not traditionally used. The P3 → P4 channel on aEEG is most anatomically similar to the C3 → C4 channel in a traditional neonatal reduced montage. The EEG data from the single channel are processed and filtered, attenuating frequencies that are outside the 2–15 Hz range and minimizing artifact that may arise from movements, pulse, sweat, etc. Data are further processed via semilogarithmic amplitude compression and displayed at a time scale of 6 cm per hour. This allows for a large amount of data to be reviewed and interpreted quickly on a single screen at the patient's bedside. Studies have proven aEEG to be valuable in providing information regarding the neonate's EEG background; however, its use for seizure detection is less predictable, with widely variable specificity and sensitivity [20, 21] (Figure 2.6).

Some neonatal ICUs use aEEG and conventional EEG simultaneously. Many times, the aEEG is displayed on the bedside monitor, for use by the primary ICU team, while the conventional EEG is interpreted remotely by the clinical neurophysiologist. This allows the bedside staff to alert the neurophysiologist to any acute concerns as they appear on the aEEG, at which time they can be confirmed on conventional EEG.

Quantitative EEG

Quantitative electroencephalography (QEEG) allows for digital trend analysis of raw EEG data. This can be particularly helpful in centers where clinical neurophysiologists may not be available for interpretation of large volumes of real-time conventional EEG analysis 24 hours per day. There are various trend techniques, which use a variety of algorithms and displays to analyze data according to frequency or amplitude

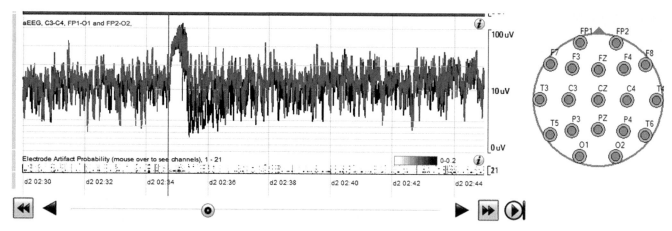

Figure 2.6 Amplitude-integrated EEG in a neonate, as displayed at the bedside.

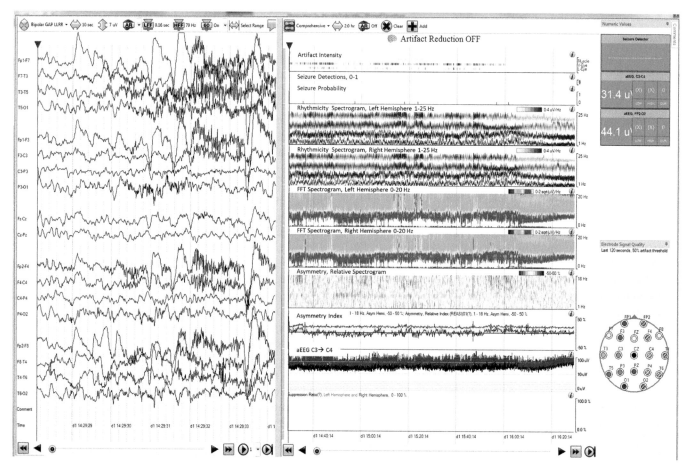

Figure 2.7 Digital trend analyses used in conjunction with conventional EEG. QEEG trends are displayed to the right of the conventional EEG. Trends included (from top to bottom): Artifact Intensity, Seizure Probability, Rhythmicity Spectrogram left and right hemispheres, FFT Spectrogram left and right hemispheres, Asymmetry Spectrogram, Asymmetry Index, aEEG.

trends, seizure or spike detection, and artifact reduction. The value of QEEG in pediatric and neonatal EEG has been less studied to date than adult QEEG, but is an area of growing interest [2, 21–23]. Importantly, review of QEEG is not intended to replace interpretation of the full EEG. Rather, QEEG complements conventional EEG and may improve reviewers' efficiency (Figure 2.7).

Frequency Trends

Color Density spectral array (CDSA) is a specific form of QEEG. Specific frequency bands (i.e., alpha, beta, delta, theta) are analyzed separately in specific channels or hemispheres and compared to the accompanying channels or opposite hemisphere. Frequency data may be displayed independently, or analyzed in proportion to the EEG voltage, which is called power. The power spectrum is the square of the voltage, which can be displayed via Fast Fourier Transform (FFT) [2, 22]. FFT is characterized by time displayed on the x-axis, and frequency on the y-axis. Power is represented on a z-axis in a color or grayscale code [2, 23]. Spectrograms can then be created and displayed to represent rhythmicity, or asymmetry between hemispheres or particular channels. A ratio of alpha to delta frequencies (the alpha-delta ratio) may be calculated using FFT and is employed to evaluate for differences in frequency bands between hemispheres, averaged over a specified period of time. Spectral analysis does not allow for analysis of waveform morphology, which is a limitation and highlights the need for co-interpretation with the raw EEG data when a suspected abnormality is detected [2, 21–23].

Amplitude Trends

Amplitude trends are intended to be combined with other EEG trends. Time is displayed on the x-axis and amplitude on the y-axis. Peak envelope-trend analysis displays a patient's median waveform amplitudes for a specified period of time. A suppression ratio calculates the percentage of time during which the EEG amplitude (in microvolts) is below a specified threshold for a specified time interval; the ratio is then typically compared between hemispheres. Akin to the power spectra, an amplitude spectrum can be analyzed by obtaining the equivalent of the square root of the power spectrum [23].

Event Detection

Event detection analysis allows for detection of particular programmed EEG patterns, such as spikes, sharp waves, or patterns concerning for seizures. It is common for false-positive patterns to be identified, and many commercially available algorithms lack sensitivity and specificity [21, 23].

Artifact Reduction

Artifact reduction is designed to identify and reduce extracerebral signals that can distort an EEG (e.g., muscle or eye movements). This technology can be helpful when the artifact source is clear, and it allows for a cleaner interpretation of the scalp EEG; however, many sources of artifact cannot be eliminated automatically, and are best identified by using extracerebral channels and video monitoring in conjunction with raw EEG data interpretation [2].

Summary

EEG monitoring is increasingly prevalent in the neonatal and pediatric ICU. Professional organizations have published recommended standards for the application, acquisition, and interpretation of EEG data. Extracerebral channels are particularly important for ICU monitoring, since sources of artifacts are ubiquitous in the ICU setting. EEG trending techniques and reduced montage approaches may enhance efficiency of ICU EEG interpretation, but they cannot replace thorough review of the raw signal by a trained clinical neurophysiologist.

References

1. Abou-Khalil B, Misulis K. *Atlas of EEG and Seizure Semiology*. Philadelphia: Elsevier; 2006.

2. Fisch B. *Fisch and Spehlmann's EEG Primer: Basic Principles of Digital and Analog EEG*, 3rd ed. Oxford: Elsevier; 1999.

3. Klem GH, Luders HO, Jasper HH, Elger C. The ten-twenty electrode system of the International Federation. The International Federation of Clinical Neurophysiology. *Electroencephalogr Clin Neurophysiol Suppl*. 1999;**52**:3–6.

4. American Clinical Neurophysiology Society. American Clinical Neurophysiology Guideline Two: minimum technical standards for pediatric electroencephalography. 2006. www.acns.org/pdf/guidelines/Guideline-2.pdf.

5. Saurabh S. Recording techniques. In Ebersole JS, Husain AM, Nordli DR, editors. *Current Practice of Clinical Electroencephalography*, 4th ed. Philadelphia: Wolters Kluwer Health; 2014.

6. Nuwer MR, Comi G, Emerson R, et al. IFCN standards for digital recording of clinical EEG. International Federation of Clinical Neurophysiology. *Electroencephalogr Clin Neurophysiol Suppl*. 1999;**52**:11–14.

7. Greenfield LJ, Jr., Geyer JD, Carney, PR. *Reading EEGs: A Practical Approach*. Philadelphia: Lippincott Williams and Wilkins; 2010.

8. Mirsattari SM, Lee DH, Jones D, Bihari F, Ives JR. MRI compatible EEG electrode system for routine use in the epilepsy monitoring unit and intensive care unit. *Clin Neurophysiol*. 2004 Sep;**115**(9):2175–80.

9. Abend NS, Dlugos DJ, Zhu X, Schwartz ES. Utility of CT-compatible EEG electrodes in critically ill children. *Pediatr Radiol*. 2015 Apr;**45**(5):714–8.

10. Berlin F, Carlile JA, de Burgo MI, et al. Technical tips: electrode application and preventing skin breakdown techniques. *Am J Electroneurodiagnostic Technol*. 2011 Sep;**51**(3):206–19.

11. Young B, Blais R, Campbell V, et al. Vapors from collodion and acetone in an EEG laboratory. *J Clin Neurophysiol*. 1993 Jan;**10**(1):108–10.

12. Falco C, Sebastiano F, Cacciola L, et al. Scalp electrode placement by EC2 adhesive paste in long-term video-EEG monitoring. *Clin Neurophysiol*. 2005 Aug;**116**(8):1771–3.

13. Clancy RR, Bergqvist AGC, et al. Normal pediatric EEG: neonates and children. In Ebersole JS, Husain AM, Nordli DR, editors. *Current Practice of Clinical Electroencephalography*, 4th ed. Philadelphia: Wolters Kluwer Health; 2014.

14. Shellhaas RA, Chang T, Tsuchida T, et al. The American Clinical Neurophysiology Society's Guideline on Continuous Electroencephalography Monitoring in Neonates. *J Clin Neurophysiol*. 2011 Dec;**28**(6):611–17.

15. Epstein CM et al. American Clinical Neurophysiology Society. Guideline two: minimum technical standards for pediatric electroencephalography. *J Clin Neurophysiol*. 2006 Apr;**23**(2): 92–6.

16. Hahn JS. Neonatal and pediatric electroencephalography. In Aminoff MJ, editor. *Aminoff's*

Electrodiagnosis in Clinical Neurology, 6th ed. Elsevier: 2012.

17. Tatum WO. Normal adult EEG. In Ebersole JS, Husain AM, Nordli DR, editors. *Current Practice of Clinical Electroencephalography*, 4th ed. Philadelphia: Wolters Kluwer Health; 2014

18. Glass HC, Wusthoff CJ, Shellhaas RA. Amplitude-integrated electro-encephalography: the child neurologist's perspective.

J Child Neurol. 2013 Oct;28(10): 1342–50.

19. Shellhaas RA, Soaita AI, Clancy RR. Sensitivity of amplitude-integrated electroencephalography for neonatal seizure detection. *Pediatrics.* 2007 Oct;120(4):770–7.

20. Hellström-Westas L, de Vries LS, Rosén, I. An *Atlas of Amplitude-Integrated EEGs in the Newborn*, 2nd ed. London: Informa Healthcare; 2008.

21. Shellhaas RA. Continuous electroencephalography monitoring in neonates. *Curr Neurol Neurosci Rep.* 2012 Aug;12(4):429–35.

22. Nuwer MR, Pedro CC, Topographic mapping, frequency analysis, and other quantitative techniques in electroencephalograph. In *Aminoff's Electrodiagnosis in Clinical Neurology*, 6th ed. Elsevier; 2012.

23. Persyst 12 On-Line User's Guide. Persyst. Version 12. San Diego, CA, USA.

Chapter 3

Logistics of Neuromonitoring

William Gallentine, Crystal M. Keller, and Brian Livingstone

Illustrative Cases

Case 1 Pitfalls in aEEG Interpretation

Case 27 Autoimmune Encephalitis

Key Points

- Starting an ICU neuromonitoring program requires in-depth logistical planning prior to initiation. Seemingly small changes to continuous EEG monitoring practices may have a striking impact on resource availability and utilization.
- Essential decisions include: what patient populations are to be monitored, for how long, as well as how often EEG data will be reviewed and by whom.
- Involving the entire team early in logistical planning – including EEG readers (attending physicians and trainees), pediatric neurologists, neonatal and pediatric intensivists and nurses, neurodiagnostic technologists, neurodiagnostic laboratory team, and hospital administrators – will help identify possible flaws in the implementation plan and avoid costly financial decisions or committing to practices that resources will not support.
- Functioning as a multidisciplinary team is essential for the long-term success of an ICU neuromonitoring program.

Introduction

Over the past decade, the utilization of continuous EEG (cEEG) monitoring in the intensive care unit (ICU) has dramatically increased. This increase has been driven predominantly by our increased awareness of the presence of nonconvulsive seizures in certain high-risk populations. With increased demand for cEEG services, the need for strong logistical planning of neuromonitoring units has become increasingly evident. Without effective planning, what may seem like small changes in cEEG monitoring protocols can result in substantial downstream effects resulting in major stressors to the care system [1, 2]. This chapter will focus on the logistics of developing a cEEG neuromonitoring unit with an emphasis on standard of care practice [3], consensus guidelines [4–6], and practical considerations.

Constructing a cEEG Neuromonitoring Team and Baseline Assessment

Forming a team early in the development of the cEEG neuromonitoring program is essential for success. Key members of the team include attending and trainee physicians (electroencephalographers, pediatric neurologists, and ICU physicians, especially those in leadership roles), neurodiagnostic laboratory technologists (NDTs) and administrators, hospital administrators, ICU nurses and physician extenders, and information technology (IT) specialists. As "buy in" is essential from each of these groups for a cEEG neuromonitoring unit to be successful, having them involved early in the planning process is invaluable and allows for early identification of potential roadblocks. Failure to identify potential problems may have substantial financial ramifications that may have been avoidable with planning.

Who and How to Monitor: Development of Institutional Guidelines

Once the team forms, a baseline assessment of resources should be performed. The following items should be considered: current monitoring practice (who is being monitored, duration of monitoring, workflow from cEEG order placement) and cEEG resources (EEG technicians – number and availability, EEG machines, electrodes, data storage, data pruning practices, EEG readers, network capacity, remote access, quantitative EEG). Understanding the hospital's commitment to growth of the unit and the possibility of future resource allocation allows for construction of realistic monitoring protocols that will not overstress the system. A checklist of infrastructure items needed for a cEEG ICU neuromonitoring unit is provided in Table 3.1.

There are many points to consider prior to starting a cEEG neuromonitoring service, perhaps none more important than identification of which patients will undergo monitoring. The American Clinical Neurophysiology Society (ACNS) has consensus statements to serve as guidelines for which pediatric and neonatal patient populations should be considered for cEEG monitoring [4–6]. As they pertain to children, these guidelines have suggested the following general indications: (1) the diagnosis of nonconvulsive seizures, nonconvulsive status epilepticus, and other paroxysmal events; (2) assessment of efficacy of treatment of seizures and status epilepticus; (3) monitoring of sedation and high-dose suppressive therapy; and (4) assessment of encephalopathy and prognostication [5]. The ACNS Neonatal guidelines propose specific high-risk neonates for which cEEG is also strongly recommended [4]. Specifics of these indications are covered in further detail in other chapters.

The ACNS guidelines provide a framework for developing institutional guidelines regarding which patients will be monitored as well as the duration of monitoring. Development of

Table 3.1 Infrastructure requirements for an ICU cEEG neuromonitoring program

Equipment

- Acquisition machines (hardwired vs. portable)
- Review station monitors
- Electrodes: consider whether to use CT/MRI compatible
- Quantitative EEG software
- Central server/network access for transfer and storage of cEEG data
- Archiving equipment
- Remote access for real-time review

Personnel

- Certified physician cEEG readers
- Neurodiagnostic technologists, with at least one ICU specialist
- Hospital and neurodiagnostic laboratory administrators
- Information technology support
- Pediatric neurology physicians
- ICU team members (physicians, physician extenders, ICU nurses)

Institutional cEEG guidelines

- Indications for monitoring and recommended duration of monitoring for each indication
- Timing of cEEG service availability and target response times for hook-up
- Protocol for ordering cEEG studies (who can order, and lines of communication)
- Outline of cEEG review frequency and reporting policy

institution-specific guidelines is very important, and should realistically accommodate institutional resources. Some institutions may already perform a combination of monitoring modalities, including amplitude-integrated EEG (aEEG) based cerebral function monitors, limited-montage cEEG, and full-montage cEEG. Agreement on when and in whom to utilize each of these modalities and when to transition from one modality to another should be part of institutional guidelines.

It is essential that institutional guidelines be co-developed by Neurology and ICU staff. At the outset, an analysis to assess anticipated cEEG volume and potential impact on other parts of the health system should be performed. This analysis will determine the adequacy of current infrastructure, including personnel and equipment, to support the implementation of the protocol. Implementation of the program in stages, by sequentially targeting specific patient populations (e.g., traumatic brain injury, hypoxic-ischemic encephalopathy, refractory status epilepticus) and limiting cEEG monitoring to specific ICUs (e.g., pediatric, neonatal, cardiac) allows for reassessment of how current resources are tolerating the added cEEG volume. The importance of ICU input in the development of the institutional guidelines cannot be emphasized

enough, as the ICU team typically identifies the patients in need of monitoring before the neurology team is involved in their care. A lack of ICU team involvement will result in unsuccessful implementation of institutional neuromonitoring guidelines.

Alongside indications for monitoring, institutional guidelines should also establish how cEEG monitoring is to be ordered and by whom (e.g., whether neurology shall be consulted prior to cEEG order), the urgency of cEEG hook-up and triage, the frequency of cEEG review and reporting, the maximum number of patients that can be monitored at a given time, and the duration of monitoring. Each of these will depend on institutional resources.

cEEG Monitoring Equipment

Electrodes

Neuromonitoring is most commonly performed using disc or cup electrodes (gold-plated silver, silver/silver-chloride, or conductive plastic) with a minimum of 16 electrodes placed according to the 10–20 International electrode system. The use of fewer electrodes decreases sensitivity for seizure detection and makes it more difficult to distinguish artifacts [5]. As patients in the ICU frequently require neuroimaging, CT and/or MRI compatible electrodes should be used when possible. Repeated removal and reapplication of cEEG electrodes for neuroimaging contributes to skin breakdown [5] and is an inefficient use of NDT time, which may be a limited resource. Subdermal single-use disposable (stainless steel) needle electrodes can be applied rapidly, but they have inferior recording quality and pose the risk of needlestick injury to staff [5]. These electrodes may cause artifact on CT and are not MRI compatible. Due to these factors, we generally do not recommend needle electrodes for cEEG recordings in the ICU. Subdermal wire electrodes offer another alternative to reduce skin breakdown and are particularly suitable for patients requiring multiday neuromonitoring. These single-use electrodes, consisting of a silver Teflon-coated wire with a silver-chloride tip, provide recording quality superior to disk electrodes, cause minimal CT artifact and can be modified to be MRI compatible [5].

Electrode cap systems can be used to facilitate EEG electrode placement by ICU staff when NDTs are not available. Drawbacks include increased risk of skin breakdown, the need for disinfection between uses, and that application can be limited by the presence of intracranial monitoring devices and head wounds [5]. As an alternative, single-use disposable templates are available to facilitate electrode application by ICU staff.

cEEG Acquisition Machines and Review Stations

Acquisition machines can be portable or fixed, with each having advantages and disadvantages. Portable units allow the flexibility of monitoring patients in different locations and present lower start-up costs as compared to fixed machines that are hardwired to a series of patient rooms or bed spaces.

However, fixed machines have advantages in the ICU environment because they do not take up valuable floor space and may provide superior camera angles and hence video quality. If portable units are to be used in the ICU, carts with small footprints are recommended to minimize the amount of floor space required.

Computers used to acquire cEEG data should have enough processing power to acquire EEG with synchronized video and simultaneously process quantitative EEG (QEEG) trends. Hard drives on acquisition machines should have the capacity to store at least 24 hours of EEG and video data. Video is an absolute necessity in identifying sources of artifact and assessing for clinical correlations to electrographic findings.

All acquisition machines should have network connectivity at a minimum speed of 100 megabits per second [5]. Hardwired Ethernet-based connections are generally preferred to ensure sufficient bandwidth to accommodate streaming EEG and video. Wireless connectivity should only be considered if the hospital's wireless network is demonstrated to be sufficiently robust, and strategic placement of wireless access points in the ICU may be required.

Review stations should be equipped with display monitors meeting the current standards of 1600 × 1200 pixels with a diagonal screen of 20 inches or more [5]. Dual monitor display facilitates concomitant review of QEEG.

Network and Remote Access

It is essential for cEEG readers to be able to access the cEEG both from numerous sites within the hospital (EEG reading room, office, clinic, wards, etc.) as well as outside the hospital while on call. Real-time remote access capabilities must be available. A robust hospital network is needed to support the transfer of EEG data and video from acquisition machines and servers to review stations. Adequate network capacity is essential to allow for appropriate EEG review speed, which is of crucial importance once a large volume of cEEG studies is performed and stored.

Neuromonitoring programs should work closely with their institution's information technology team to ensure the protection of all personal health information, on both wireless networks and through remote access. Options for remote access include a virtual private network (VPN) connection to the institution, server-based remote desktop environments such as Citrix, or third-party secure remote desktop connections [5].

Data Storage

Continuous EEG is typically stored on a central hospital server using database software supplied by the EEG vendor. Servers must have adequate storage capacity, taking into consideration the following variables: the amount of video and EEG data generated by each acquisition machine per day (typically about 12 gigabytes), the number of acquisition machines in operation, and the number of days that EEG data will be stored prior to pruning and archiving [5]. Ideally, acquisition units will upload video cEEG data to the central server in real time,

with fallback to storage on a local hard drive in the event of an interruption in network connectivity. Storing data on a central server allows for high-speed access as well as multiuser access to the same file from multiple different sites. The servers hosting patient data should be routinely backed up for redundancy to protect against data loss.

Video cEEG data can be digitally archived to DVDs, external hard drives, archive servers, or network attached storage devices [5]. Ease of access should be taken into consideration, as comparison of newly acquired cEEG and archived cEEG recordings is commonly necessary. To save storage space before archiving, video data are usually clipped to include only pertinent clinical events. The cEEG data may be retained in their entirety or clipped. Clipped file samples should provide an adequate representation of what is described in the report, such as clinical events and relevant samples of background, interictal discharges, periodic discharges, and electrographic seizures. Quantitative EEG trends used in cEEG interpretation should also be stored. Although legal requirements vary by jurisdiction, EEG data must typically be stored for 7–10 years or 2–10 years after a pediatric patient's 18th birthday.

Quantitative EEG

Over the past several years, use of QEEG in the ICU has become more commonplace. QEEG has proven quite useful in detection of electrographic seizures, and more recently as a bedside monitor of cerebral function. QEEG may be part of a vendor's cEEG platform, or separate commercially available software may be purchased and integrated into an institution's cEEG system. Software packages vary in types of monitoring trends and seizure detection algorithms, and some have multi-patient display capabilities. QEEG helps reduce cEEG review time and may reveal slowly evolving changes in the cEEG background over long periods, which may not be as evident on raw EEG review [5]. QEEG should not be used in isolation because some seizures are likely to be missed. Furthermore, QEEG findings should always be confirmed on the raw EEG to avoid misinterpretation of artifact. Commonly used QEEG techniques display amplitude (as in aEEG), rhythmicity, symmetry, frequency, and/or power over a compressed time scale. QEEG trends can be combined to create more sophisticated multiple-trend panels (Figure 3.1). Some trends may be more useful in certain patients, while not as helpful in others. The choice of QEEG trends can be tailored to individual patients, and custom trends or trend panels can be created. QEEG trends are most commonly generated using a hemispheric average of electrodes, which allows for right–left comparison of a given trend. However, QEEG trends for individual EEG channels may also be displayed. A basic QEEG panel would often include bi-hemispheric amplitude-integrated EEG (aEEG), color density spectral array (CDSA), asymmetry index, and a rhythmicity spectrogram or envelope trend.

The current standard of care for ICU cEEG monitoring is continuous EEG data acquisition with intermittent EEG review [5]. Although this model is certainly superior to no cEEG monitoring at all, intermittent review does create the

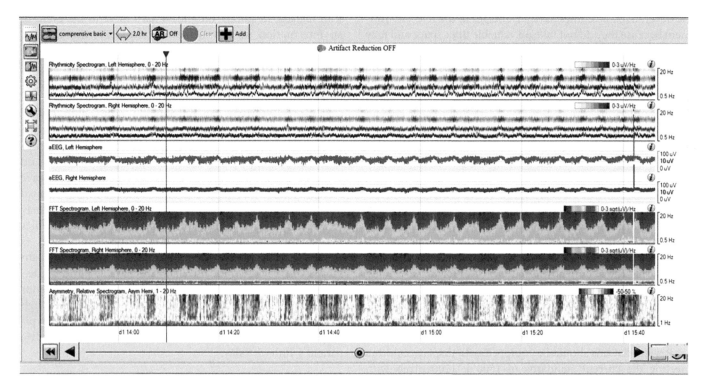

Figure 3.1 Basic quantitative EEG panel. QEEG trends include rhythmicity spectrogram (rows 1 & 2 from top), amplitude-integrated EEG (rows 3 & 4), fast Fourier transform (FFT) spectrogram, also known as color density spectral array (CDSA) (rows 5 & 6), and asymmetry index (bottom).

possibility that seizures may go undetected for several hours (see Case 1 in Part V).

Excitingly, QEEG does offer the possibility of enabling ICU staff without EEG expertise to identify changes in the cEEG, thereby providing real-time bedside neuromonitoring. In just a few quick training sessions, ICU staff are typically able to identify common patterns of concern, most notably electrographic seizures. However, these patterns should not be acted upon by the ICU without confirmation on the raw EEG by properly trained staff. This safeguards against misinterpretation of artifact and resultant overtreatment. In addition to QEEG, the raw EEG should also be displayed at the bedside to allow the ICU team to see if something technically has gone wrong that could influence what is seen on the QEEG, most commonly, poorly connected electrodes (Figure 3.2). Finally, some QEEG systems include computerized seizure detection algorithms which can be linked to audible or email alarms to alert EEG readers or bedside practitioners. However, the relatively high false positive rates of current algorithms have limited their adoption. QEEG is increasingly used as a bedside monitor, in hopes that those patients with electrographic seizures may be more rapidly identified and treated.

Personnel

Neurodiagnostic Technologists (NDTs)

Per ACNS guidelines, all ICU cEEG recordings should be performed by trained and certified neurodiagnostic technologists (NDTs), with at least one technologist on the team

meeting criteria as an NDT ICU specialist [5]. These NDTs should have at least 3 years of experience (including 1 year of cEEG) and should receive special training in cEEG equipment management and troubleshooting, with emphasis on electrical safety, infection control, and data acquisition [5]. They should also receive added training in the recognition of ictal/interictal EEG patterns, artifacts, clinical seizures, seizure related-medical emergencies, and QEEG analysis [5].

Impact of Neuromonitoring Program on NDTs

Ideally, ICU cEEG services would be available 24 hours per day, 7 days per week. A large obstacle for many programs is the evening and weekend availability of NDTs. In a 2013 study looking at the resources available across pediatric centers in the United States and Canada, cEEG electrodes were placed by NDTs in 89% of recordings [3]. Only 28% of centers had 24/7 in-house NDT coverage, 51% always had NDTs available but at times only through emergency call-back, and 21% had times when NDTs were not available at all [3].

Starting a cEEG neuromonitoring unit can have a significant impact on NDTs. First, the added volume of cEEGs has the potential to significantly increase workload. Furthermore, the urgency with which cEEG studies are requested to be hooked up may pose additional stress. Shifting to a 24/7 operation from a 9-to-5 operation may mean changing from daytime hours to shift work, which may further add to stress. During the development of institutional neuromonitoring guidelines, it is important to set expectations on how quickly patients can be hooked up during the daytime

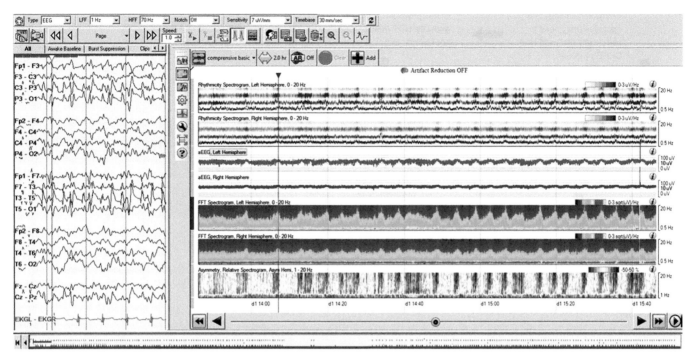

Figure 3.2 Example of bedside QEEG display with 3 seconds of raw EEG also displayed (left) in a patient having frequent electrographic seizures. This allows for potential identification of electrographic seizures vs. artifact from disconnected electrodes.

and after hours. A shared understanding between neurology, EEG, and ICU may reduce frustration across the team. Planned expansion of the number NDTs to ensure adequate coverage is essential in preventing NDT burnout.

EEG Readers

The ACNS guidelines recommend the cEEG team be supervised by a physician with expertise in ICU cEEG [5]. Reviewing practices vary among centers [3]. Some centers rely solely on physician cEEG review, while others rely on NDT review prior to physician review [3]. Other programs have clinical neurophysiology or epilepsy fellows providing the initial review, followed by an attending physician. Continuous EEG studies are most commonly reviewed twice per day with results provided via written report once per day [3], but verbal reports may be conveyed to the ICU more frequently depending on the findings. Continuous physician review of cEEG is uncommon, but in some centers NDTs perform continuous cEEG review [3]. In patients with active seizures, physician review typically becomes more frequent. It is important for the ICU team to know how often studies will be reviewed, so including expected review frequency in the institutional guidelines is recommended. The impact on cEEG readers also needs to be taken into consideration when developing institutional guidelines. Specifically, the following questions should be considered: (1) Will the readers be able to keep up with the additional cEEG volume? (2) Will the cEEG readers be able to review data remotely, including with QEEG availability? These very important questions need to be addressed in planning your neuromonitoring unit; these issues may limit the growth of the program without adequate support.

Information Technology Support

Strong information technology support (IT) is imperative for the long-term success of a cEEG neuromonitoring program. Having a designated IT support person for the unit is strongly encouraged as technical issues with acquisition machines, the server, the network, QEEG, and so on are inevitable and often require rapid intervention so that they do not negatively impact the clinical activities of the NDTs working in tandem.

Importance of Communication within the cEEG Neuromonitoring Team

The process of actually getting a child in need of a cEEG hooked up, EEG video data acquired, and then the data interpreted is typically quite complicated and requires a significant amount of communication and coordination among team members. A commonly used paradigm is described in Figure 3.3. Depending on the number of steps an institution has in its cEEG guidelines, significant delays can occur as a result of numerous communications required. Institutions should strongly consider streamlining the number of communications needed to obtain a cEEG. In addition, institutional guidelines can facilitate more streamlined communications.

Conclusion

Continuous EEG monitoring has become an essential tool in the management of children in the ICU. Development of a neuromonitoring program takes careful consideration in

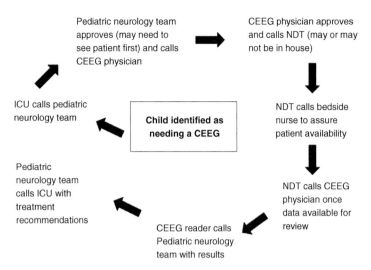

Figure 3.3 Diagram of a commonly used cEEG paradigm illustrating the potential for communication complexities. With each added layer of required communication, a potential delay in time as well as the potential for communication error exists. When developing institutional guidelines, one should strongly consider streamlining the number of communications in order to maximize efficiency.

regard to institutional cEEG monitoring guidelines and available resources. Intensive care unit cEEG neuromonitoring programs require specialized equipment and personnel, along with substantial institutional infrastructure. Although standard practice is intermittent review of continuously acquired cEEG data, bedside display of QEEG trends offers the possibility for real-time neuromonitoring by ICU caregivers. The long-term success of an ICU cEEG program is contingent upon strong communication between all members of the neuromonitoring unit team.

References

1. Abend NS, Topjian AA, Williams S. Could EEG monitoring in critically ill children be a cost-effective neuroprotective strategy? *J Clin Neurophysiol.* 2015;**32** (6):486–94.

2. Gutierrez-Colina AM, Topjian AA, Dlugos DJ, Abend NS. Electroencephalogram monitoring in critically ill children: indications and strategies. *Pediatr Neurol.* 2012;**46** (3):158–61.

3. Sanchez SM, Carpenter J, Chapman KE, et al. Pediatric ICU EEG monitoring: current resources and practice in the United States and Canada. *J Clin Neurophysiol.* 2013;**30**(2):156–60.

4. Herman ST, Abend NS, Bleck TP, et al. Consensus statement on continuous EEG in critically ill adults and children, part I: indications. *J Clin Neurophysiol.* 2015;**32**(2):87–95.

5. Herman ST, Abend NS, Bleck TP, et al. Consensus statement on continuous EEG in critically ill adults and children, part II: personnel, technical specifications, and clinical practice. *J Clin Neurophysiol.* 2015;**2**(2):96–108.

6. Shellhaas RA, Chang T, Tsuchida T, et al. The American Clinical Neurophysiology Society's Guideline on Continuous Electroencephalography Monitoring in Neonates. *J Clin Neurophysiol.* 2011;**28**(6):611–17.

Nursing Considerations in Neuromonitoring

Kathi S. Randall and Diane Wilson

Illustrative Case

Case 1 Pitfalls in aEEG Interpretation

Key Points

- Neuromonitoring devices can be divided in to two broad categories: monitors of cerebral function and cerebral perfusion.
- Neuromonitoring is a shared responsibility in the ICU with several key roles for bedside nursing staff, including the identification and reporting of trends.
- Nursing staff should be familiar with equipment and supplies needed for neuromonitoring as well as troubleshooting common artifacts and problems.
- Guideline development and ongoing education are essential to the success of any neuromonitoring program.

Introduction

Over the past decade, continuous neurophysiological monitoring has become more common in intensive care units (ICUs). For many pediatric patient populations neuromonitoring is now the standard of care [1]. Since bedside neuromonitoring is frequently applied, maintained, and reviewed by the bedside nurse, it is critical that nurses are fully aware of the technical aspects of how to use the devices, the rationale for their use and the potential benefits of monitoring.

This chapter provides suggested pathways for integrating bedside neuromonitoring into clinical practice and discussion of day-to-day nursing roles and responsibilities related to bedside monitoring. Because there is limited published experience in nursing roles related to neuromonitoring [2, 3], the recommendations in this chapter primarily come from the authors' experiential knowledge of monitoring trends, equipment, and troubleshooting. Adjustments for the needs and resources in other settings may be warranted.

Neuromonitoring at the Bedside

Types of Monitors

Bedside brain monitors currently available for use in the ICU fall into two broad categories: brain function monitors and brain perfusion monitors.

Brain function monitors utilize the familiar electroencephalography (EEG) technology, but their bedside display relies heavily on trending software that allows those not formally trained in reading "raw EEG" to quickly assess brain activity. In pediatric patients, brain function monitoring typically is performed using video continuous EEG (cEEG) recording with quantitative EEG (QEEG) trends displayed at the bedside. The QEEG algorithms digitally separate the complex EEG signal into its more basic components and compress the recorded data over time, allowing display of several hours of EEG data on a single screen. Although the raw EEG is reviewed in detail by a neurologist or neurophysiologist who is usually remote from the bedside, the QEEG trends can be viewed by bedside caregivers to assess real-time changes in brain activity. See Box 4.1 for a list of commonly used QEEG trends.

The most common EEG trend used at the bedside in the neonatal ICU (NICU) is amplitude-integrated EEG (aEEG), which may be processed from the full array of electrodes used in simultaneous cEEG recording, or may be recorded from a reduced number of electrodes typically applied by NICU staff instead of EEG technologists [4]. Both aEEG and other QEEG trends can be used to assess the presence of sleep–wake cycling, to screen for seizures, and to evaluate for suppressed or asymmetrical brain activity [5, 6]. It is important to emphasize that while aEEG and QEEG trends do not replace the need for a comprehensive review of the cEEG recording by a neurologist or neurophysiologist, these trends have been shown to be useful for an initial screening or periodic review of baseline EEG activity at the bedside, and have the benefit of ready availability day or night [7]. For the NICU population, aEEG is available both through stand-alone monitors and as a display option in conjunction with cEEG monitoring. Other QEEG trends (such as % suppression and CDSA) are similarly available as a bedside display option when recording cEEG on many commercially available systems. The various commercial monitors all have easy-to-use, skin-friendly sensor options available in pediatric and neonatal sizes.

For brain perfusion monitoring, the most commonly used technology in both pediatric and neonatal ICUs is near-

Box 4.1 Commonly Used QEEG Trends

1. aEEG
2. Asymmetry
3. % Suppression
4. Inter-burst interval
5. Color density spectral array (CDSA/DSA)
6. Spectral edge frequency
7. Peak envelope amplitude

infrared spectroscopy (NIRS). These monitors can be used to trend brain perfusion over long periods, evaluate cerebral autoregulation, and assess regional oxygen saturation, extraction, and utilization during interventions [8–11]. NIRS monitors are most typically stand-alone monitors and rarely integrated within other physiological or neuromonitoring devices.

Roles for Nurses

There are several essential roles that ICU nurses play in bedside brain monitoring (Box 4.2).

When first introducing neuromonitoring to a unit, a stepwise implementation strategy is recommended to ease the stress of integrating a new technology into the ICU and to facilitate the adoption of new nursing roles. For example, the first skills and responsibilities that nurses might assume related to bedside brain monitoring might be sensor application, maintenance, and documentation. Then, after a predetermined period of weeks or even months, nurse responsibilities might expand to include troubleshooting, reporting artifacts, and identifying unusual findings. Later phases could include more detailed interpretation and classification of normal versus abnormal findings. Development of neuromonitoring guidelines that reflect each unit's intended use, availability of support personnel and level of expertise is essential to the success of any neuromonitoring program. Guidelines should include detailed instructions for not only device application but also troubleshooting of equipment issues. As with any practice change, real-time support is essential to success. Selection and training of nursing champions for each daytime, evening, and weekend shift who can aid new users, act as resources, answer questions, or listen to concerns will contribute to the program's success and facilitate nurses' role acquisition.

Role #1: Application and Equipment Set-Up

Equipment Selection

There is a growing number of options on the market worldwide for bedside brain monitors, and prices vary considerably depending on the brand and features chosen. To make the best choice for an institution, it is important to solicit input from the various disciplines and departments that may use, or support, these devices in the ICU.

Box 4.2 Potential Roles for Nurses during Neuromonitoring

1. Application and Equipment Set-Up
2. Sensor Maintenance and Clinical Event Marking
3. Recognition of Normal Patterns (aEEG/QEEG)
4. Notification of Abnormal Patterns
5. Parent Education
6. Facilitate Interprofessional Communication
7. Documentation of Brain Monitoring in the Patient Record
8. Nursing Education

Neurology and neurophysiology team members may already be using similar devices in other parts of the hospital; compatibility of equipment and need for additional training with new systems may be a consideration. The ICU nursing team will have specific needs based on space constraints and compatibilities with other devices at the bedside. The ICU and/or neurology team may have the need for network integration for remote viewing and file storage, along with plans for ongoing or future research. Data management workflows and storage solutions should be considered as part of the overall strategy. From a purely financial point of view, the hospital may have existing purchasing agreements and service contracts with vendors, and this may make one device more competitive over another. Another critical point of consideration prior to choosing a bedside brain monitor is the ability of the vendor to provide adequate technical and clinical support during and after installation of the device. Consideration of all these needs will be vital to selecting the best monitors for your ICU.

Procurement of Supplies

Since there are multiple vendors for monitoring devices, it is important to find the right fit for the individual program with input from all stakeholders. A request for proposal (RFP) cycle is the best way to ensure that the monitors purchased will meet the needs of both pediatric and neonatal patients. All RFPs should include a wish list indicating essential as well as optional features. Speaking with various vendors to understand their business model and equipment servicing standards is an essential part of procurement. Considerations such as the ordering of additional sensors or electrodes is best served at the beginning of procurement of monitoring devices.

Storage of Supplies

Monitoring devices should be kept near the ICU with easy access to supplies for overnight and weekend hook-ups. Sensors and electrodes should be clearly labeled and kept with other monitoring equipment. Since some electrodes are disposable and others are not, it is important to have this information posted (ideally on the machine) so that the users are aware.

Creation of Order Sets and Nursing Protocols

Local guidelines for monitoring should establish not only how to apply sensors but also when and who to monitor. As a general rule, neuromonitoring should be considered as important as monitoring any other vital sign; it should be initiated as quickly as possible after admission or after the need has been identified. However, there may be competing priorities, and the initiation of brain monitoring may need to be delayed until other critical procedures (such as stabilization of airway and vascular access) are complete. Similarly, monitoring may be postponed until after any emergent brain imaging has occurred.

Clear guidelines include identification of pediatric and neonatal patients eligible for aEEG, QEEG, and/or NIRS by diagnosis and/or symptomatology (e.g., a diagnosis of hypoxic-ischemic encephalopathy or clinical seizures). Guidelines should cover topics such as machine set-up, electrode placement, monitoring and charting parameters, and the expected frequency of monitoring and charting (e.g., hourly, each shift, or daily). A quick reference chart for interpretation of tracings is often helpful and can be posted at the bedside and throughout the unit in easily accessed areas. Troubleshooting machine-specific issues is also an essential element of protocols and ongoing training. Where possible, an online learning module is very helpful, with examples of various tracings and application troubleshooting. Finally, guidelines should also include a section on when discontinuation of monitoring is appropriate, and/or when escalation from trend-only monitoring (i.e., aEEG) to continuous video-EEG is appropriate (Figure 4.1).

Sensor Selection and Application

When training a team on sensor application, it is helpful to choose initially only a small group of users so that they can master the skill more quickly, while keeping in mind the equal importance of training at least some staff from all shifts so that someone trained is available at all times. Bedside nurses are the obvious choice for training to apply neuromonitoring sensors since they are at the patient bedside 24 hours a day [3]. However, when admitting or caring for a critically ill patient there are often many competing urgent priorities and, depending on the type of sensors used, application may be time consuming. In such cases, it may be beneficial to assign the time-sensitive task of initiating neuromonitoring to support personnel instead of the bedside nurse. Thus, to ensure that brain monitoring can begin quickly at any time, day or night, training should include additional personnel, such as the charge nurses, transport nurses, physicians, nurse practitioners (NPs), EEG technologists, and respiratory therapists (RTs). In general, any nursing and allied health professionals such as NPs and RTs and physicians could be responsible for setting up bedside aEEG and NIRS. Other bedside QEEG trends are typically started by trained EEG technologists in conjunction with the initiation of continuous EEG, due to the complexity of the monitoring system and placement of multiple electrodes for both neonatal and pediatric montages.

Various types of sensors are available. Selection for use within an ICU and for an individual patient should be based on availability of trained staff, expected length of monitoring, how quickly the sensors need to be placed, and other clinical factors, such as the patient's skin condition, patient age, and the acuity of the patient [12]. There are several types of electrodes available for aEEG/cEEG monitors; a list of pros and cons for each can be found in Table 4.1. NIRS monitoring usually offers two sizes of sensors, one for neonatal/pediatric patients (<40 kg) and a larger option for pediatric/adult patients (>40 kg).

Regardless of what kind of sensor is used, there are some basic steps that are required for every application procedure. See Box 4.3 for steps.

An important consideration when choosing a type of sensor is whether or not the patient is likely to need MRI or CT in the near future, in which case the use of commercially available MRI- and CT-compatible sensors for cEEG/QEEG can be used. MRI- and CT-compatible electrodes are

Box 4.3 Steps for Sensor Application

1. Select sensor.
2. Determine location(s).
3. Disinfect, exfoliate, or cleanse the skin (based on sensor type and gestational age).
4. Apply or insert sensor.
5. Secure using skin-friendly adhesives or elastic bandage.
6. Ensure quality signal and low impedance.
7. Begin monitoring.

TIP: When applying NIRS sensors to extremely premature infants, a transparent dressing can be applied to the skin before applying the NIRS sensor without risk of diminished signal quality.

now available for both pediatric and neonatal patients and are used as the standard of practice in many institutions.

Collaboration with Technologist for Patient Positioning and Transport Considerations

In the intensive care setting, monitoring may need to be interrupted for various reasons, such as procedures or neuroimaging. If this is anticipated before monitoring is started, it should be communicated and considered prior to initiation of monitoring, because it may affect choice of monitor, choice of electrode, and/or timing of application. Meticulous attention to patient repositioning is essential during neuromonitoring to reduce the risk of pressure sores and skin breakdown.

Role #2: Sensor Maintenance and Clinical Event Marking

Once the sensors are applied, the bedside nurse will assume the primary responsibility for ongoing management of the device, as well as the sensors (Figure 4.2).

Care guidelines should address the frequency of assessment for:

1. **Sensor position:** Dislodged or poorly positioned sensors will lead to erroneous readings. Frequent reassessment of sensor location is required. Hydrogel sensors can migrate during patient repositioning. If sensors are not placed appropriately, artifact may cause misinterpretation of the data. During neuromonitoring, electrodes may need to be removed briefly for procedures like cranial ultrasound. Brief removal of one or two electrodes during the use of a full montage will often not affect the overall recording, and whether recording can continue with temporary electrode removal should be discussed with the EEG technologist. NIRS sensors are placed over the forehead for cerebral oxygen saturation and over the flank for somatic oxygen saturation and do not often interfere with procedures or imaging.

2. **Sensor symmetry:** Proper placement of electrodes symmetrically and equal distance apart often requires measurement with a specialized measuring tape. Symmetry of electrodes in the central and parietal head regions

---

STOP: ENSURE ASSESSMENT OF ALL ASPECTS PRIOR TO PROVIDING ANTICONVULSANT MEDICATIONS

aEEG Routine Assessment and DURING SEIZURE ACTIVITY

---

1. **CHECK IMPEDANCE** (quality of electrode contact). **Is the impedance line flat between 0 and 5 μV?**

---

2. **ARE ALL SCALP LEADS WELL CONNECTED?**
   Abrupt changes in the absence of clinical concerns may represent lead disconnection.

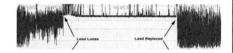

---

3. **CHECK FOR ARTIFACT OR OTHER CONDITIONS THAT CAN INFLUENCE THE aEEG TRACING?**
   a. **Is the live aEEG wave the same frequency as the heart rate (ECG tracing), HFO, or breathing?**
      If so and if there are no clinical manifestations of seizures (i.e., abnormal movements. change in heart rate, breathing, blood pressure, oxygen saturations), *the changes on aEEG may represent artifact rather than seizures.*
   b. **Potential causes of an elevated background voltage:** ECG tracing, muscle activity, HFO, gasp artifact, interventions resulting in repetitive movements (i.e., patting)
   c. **Potential causes of a depressed background voltage:** scalp edema, leads too close together, sedation

---

4. **EXAMINE THE TRACING OVER A PERIOD OF TIME**
   a. If there are suspected seizures, ensure to assess the tracing prior to the onset of seizures. If there is an unexplained abrupt change in the tracing *without clinical seizures,* assess for artifact or lead disconnection.
   b. Do the lower and upper margins seem to flow in parallel?
   c. Is the lower margin above 5 μV?
   d. Is the upper margin above 10 μV?
   e. Is their regular widening and narrowing of the trace within the above margins (Sleep Wake Cycling, SWC)?

Normal trace (continuous with cycling)
- Upper margin > 10 μVolts
- Lower margin < 5 μVolts
- Widening and narrowing of the trace [sleep wake cycling (SWC)]

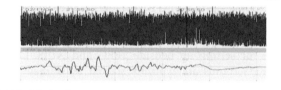

Moderately abnormal trace (discontinuous pattern)
- No evidence of sleep/wake cycling
- Upper margin > 10 μVolts
- Lower margin < 5 μVolts
- Increased variability (trace is broad)

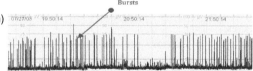

Severely abnormal (inactive, flat trace)
- May be accompanied with brief bursts of higher voltage (burst suppression)
- No evidence of sleep/wake cycling
- Upper margin < 10 μVolts
- Greatly reduced variability

Seizures
- Seizure onset shows continuous high activity
- Causes tracing to narrow and rise up
- Frequent and prolonged periods of elevation in both the lower and upper margins that coincide with an EEG repetitive rhythmic pattern.

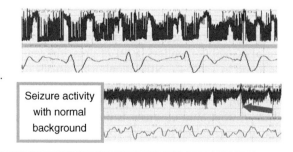

Seizure activity with normal background

Figure 4.1 aEEG assessment tool, courtesy The Hospital for Sick Children.

Table 4.1 Advantages and disadvantages of EEG electrode types

Electrode type	Advantage	Disadvantage
Subdermal needles	Quick application Stable, low impedance Low maintenance for staff	Invasive Risk for needle-stick injury
Hydrogel ("Peel & Stick")	Gentle adhesive Noninvasive	Skin preparation can be time consuming and may cause minor excoriation. Maintenance required
Reusable cups/discs	Less waste Compatible across most devices	Skin preparation can be time consuming and may cause minor excoriation. Higher cost Reprocessing costs Restocking system required
Disposable cups/discs	Inexpensive Compatible across most devices	Skin preparation can be time consuming and may cause minor excoriation. Risk for pressure injury with long-term use

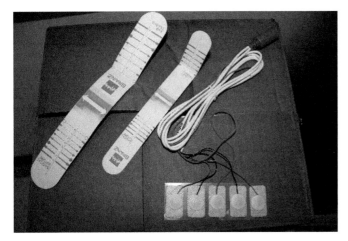

Figure 4.2 (a) Measuring guides for sensor placement.

ensures that the tracing is reliable and in the most sensitive areas for seizure detection. Generally, the measurements are half the distance between the tragus of the ear and the central point on the top of the skull for aEEG. Specialized measuring tapes may be used to help improve consistency in electrode distance during application. Measuring and application techniques are more complex for cEEG/QEEG electrode placement and therefore are typically applied by a trained EEG technologist.

Future Directions: As the demand for continuous brain monitoring has increased, products such as premeasured electrode caps have been developed in pediatric and neonatal sizes to simplify electrode application and decrease variability in positioning between users. These tools may allow bedside providers to apply more complex electrode arrays in the future without requiring an EEG technologist.

3. **Signal quality** and **skin impedance:** Some EEG monitors have automated systems to evaluate signal quality and

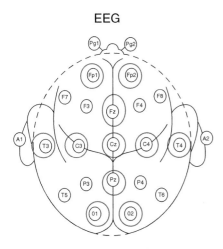

EEG

10–20 system, modified for neonates

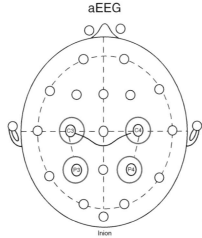

aEEG

Inion

Dual channel (C3→P3, C4→P4)

Figure 4.2 (b) 10–20 electrode montage.

impedance. Signal impedance is normally shown in a separate display and ideally should be less than 5 kΩ, not exceeding 10 kΩ. The closer the impedance is to zero, the better the quality of the signal will be. NIRS monitors use built-in alarms to alert the user of poor signal quality.

4. **Skin integrity**: Assess for redness or any sign of breakdown around sensors at regular intervals during monitoring, usually every 3–4 hours. If redness occurs, remove the leads and replace them close to their previous location. In rare instances, brain monitoring may need to be modified or even discontinued in order to provide the scalp with rest before monitoring can be resumed.

Clinical Event Marking on Brain Monitors

Routine clinical interventions can have a significant impact on brain function and brain perfusion. Unfortunately, bedside brain monitors do not interface directly with the patient's electronic medical record, so significant "clinical events" such as seizure-like movements, changes in vital signs, and medication administration are not automatically marked in the brain monitor recordings. The notation of these clinical events and interventions are of extreme value when interpreting a recording; this requires manual addition of comments and notations during relevant events at the bedside. When event marking it performed through the recording device, efficient notations may be made through device-specific features. These may include event-notation push buttons, predefined event keys, free text keyboard entry of comments in real time, or voice marking via microphone. Many systems allow users to create for each unit or even each patient a customized, high-priority list of events that can be easily accessed from the main recording screen of the device.

Some of the significant events that should be marked during bedside brain monitoring include:

• Changes in vital signs, such as apnea/bradycardia or sudden elevations in heart rate and blood pressure, which may signify subclinical seizures
• Changes in ventilation methods, especially from convention to high frequency, which may create artifact that falsely elevates the aEEG background trend
• Medications, especially those that may affect the brain, specifically sedation and anti-epileptic medications
• Any clinical observations of seizures, or seizure-like behaviors, such as staring, arching, eye deviations, rhythmic jerking of limb(s), lip smacking, tongue thrusting
• Hands-on care, patting, rocking, and repositioning the infant should be noted, because it creates artifacts on the tracing that may be mistaken for seizure
• Any time the sensors are manipulated, replaced, or repaired
• For NIRS: Escalation or changes in vasopressor support and blood transfusion should be noted

Just as event marking is crucial for interpretation of recordings, optimization of accompanying video recordings can be very helpful. Bedside nurses should periodically assess camera position and adjust camera angles if the patient is no longer visible on camera. Whenever possible within the limits of clinical care, patients undergoing recordings with video should not be covered with a blanket or bundled in order to preserve visualization of any clinical events captured.

Role #3: Recognition of Normal Patterns (aEEG/QEEG)

Depending on the neuromonitoring device in use, data may be available for review within minutes of application. In other situations, it may require an hour or more to establish a baseline trend. In order to quickly recognize issues and report potential problems, bedside nurses must be knowledgeable of the expected and normal patterns, values, and readings. A brief summary of normal values is included below and discussed further in Chapter 5.

aEEG

In order to classify normal and abnormal aEEG patterns, voltage normative values have been established. As way of a very brief overview, there are five basic aEEG patterns typically displayed in neonates (Figure 4.3) [5].

Hellstrom-Westas [6] has provided guidelines for normal aEEG patterns in both term and preterm infants. Term infants (greater than 36 weeks) should have continuous aEEG patterns, premature infants (less than 36 weeks) will typically have discontinuous patterns and extremely premature infants (less than 29 weeks) often exhibit an extremely discontinuous pattern resembling bust suppression. Low-voltage and isoelectric (or flat) patterns are considered pathological regardless of gestational age and can be highly predictive of significant brain injury and poor long-term outcomes. Of note, the voltages used in this system and listed in Figure 4.3 all refer to cross-cerebral aEEG (with electrodes at P3-P4). An aEEG using electrodes in other locations (such as hemispheric aEEG) will have different resulting voltages that cannot be classified using this system.

Premature infant considerations: Extremely premature infants (less than 29 weeks) may exhibit an aEEG pattern that resembles "burst suppression" but will possess more variability of the lower margin than a true burst suppression pattern. In this case, the aEEG pattern is considered as expected or normal for age, although a similar pattern in a term infant would be considered severely abnormal [6].

QEEG

Many QEEG trends are available and vary in usefulness with age. Trends such as inter-burst interval are useful in premature infants [6], whereas trends such as density spectral array (DSA) are useful in pediatric patients [7]. It is important to remember that EEG background patterns change with age; as a general rule, the older the patient, the more continuous the EEG background pattern should be. Discontinuous EEG activity can manifest when the brain has been injured or influenced by medications, such as sedatives or some anti-epileptics. A careful review of the patient's recent medication administration record will be helpful in determining if a lack of continuous EEG activity is due to injury or is an expected side effect of a medication (Figure 4.4).

BACKGROUND PATTERNS

A characteristic aEEG/CFM is shown on the left, and a schematic view is shown on the right.

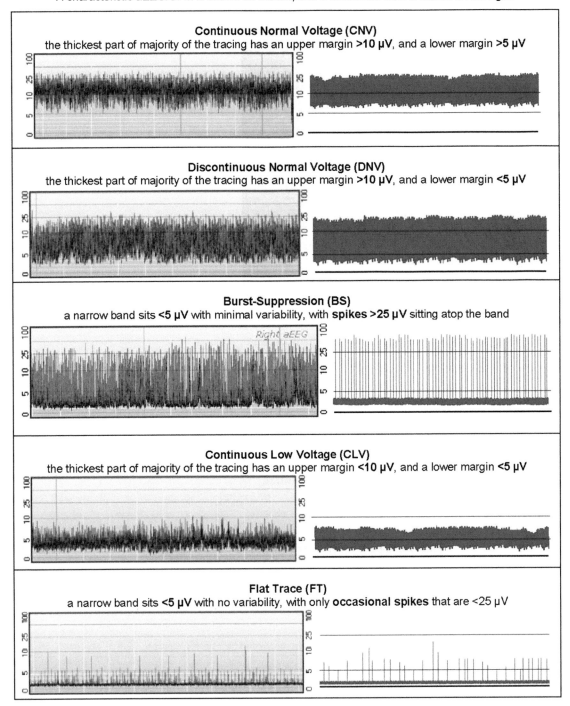

Continuous Normal Voltage (CNV)
the thickest part of majority of the tracing has an upper margin **>10 µV**, and a lower margin **>5 µV**

Discontinuous Normal Voltage (DNV)
the thickest part of majority of the tracing has an upper margin **>10 µV**, and a lower margin **<5 µV**

Burst-Suppression (BS)
a narrow band sits **<5 µV** with minimal variability, with **spikes >25 µV** sitting atop the band

Continuous Low Voltage (CLV)
the thickest part of majority of the tracing has an upper margin **<10 µV**, and a lower margin **<5 µV**

Flat Trace (FT)
a narrow band sits **<5 µV** with no variability, with only **occasional spikes** that are **<25 µV**

Figure 4.3 Classification of aEEG background patterns. Courtesy of the Hospital for Sick Children.

Sleep

Sleep is an important feature of a healthy brain and can be identified with relative ease on bedside aEEG and QEEG trends. Generally, the background pattern of EEG will slow during sleep. In newborns, the background may become less continuous. Sleep spindles are a distinct feature seen on pediatric EEG and develop around 2 months of age. Neonatal patients begin to develop sleep–wake cycling patterns around 32 weeks' gestation. Although not well defined initially, this feature can be seen emerging in the aEEG trend in healthy preterm neonates with increasing conceptional age. Sleep–wake cycling becomes more obvious and regular as the neonate reaches term-equivalent age. The aEEG trend has a characteristic alternating "thin-thick" pattern as sleep–wake cycling matures (Figure 4.5).

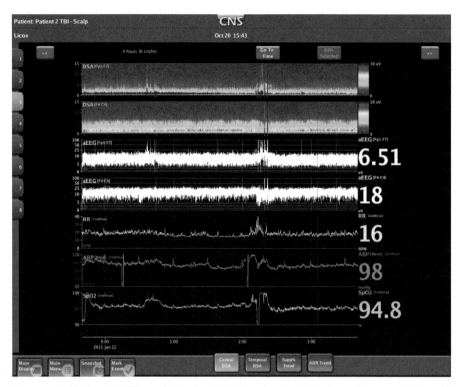

Figure 4.4 Multimodal QEEG trend with physiological monitoring display. Image Courtesy of Moberg ICU Solutions.

Steps to aEEG Interpretation

Question and Analysis

Ensure that areas of the trace being read have a white background to them (not yellow or red that show marginal to poor impedance).

Examine the aEEG strip as a whole.

- **Is it a gentle wave?** *YES*
- **Do the lower and upper margins seem to flow in parallel?** *YES*
- **Is the lower margin above 5 μV?** *YES*
- **Is the upper margin above 10 μV?** *YES*
- **Is their regular widening & narrowing of the trace, within the above margins (Sleep Wake Cycling)** *YES*

This is classified as a normal or Continuous Normal Voltage (CNV) pattern and in most cases is a good prognostic sign. Early return of **SWS** after hypoxic-ischemic insult is also a good prognostic sign.

Illustration

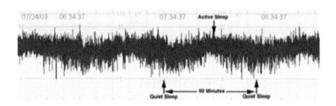

Normal trace (CNV): Upper margin is > 10 μV & lower margin is > 5 μV. The widening and narrowing of the trace implies periods of wakening and sleep i.e. sleep wake cycling (SWS).

Figure 4.5 Steps to identify sleep wake cycling.

Symmetry

It is important for bedside nursing staff to recognize asymmetrical patterns, and if they are persistent, to ensure that leads are appropriately placed. Asymmetry is common in newborn infants who have had prolonged delivery and is often related to scalp molding, which resolves over time. Asymmetry could also be an indication of a focal brain lesion, such as stroke. Many cEEG monitors display a trend of asymmetry. Asymmetry is displayed as a linear graph derived from a calculation of average amplitude between right and left cerebral hemispheres. The midpoint of the line graph is zero, which represents no difference in brain activity between hemispheres. If the line trends up or down, then this indicates that an asymmetry in brain activity exists in the direction identified by the monitor. When combined with other QEEG trends and a review of the raw EEG, this QEEG feature of may assist in the timely recognition of a new or evolving focal injury.

NIRS

Normal values for cerebral regional tissue saturation, expressed as rSO_2, range in neonates from 66% to 86%, depending on conceptional age. The critical levels for cerebral saturations are those sustained at less than 40% [10]. In pediatric patients, the generally normal range is 60%–80%, with less than 50% representing a critically low reading.

See Table 4.2 for normal values of cerebral saturations for pediatric, term, and preterm infants.

Role #4: Notification of Abnormal Patterns

Reporting Abnormal Findings

Electroencephalogram trends such as aEEG and CDSA (also sometimes called CSA or DSA) were developed to facilitate interpretation of prolonged EEG recordings by neurologists and neurophysiologists, but have become especially useful in the identification of abnormal background patterns and potential seizures by bedside care providers without formal training in EEG [7]. During bedside neuromonitoring, several situations warrant bedside nurses bringing changes to the attention of the ICU medical team [2, 5] or other available on-unit resources as appropriate (Figures 4.6 and 4.7).

1. **Elevated impedance** (>10 kΩ) can have several causes and can make interpreting the aEEG pattern nearly impossible. The two most common reasons for elevated impedance are the electrode adhesive drying out and the electrodes becoming dislodged from the skin. If adhesive has dried, sparing hydration may resolve the problem. If electrodes

are dislodged, they should be replaced. If the impedance is high at the onset of monitoring, it is likely due to inadequate skin preparation. In those cases, the skin preparation procedure should be repeated until acceptable impedance is achieved. Another cause for elevated impedance is scalp edema; this is important to recognize because in this case additional skin preparation will not reduce the impedance values. In situations when the bedside nurse is unable to troubleshoot or resolve unacceptable impedance issues, the high impedance should be reported to the medical team, and a decision made whether to discontinue monitoring or suspend monitoring until resources are available to resume monitoring with acceptable impedances.

2. **Abnormal aEEG background pattern** or any pattern that is unexpected or inconsistent with the patient's age and state should be brought to the attention of the medical team. Examples of abnormal background patterns include: reduced upper margin voltage on the aEEG band < 10 microvolts, sustained drift in the lower margin of the aEEG band below 5 microvolts in term infants, a lack of sleep–wake cycling in infants > 35 weeks conceptional age, and lack of symmetry between cerebral hemispheres.

3. **A sudden change in the aEEG or CDSA band** that is not explained by patting or other bedside patient manipulation should be reported to the medical team as soon as it is identified, as this type of pattern may be suspicious for seizures. On aEEG, a suspicious pattern for seizures consists of a sudden rise in the upper and lower margins as well as narrowing of the activity band. In older patients undergoing cEEG, QEEG trends such as CDSA may provide an early indicator of the presence of a subclinical seizure in a sedated or paralyzed patient. A classical representation of seizure on CDSA would include both a sudden upward arch on the y-axis of the displayed band (caused by an increase in the patient's EEG amplitude and frequency) along with a change in the band to warmer colors (red) (which represents increased EEG power).

Although nurses can review the raw EEG recording to look for potential artifacts, the medical team should be notified of areas suspicious for seizures on the aEEG/QEEG and a timely review should be completed to determine whether additional monitoring or consultation is warranted or whether the treatment plan needs to be modified. Several seizure-detection algorithms are now commercially available and can aid in the identification of areas that are highly suspicious for seizures and that warrant additional review by the medical team.

4. **Artifacts** are common in the ICU and can significantly interfere with the recording, making interpretation of the background pattern and identification of seizures nearly impossible. The most prevalent artifacts include: movement artifact (e.g., patient handling during cares, patting and rocking an infant after feedings); electromyogram (EMG) or muscle artifacts (e.g., eye movement, sucking, crying); high-frequency ventilation;

Table 4.2 Normal NIRS values [9,13]

	Cerebral saturation range
Term infants	70%–86%
Preterm infants	66%–83%
Pediatric	60%–80% (<20% from baseline)

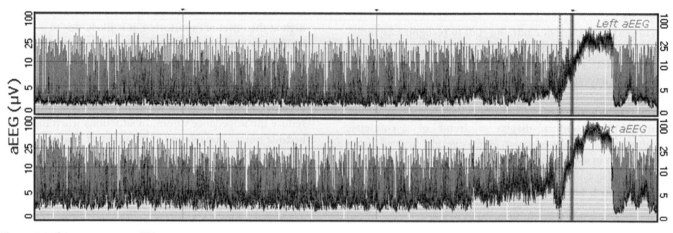

Figure 4.6 Seizure pattern on aEEG.

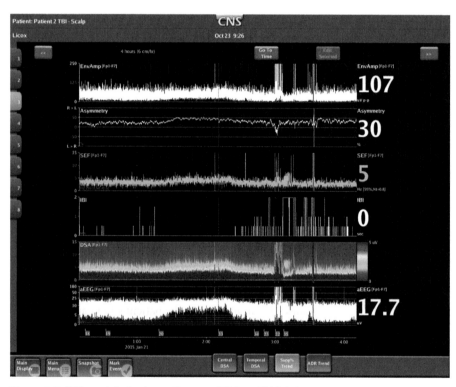

Figure 4.7 DSA trend display. Image Courtesy of Moberg ICU Solutions.

electrocardiogram (ECG); and electrical noise in the environment from ventilators and IV pumps. Frequent review for these common artifacts can facilitate quick identification and allow early corrective action to minimize their presence whenever possible.

While cEEG and associated trends are typically reviewed remotely by a neurophysiologist and/or EEG technologist, review is most often done periodically, not in real time, and with less frequency overnight. Real-time, continuous review of cEEG/QEEG or aEEG trends by neurophysiologists or technologists is rare in current practice. Therefore, in addition to the above findings that should prompt an alert to the ICU team, there are important findings that should be reported to the ICU medical and

neurophysiology team if they are identified by bedside clinicians (Figure 4.8):

1. **Loss of connection.** Normally cEEG/QEEG is connected to the hospital network for remote review by a neurophysiologist. If there are network issues causing a loss of bedside display or indicators that network connectivity is interrupted, this should be reported immediately to the information technology staff available. Similarly, there are instances of monitoring failure due to interruption of the power source (e.g., due to cables accidentally dislodged or failure to switch from battery to outlet power after patient transfer). In these cases, quick recognition at the bedside and notification of the ICU and neurophysiology teams can allow recording to resume promptly.

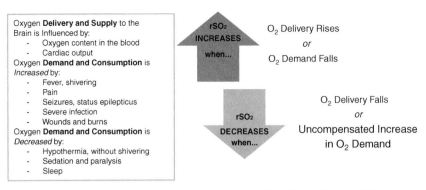

Oxygen **Delivery and Supply** to the Brain is Influenced by:
- Oxygen content in the blood
- Cardiac output

Oxygen **Demand and Consumption** is *Increased* by:
- Fever, shivering
- Pain
- Seizures, status epilepticus
- Severe infection
- Wounds and burns

Oxygen **Demand and Consumption** is *Decreased* by:
- Hypothermia, without shivering
- Sedation and paralysis
- Sleep

rSO₂ **INCREASES** when...

O₂ Delivery Rises
or
O₂ Demand Falls

rSO₂ **DECREASES** when...

O₂ Delivery Falls
or
Uncompensated Increase in O₂ Demand

Figure 4.8 Bedside NIRS troubleshooting guide, courtesy of The Hospital for Sick Children.

2. **Clinical seizures.** These should be reported immediately to the ICU team and consulting neurology team and marked on the tracing at the time witnessed. The events can then easily be correlated with the EEG tracing and video recording through remote review by the neurophysiologist to confirm they are seizures or clarify if they are seizure mimics.

For NIRS, there are similar situations that should be of concern to bedside caregivers [8, 11, 13, 14].

1. **Loss of signal quality or connection.** Possible causes of poor signal quality may include the patient's position, lack of adhesion between the skin and the sensors, excessive ambient light, especially from phototherapy, or excessive humidity in the microenvironment. Nurses should work to resolve this situation as quickly as possible by examining the sensor and skin integrity, applying gentle pressure, ensuring quality connection between the sensor cable and the device, or by changing the NIRS monitor itself if the sensors appear to be well applied. If unable to correct the issue, the nurse should notify the medical team to decide if monitoring can be suspended until other resources are available to troubleshoot the signal quality or discontinue monitoring based on the infant's condition.

2. **A change of 10%–15%** above or below the infant's baseline NIRS trend is significant and should be reported to the medical team.

3. **Cerebral saturation <50%.** A small number of studies have shown the risk for brain injury is increased when cerebral saturations are sustained at less than 40%. By using 50% as a cutoff, there will be time to notify the medical team and take corrective action before reaching the point where the potential for injury is increased.

Nursing policies and clinical guidelines should outline which aEEG, QEEG, and NIRS findings should be reported to the medical team, who should be notified, and how quickly. Unless otherwise arranged, the ICU medical team will determine when the neurology or neurophysiology teams will be consulted based on the findings from bedside brain monitoring devices; this consultation is typically not the responsibility of the bedside nurse.

Role #5: Parent Education

While parent education is a shared responsibility, bedside nurses frequently explain and reassure parents about devices in use at the bedside. Brain monitoring devices can cause additional stress and anxiety for some families. Thorough and consistent education along with well-written materials can help to minimize stress and maximize parental understanding of the need for brain monitoring. Parent education can be accomplished any number of ways and might include a pamphlet or information on an ICU website. During the creation of such educational materials, parental input helps ensure that information is clear and meaningful.

Components of parent education should at a minimum address the following common questions: why the device is in use, whether it causes pain, can they hold their baby, how often it is read, who is reading it, what value it provides to the care of their baby, and how long will it stay on.

Role #6: Facilitate Interprofessional Communication

The information gathered by neuromonitoring devices can help bedside clinicians manage the daily needs of a patient, or it may help to identify and justify the need for urgent consultations, additional neuroimaging, and other types of evaluations or therapeutic interventions. Daily rounding, discussion, and collaboration between nursing, intensivists, and neurologists regarding neuromonitoring is ideal and has become the standard in many ICUs [1, 5, 9, 15, 16]. Part of the patient care discussion should focus on the need to continue brain monitoring and the clinical value it will offer if continued. It is important that these discussions happen daily in order to maximize the use of the equipment, minimize strain on bedside resources, and contain patient costs. As in all areas of patient care, the nurse can facilitate clear communication, both by providing details of the bedside perspective and in helping to identify any gaps in communication observed.

Role #7: Documentation of Brain Monitoring in the Patient Record

At a minimum, nurses should document in the patient's medical record the type of brain monitors in use and record patient values at specified intervals (e.g., every 3 hours). To meet the individual needs of each unit, documentation may be in the electronic medical record or recorded on a paper flowsheet.

Customized fields for documenting about the patient experience with a bedside brain monitor could include:

- Monitor type in use
- Sensor type, location, and number
- Displayed values or patterns from the device

  ○ For aEEG:

    · Upper and lower margin of aEEG (either numerical values or categorical normal/abnormal)
    · Sleep–wake cycling on aEEG (present or absent)
    · Suspected seizures on aEEG (noting if present, the times identified)
    · Suspected artifacts on aEEG (noting if present, the times identified)
    · Impedance and interventions to improve when >10 kΩ

  ○ For cEEG/QEEG

    · Abnormal background changes, including:
    · Asymmetry
    · Sustained periods of suppressed background (% suppression)
    · Presence or absence of seizures
    · Impedance

  ○ For NIRS:

    · Baseline or average values for each site (when available)
    · Current values for each site monitored
    · Signal quality

- Adjustments or changes made to sensors
- Skin condition, during monitoring and upon removal of sensors
- Any network or other IT issues
- Notifications made to the medical team

Role #8: Nursing Education

It is essential that nurses have adequate initial and ongoing education on the rationale for, proper use of, and troubleshooting with bedside brain monitoring. In-person education and conferences are ideal. Online courses may offer an alternative with more flexibility. Online, digital, and print materials with well-designed content and self-assessments can offer initial and ongoing education with maximal flexibility [2, 3].

Training materials and courses can be developed by the individual ICUs or are available through various individuals or groups. Training should include both the underlying principles of brain monitoring and also offer practical case examples with illustrative images from commonly used devices (Box 4.4) [3, 12].

Box 4.4 Nursing Education Curriculum

1. Clinical utility of brain monitoring and predictive value
2. Normal values and trend patterns
3. Age-dependent variations
4. Unit-specific protocols or guidelines – including whom to monitor, when to monitor, and how long to monitor
5. Case studies to practice classification of presented patterns and values
6. Scenarios of when to notify the medical team or on-unit resource team
7. How to apply and troubleshoot sensors and devices
8. Parent education examples and role-play

Quality Improvement

Quality improvement (QI) is the process of examining the gap between the ideal practice and reality in order to find ways to make the care itself or the delivery system better [17]. When implementing a new practice, like bedside brain monitoring, there are opportunities to establish a vision of what the ideal practice could look like for an ICU. As implementation moves forward, the QI team can periodically check in with how the practice is actually going and make adjustments that will move the unit closer toward its goals.

For example, if a unit purchased a bedside aEEG monitor, quality measures to follow might include: frequency of use per month, variance of use from established protocol, identification of any patients who should have been monitored but were not, the time needed to place sensors, incidence of skin issues, and the impact monitoring had on the number of consults or ordering of additional tests. By evaluating actual practice, a unit can either expand practice if the implementation is going well, or take a step back and refine the practice if the team has not yet met goals or identifies system issues.

Summary

1. Bedside brain monitors can evaluate brain function or brain perfusion.
2. aEEG, QEEG, and NIRS are the most common bedside brain-monitoring modalities in the ICU.
3. Nurses can have many roles related to bedside brain monitors. Their primary responsibilities typically include proper application of skin sensors, maintaining a quality signal to ensure a readable recording, and notifying the medical team of any unexpected values or trends.
4. Everyday interventions and medications can have a significant effect on brain function and brain perfusion.
5. Parent education on the use of bedside brain monitors will help to alleviate stress and improve understanding of its importance.
6. Bedside brain monitoring is a new practice for many ICUs and offers quality improvement opportunities.

Conclusion

In the ICU, it is standard of care to initiate monitoring of the patient's respiratory rate, heart rate, oxygen saturations, temperature, and blood pressure both invasively and noninvasively. Bedside brain monitors, such as aEEG and NIRS, are noninvasive bedside tools that expand our assessment capabilities in real time and have the advantage of being started by ICU staff at any time. These monitors should be considered primary screening or trending tools that complement gold-standard assessments such as conventional cEEG and imaging.

The future of bedside brain monitoring is bright due to increasing interest and use, with an abundance of ongoing research. Bedside brain monitors can guide nursing care and provide a deeper understanding of the real-time impact of common bedside procedures, medication, and interventions on cerebral function and perfusion.

Defining and dividing the responsibilities related to brain monitoring and offering thorough and ongoing education for all members of the ICU team create an environment in which this new technology can be accepted into everyday practice with minimal difficulties.

References

1. Shellhaas RA, Chang T, Tsuchida T, et al. The American Clinical Neurophysiology Society's guideline on continuous electroencephalography monitoring in neonates. *J Clin Neurophysiol.* 2011;**28**:611–17.

2. Foreman SW, Thorngate L. Amplitude-integrated electroencephalography: a new approach to enhancing neurologic nursing care in the neonatal intensive care unit. *NAINR.* 2011;**11**:134–140.

3. Zoet-Lavooi J, van Rooij LGM, Brouwer AJ, Lemmers P, de Vries LS. Neuromonitoring: how to train your nursing staff. Paper presented at the 5th Congress of the European Academy of Paediatric EAPS 17–21, Barcelona, Spain, October 2014.

4. McCoy B, Hahn CD. Continuous EEG monitoring in the neonatal intensive care unit. *J Clin Neurophysiol.* 2013;**30**:106–14.

5. Shah NA, Wusthoff CJ. How to use: amplitude integrated EEG (aEEG). *Arch Dis Child Educ Pract Ed.* 2015;**100**:75–81.

6. Hellstrom-Westas, L. The electrocortical background, its normal maturation, classification, and effects of medication. In de Vries LS, Rosen I, Hellstrom-Westas L, editors. *Atlas of Amplitude-Integrated EEGs in the Newborn,* 2nd ed. London: Informa Healthcare; 2008, pp. 17–42.

7. Pensirikul AD, Beslow LA, Kessler SK, et al. Density spectral array for seizure identification in critically ill children. *J Clin Neurophysiol.* 2013;**30**:371–5.

8. Marin T, Moore J. Understanding near-infrared spectroscopy. *Adv Neo Care.* 2011;**11**:382–88.

9. Bernal NP, Hoffman GM, Ghanayem NS, Arca MJ. Cerebral and somatic near-infrared spectroscopy in normal newborns. *J Pediatr Surg.* 2010;**45**:1306–10.

10. McNeill S, Gatenby JC, McElroy S, Engelhardt B. Normal cerebral, renal and abdominal regional oxygen saturations using near-infrared spectroscopy in preterm infants. *J Perinatol.* 2011;**31**:51–7.

11. Toet MC, Lemmers PM. Brain monitoring in neonates. *Early Hum Dev.* 2009;**85**:77–84.

12. Whitelaw A, White RD. Training neonatal staff in recording and reporting continuous electroencephalography. *Clin Perinatol.* 2006;**33**:667–77.

13. Chock VY, Davis AS. Bedside cerebral monitoring to predict neurodevelopmental outcomes. *NeoReviews.* 2009;**10**, e121–e129.

14. McNeill S, Gatenby JC, McElroy S, Engelhardt B. Normal cerebral, renal and abdominal regional oxygen saturations using near-infrared spectroscopy in preterm infants. *J Perinatol.* 2011;**31**:51–7.

15. Glass HC, Wusthoff CJ, Shellhaas RA. Amplitude-integrated electro-encephalography: the child neurologist's perspective. *J Child Neurol.* 2013;**28**:1342–50.

16. Glass HC, Bonifacio SL, Peloquin S, et al. Neurocritical care for neonates. *Neurocrit Care.* 2010;**12**:421–9.

17. Duke University, QI Department, School of Medicine. *Patient Safety Education.* 2016. http://patientsafetyed .duhs.duke.edu/module_a/introduc tion/contrasting_qi_qa.html

Normal Neurophysiology, Benign Findings, and Artifacts

Sylvie Nguyen The Tich and Emilie Bourel-Ponchel

Key Points
- Recognizing a normal recording is the first, but not the simplest, step of EEG analysis.
- Normal EEG patterns evolve in a predictable, age-dependent manner.
- Clinicians should recognize common artifacts on EEG that may mimic seizures or other abnormalities.

Introduction

Continuous electroencephalography (EEG) is used in the intensive care unit (ICU) to answer specific questions: are there any markers of brain injury? Are there seizures? How is brain function changing over time? Clinicians are challenged to recognize abnormalities and distinguish them from normal findings and artifacts. To do this, we advise simultaneously using bedside display of quantitative EEG (QEEG) (at least two and up to eight channels) interpreted by the ICU provider, at the same time as conventional EEG (cEEG) is recorded and interpreted by the neurophysiology team [1, 2]. While QEEG interpretation requires training and experience, this combined approach has the benefit of providing real-time neurophysiological data in the form of QEEG that is accessible 24/7 to the ICU team. At the same time, cEEG is available for detailed review by the neurophysiologist to confirm any possible abnormalities identified on QEEG and to look for features not seen on QEEG. This joint approach can improve the speed and accuracy of analysis of neonatal and pediatric EEG in the ICU [3, 4].

This chapter provides a guide for practitioners reviewing neonatal and pediatric EEG to help recognize normal tracings. While a comprehensive discussion of all normal variants is beyond the scope of this chapter, recognition of expected normal features and common artifacts makes the identification of disease-specific abnormalities much easier.

The Approach to EEG and QEEG Analysis

The approach detailed below describes identification of normal EEG in neonates and children using full-array continuous EEG. These principles may also apply to identifying normal features in reduced-array, source (or "raw") EEG recordings used to derive QEEG.

Contextual Information

Before reviewing a tracing, the following information is required:
- Chronological age and, for newborns, conceptional age (CA)
- Drugs received before and during the EEG, specifically sedative and anticonvulsive medications
- Body temperature (whether hypothermic or normal)
- Events that occurred immediately before and during the EEG, ideally directly noted on the tracing: suspected seizures, nursing cares, etc.

Any analysis should start by first checking that the technical quality of the recording is sufficient for reliable analysis. Any documentation of recording interpretation should state whether there were limitations in recording quality as well as the technical and behavioral conditions of recording (alertness, agitation, number and location of electrodes, duration of the recording, etc.).

Methodology

From term-equivalent age onward, normal EEG is characterized by background activity with continuous and symmetric waveforms that vary with time, according to sleep or wake state. The two main pitfalls in identifying normal neonatal and pediatric EEGs are recognizing background activity that is normal for age and distinguishing physiological patterns or artifacts from epileptiform activity.

A systematic approach can be helpful in determining whether EEG is normal. The following questions should be successively checked (Figure 5.1):
1. Global analysis of background activity: Is the background continuous? Is the amplitude normal for age? Is the background symmetrical? Is the background normally reactive and variable?
2. Are appropriate physiological features for age recognizable?
3. Analysis for abnormal features: Are there sharp waves, epileptiform discharges, and/or other superimposed abnormalities? Are there seizures or seizure mimics?

Global Analysis of Background Activity

Is the Background Continuous?

A continuous tracing displays activity without any interruption. Activity that falls below normal amplitude for age is an interruption, and is sometimes described as the "inter-burst

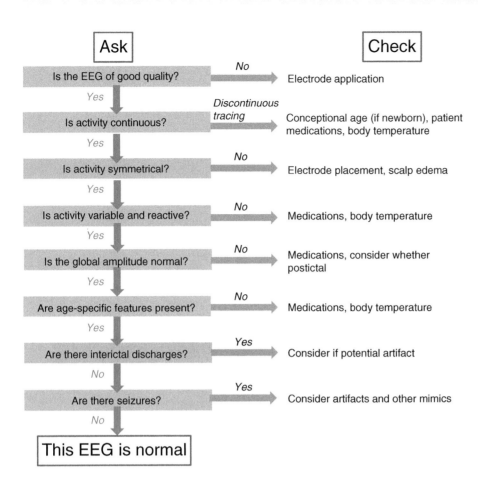

Figure 5.1 Suggested approach to analyzing EEG.

interval" (IBI). Normal amplitudes vary by age. In a neonate, continuous activity is defined as always having peak-to-peak amplitude above 25 μV. A neonatal tracing is discontinuous if activity is frequently interrupted by periods of peak-to-peak amplitude below 25 μV lasting longer than 2 seconds. The degree of discontinuity is usually quantified by the typical or most prevalent duration of the IBI. The presence of IBIs is normal in preterm infants (such as in the pattern called "tracé discontinu"), with expected IBI duration varying with conceptional age and behavioral state (see below). In older infants and children, the background should always be continuous, although normal continuous activity in older children may have amplitudes as low as 10 μV.

Discontinuity can be provoked by anesthetics, sedatives, or by very low body temperature (≤32°C) [4]. Therefore, before concluding that a discontinuous EEG reflects brain abnormality, it is essential to confirm the conceptional age in neonates and assess for drug exposure and body temperature in all patients.

Amplitude-integrated EEG (aEEG) is the most common type of QEEG used to assess background continuity, typically in newborns. See Chapter 2 for details on the acquisition of aEEG. In brief, aEEG displays the amplitudes of the recorded EEG on a logarithmic y-axis, against time on a linear x-axis. In the generation of aEEG, recorded activity is filtered, typically to minimize the display of very low- or high-frequency activity. Waveforms are also rectified, meaning amplitudes are measured not from peak-to-peak but, rather, as an absolute amplitude from baseline. The aEEG display consists of a series of juxtaposed vertical lines – each line reflects on the y-axis the lowest amplitude and highest amplitude recorded during a brief time window (typically around 10 seconds). The pattern created by a series of these vertical lines over time is the "activity band." Visualization of the activity band is a rapid way to assess the overall amplitudes of activity during a given time window (Figure 5.2).

On aEEG, continuity appears as activity with amplitudes always in the normal range. In term newborns, the lower margin of an activity band (the minimum amplitude sampled) is always >5 μV, and the upper margin of the activity band (the highest amplitude sampled) is always >10 μV, often much higher. Of note, these minimal amplitudes differ from that used in analysis of conventional EEG: on aEEG the activity band need only to have a lower margin >5 μV and an upper margin >10 μV to be deemed continuous, while conventional EEG requires amplitudes >25μV. This is in part due to the signal filtering in aEEG display, but primarily due to the differences in how amplitudes are measured between the two techniques. An aEEG measures amplitudes of rectified waveforms, in which the amplitude is the absolute value of the wave peak from the baseline. In conventional EEG, however, amplitudes are measured peak-to-peak, from the lowest point of a wave from to the highest peak of the following wave. Thus, the amplitude criteria for a normal tracing differ between aEEG and conventional EEG.

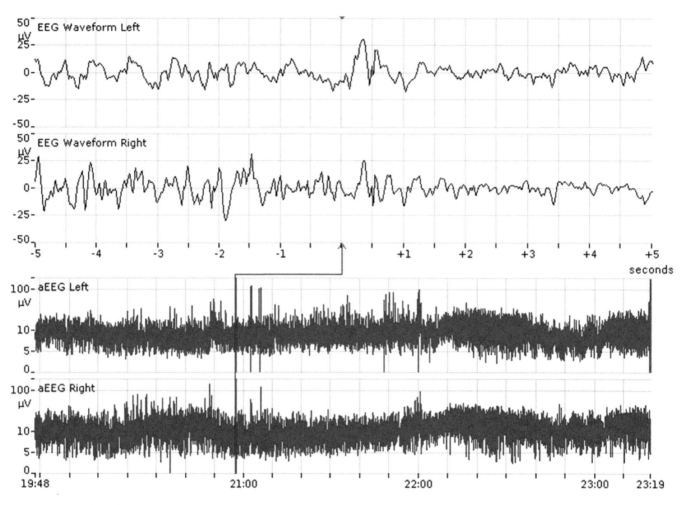

Figure 5.2 Two-channel EEG with corresponding aEEG from a normal term newborn. The top two panels display left-hemisphere (C3-P3) and right-hemisphere (C4-P4) EEG recording. The bottom two panels display the corresponding time-compressed aEEG for the left and right channels. The dense blue activity band displays the highest and lowest amplitudes over time against a logarithmic y-axis. The red cursor indicates the corresponding point on the EEG and aEEG traces.

In aEEG, the upper and lower margins of the activity band are used to assess overall amplitudes and check for continuity in a tracing. These margins may also be affected by noncerebral factors, such as interelectrode distance and scalp edema, and by extracerebral artifacts such as those from ECG and high-frequency ventilation. In case of ECG or high-frequency ventilation, artifacts may artificially increase the lower margin, which may make a truly discontinuous aEEG falsely appear normal (Figure 5.3).

In older children, and in cases where the abnormal pattern of burst suppression is present, the degree of discontinuity may be characterized by a QEEG trend, the burst suppression index. Burst suppression is discussed further in Chapter 6.

Is the Amplitude Normal for Age?

Normal amplitudes in term newborns and young children can range broadly from 25 to 150 µV and from 25 µV to over 300 µV in preterm neonates. In older children and adults, normal amplitudes may range from 10 to 100 µV.

The maximal amplitude varies with age and state. In children, the highest amplitudes are observed during non–rapid eye movements (non-REM) sleep with high-voltage delta

waves up to 200 µV that disappear with awakening. In preterm neonates, high-voltage waves are observed during quiet sleep (or its precursor in extremely preterm infants). If the maximal amplitude values are constantly around 200 µV, particularly in states other than non-REM sleep, this is abnormal.

Quantitative EEG and aEEG are complementary tools to cEEG for analyzing amplitude range and its slow variations with time. This is particularly helpful in evaluating for the amplitude variations that characterize sleep–wake cycling (Figure 5.4). As amplitudes are higher and more varied in quiet sleep states for neonates, aEEG shows an elevated, broader activity band during quiet sleep. This alternates with a slightly lower, narrower activity band during the lower amplitude activity present in wakefulness. Similarly, QEEG trends reflect the higher amplitudes found in non-REM sleep in older children, with lower amplitudes while awake and in REM sleep.

One form of QEEG, the envelope trend, is similar to aEEG in displaying waveform amplitudes as a function of time (Figure 5.5). In the envelope trend, rather than an activity band representing the lowest and highest amplitudes in each time window, a linear output graphs the median amplitude for

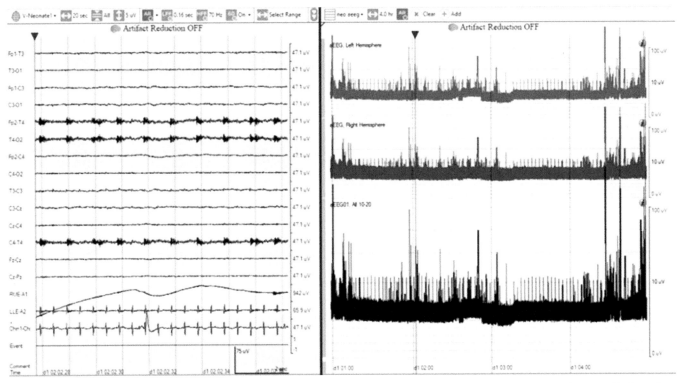

Figure 5.3 Abnormal cEEG with aEEG with activity band elevated by artifact. The EEG on the left shows minimal discernable activity, but is notable for artifact, particularly seen at T4. The aEEG on the right appears to have a lower margin above 5 μV in each panel, which does not reflect cortical activity, but rather artifact.

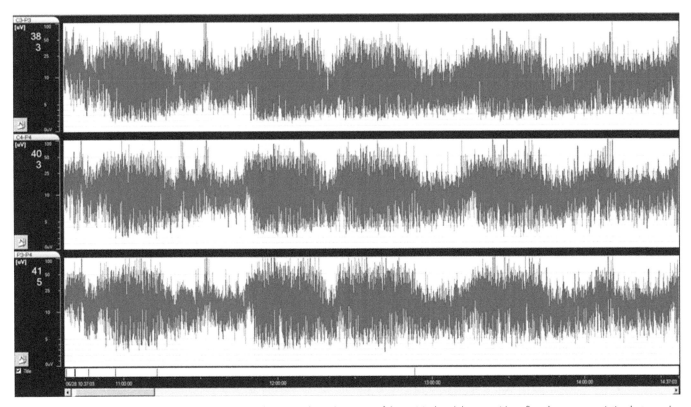

Figure 5.4 aEEG displaying sleep–wake cycling in a normal term newborn. Segments of the activity band that are wider reflect the greater variation between low and high amplitudes in quiet sleep. Narrowing reflects the consistently lower amplitudes of active sleep.

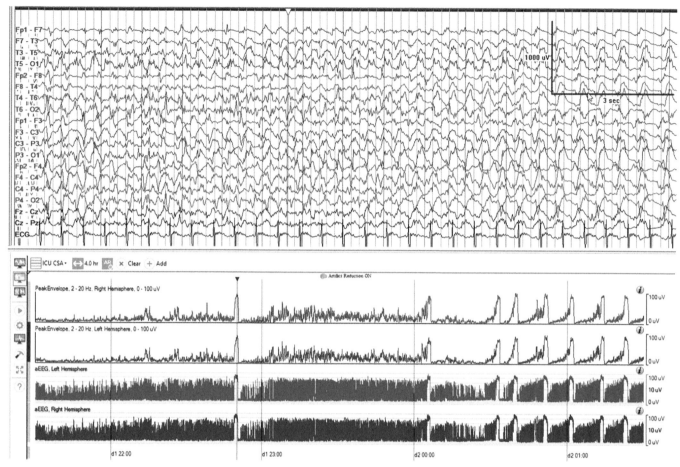

Figure 5.5 EEG from a 9-month-old infant with GMPPB-related dystroglycanopathy (muscle-eye-brain disease) who presented in refractory status epilepticus. A series of generalized seizures are seen on raw EEG (top panel), envelope trend (middle two panels), and aEEG (bottom two panels).

each time point. This results in a simple line trend that allows clear visualization of amplitude changes over time.

Is the Background Symmetrical?

A normal cEEG is symmetrical; there is no significant or persistent difference in the frequency or amplitude between the two cerebral hemispheres. Asymmetry suggests lateralized brain dysfunction. In cases of apparent asymmetry, electrode placement and local conditions such as focal edema of the scalp should be carefully considered to exclude these as noncerebral causes.

On QEEG, asymmetry cannot be evaluated when only three electrodes (generating a single cross-cerebral channel) are used. At least five electrodes (generating independent left and right channels) should be used along with display of the raw EEG tracing in order to check for symmetry. In aEEG, displays showing a right-hemispheric trend alongside a left-hemispheric trend may facilitate comparisons for symmetry. This is also true for other QEEG trends, such as color density spectral array (CDSA) and envelope trends.

Some QEEG trends are specifically designed to identify differences between hemispheres. Envelope trends may superimpose the tracings of the left and right hemispheres to allow direct comparisons of amplitudes from each side. Asymmetry indices use formulas to quantify the difference in EEG power

between hemispheres (Figure 5.6). These may be set up to display absolute asymmetry or relative asymmetry values.

Is the Background Normally Reactive and Variable?

Normal variations in EEG background reflect physiological, internally, or externally driven changes in cerebral activity. These can be more specifically expressed as "variability" and "reactivity." Variability represents the spontaneous, internally driven changes that correlate with behavioral states including wakefulness and sleep. Reactivity represents response to stimulation, or externally driven changes. Both are important features of normal EEG. Some overlap exists between reactivity and variability, as internal arousal may be provoked by external stimulation.

In standard EEGs, reactivity is tested during the recording by performing sensory stimulation such as making noise or touching. Reactivity testing should also be performed during cEEG in the ICU, preferably at least daily. During unsupervised monitoring, external stimulations such as nursing care or patting may also provoke reactivity. The normal response to stimulation is attenuation of the background activity or a decrease in amplitude.

Variability is most easily appreciated on QEEG over periods up to several hours. QEEG and aEEG trends allow easy

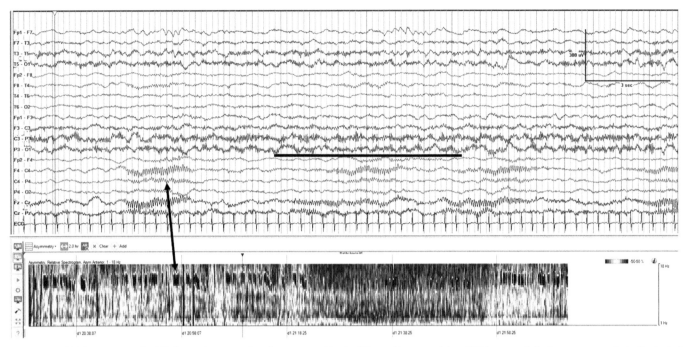

Figure 5.6 EEG from a 5-month-old infant with nonaccidental trauma, resulting in diffuse white matter injury. EEG (top panel) displays asymmetry, including lack of left-hemisphere sleep spindles. Note muscular artifacts on left side [underlined]. This is evident on relative asymmetry spectrogram (lower panel). Red indicates increased frequency-dependent power on right, whereas blue indicates increased power on left. Note periodic bands of red in the 12–14 Hz frequency range corresponding to right-sided sleep spindles [arrow].

identification of sleep–wake cycling and other variations that may reflect reactivity. A normal sleep/wake organization over time is a good marker of normality.

Are Appropriate Physiological Features for Age Recognizable?

The main differences between neonatal and pediatric EEG as compared to adult EEG are the maturational changes present during childhood. Some specific features (such as encoches frontales, spindles, or vertex waves) are good markers of normality. Furthermore, some sharp features need to be recognized as normal and physiological at certain ages, such as trains of vertex waves, sharp bursts of theta at sleep onset, and frontal and anterior slow waves in newborns.

For the purpose of this chapter, we discuss separately preterm and term-born neonates, infants up to 2 years, children between 2 and 5 years, 5 and 10 years, and older than 10 years. Age-specific EEG features during wakefulness, sleep onset, and REM and non-REM sleep are detailed below.

Identification of physiological features is not possible on QEEG trends, though they may sometimes be seen on the accompanying source or "raw" EEG tracing.

Are There Any Abnormal Features?

After comprehensive evaluation of the background to confirm normal features are present, the EEG should be reviewed to consider whether abnormal features are present, such as sharp waves, epileptiform discharges or focal or diffuse slowing. Abnormal EEG is discussed further in Chapter 6. For each apparent abnormality, the first step is to make sure that these findings are not actually artifacts (see below).

Are There Normal or Abnormal Sharp Waves?

Abnormal discharges are described in detail in Chapter 6. Of note, normal EEG at some ages includes some sharply contoured activity that is normal. This includes trains of vertex waves, sharp bursts of theta at sleep onset, and frontal and anterior slow waves in newborns (see below). These normal sharp waves need to be recognized as physiological in order to avoid misinterpretation and potential overdiagnosis.

Sharp waves are not visible on QEEG and are only visible on the source EEG tracing.

Are There Seizures or Seizure Mimics?

A seizure is defined on EEG as abnormal rhythmic activity with abrupt onset and offset with evolution in morphology, frequency, or amplitude. By convention, it must last for more than 10 seconds, unless there is a clear clinical correlate. Seizures are always abnormal and must be distinguished from rhythmic artifacts that may create close mimics.

During QEEG monitoring, seizures may appear as abrupt changes in the trend display. Seizures appear on aEEG as an abrupt elevation of the lower margin, particularly if the seizure is of higher amplitude than the surrounding background. On CSA, seizures may appear as changes in frequency content. Unilateral seizures may appear as paroxysmal asymmetry evident on envelope trend or asymmetry index. A careful analysis of the accompanying source EEG is required to make sure suspected seizure on QEEG is not a rhythmic artifact (e.g., patting, respiratory artifact).

Identification of seizures is discussed further in Chapter 6.

Age-Specific Aspects

Preterm and Full-Term Newborns

Overview

Conventional EEG

Background EEG activity in preterm babies has very specific aspects and changes very quickly from week to week during the period of prematurity (Tables 5.1 and 5.2).

Sleep organization differs from that observed in term newborns. Before 26–27 weeks conceptional age, sleep and awake states may be distinguished mainly by behavior. From 28 to 30 weeks conceptional age onward, organization into three states (wakefulness, active and quiet sleep) emerges. Active sleep is a precursor of what will later become rapid eye movement (REM) sleep. Active sleep is characterized behaviorally by periods of rapid eye

movements, small and large body movements, and irregular respirations. In active sleep the EEG varies by conceptional age but is similar to that of wakefulness. In contrast, quiet sleep is characterized by slow, regular respirations, and less body movement (except sucking). Quite sleep is characterized by a more discontinuous EEG (see Table 5.1). The patterned progression from awake to active sleep to quiet sleep is the sleep cycle. The duration of sleep cycle increases with conceptional age from approximately 25 minutes of active sleep and 10 minutes of quiet sleep at 27 weeks, to 40–70 minutes of total sleep (with at least half in active sleep) by term [5, 6]. A specific characteristic of neonatal sleep organization is that sleep onset is into active sleep rather than first to quiet sleep, as would be seen in older infants and children.

In extremely (<28 weeks) and very preterm (28–32 weeks) neonates, the background EEG activity is physiologically discontinuous with bursts of activity often exceeding 300 µV

Table 5.1 Age-related specific background activity on conventional EEG in normal premature and full-term infants

Conceptional age	Sleep–wake cycling	Background activity			Appearance of reactivity	
		Awake	Active sleep (AS)	Quiet sleep (QS)	From active sleep (AS)	From quiet sleep (QS)
24–27 weeks	Resting and active behavior states, +/– EEG variation	Discontinuous (with lability of the discontinuity period) IBI: up to 60 sec			Rare	Rare
28–31 weeks	Emerging: Awake-AS-QS	Discontinuous IBI: up to 35 seconds	Discontinuous	Discontinuous "Tracé discontinu"	28–29 weeks: inconsistent 30–31 weeks: decrease of amplitude	28–29 weeks: inconsistent 30–31 weeks: transient appearance of continuous
32–35 weeks	Present: Awake-AS-QS	Increasingly continuous IBI: up to 20 seconds until 33 weeks IBI: up to 10 seconds until 35 weeks	Discontinuous, becomes increasingly continuous with age	Discontinuous "Tracé discontinu"	Present: Diffuse transient decrease of amplitudes	Inconsistent: Transient appearance of continuous slow wave activity
36–37 weeks	Present: Awake-AS-QS-AS	Continuous "Activité moyenne" IBI: up to 6 seconds	Continuous	Semi-continuous or "Tracé alternant"	Present: Transient decrease in EEG activity	Present: Lengthening of IBI or slow wave burst
38–40 weeks	Present: Awake-AS-QS-AS	Continuous "Activité moyenne"	Continuous	Semi-continuous or "Tracé alternant"	Present: Attenuation of background activity	Present: Attenuation of background activity

AS = active sleep, IBI = interburst interval, QS = quiet sleep

Table 5.2 Age-related specific cEEG features in premature and full-term infants

Conceptional age	Graphoelements	Morphology	Amplitude	Frequency	Spatial localization
24–27 weeks	Slow delta waves +++	Mono- or diphasic Smooth, or with sparse superimposed theta/alpha rhythms Isolated, or in short monorhythmic sequences	Up to 300 μV	0.3–1 Hz	Occipital – central – frontal bilateral/ synchronous or unilateral
	Theta waves ++	Mono-Diphasic, in bursts of sharply contoured waves +/– delta wave	Up to 200 μV	4–7 Hz	Diffuse or predominate in temporal areas
28–31 weeks	Theta waves (temporal theta) +++	Mono-Diphasic, in bursts of sharply contoured waves +/– delta wave mainly observed in QS	>300 μV	4–7 Hz	Diffuse or predominate in temporal areas
	Delta brushes ++	Mono- or diphasic, with superimposed faster rhythms, Isolated or in short sequences Notable in AS and QS	50–2500 μV	0.3–2 Hz	Predominate in occipital areas
32–35 weeks	Delta brushes +++	Mono- or diphasic, with superimposed faster rhythms, Isolated or in short sequences Notable in AS and QS	50–250 μV	0.3–2 Hz	Temporal and occipital
	Temporal theta +/–	Mono-Diphasic, in bursts of sharply contoured waves +/– delta wave mainly observed in AS until 32 weeks and QS until 33–34 weeks	Up to 120 μV	4–7 Hz	Predominate in temporal areas
	Frontal sharp transients +/–	Immature, smooth incomplete, asymmetric		1–2 Hz	Frontal
36–37 weeks	Delta brushes +/–	Mono or diphasic, with superimposed faster rhythms, Isolated or in short sequences	50–200 μV	0.5–2 Hz	Occipital

Table 5.2 (cont.)

Conceptional age	Graphoelements	Morphology	Amplitude	Frequency	Spatial localization
	Frontal sharp transients ++	Diphasic (negative deflection followed by positive deflection) More frequently in AS and onset QS	50–150 µV	1–2 Hz	Frontal, unilateral, or bilateral
	Slow anterior dysrhythmia +/–	Short bursts of monomorphic delta waves	50–100 µV	1–3 Hz	Frontal
38–40 weeks	Frontal sharp transients +++	Diphasic (negative deflection followed by positive deflection) More frequently in AS and onset QS	50–150 µV	1–2 Hz	Frontal, unilateral, or bilateral
	Slow anterior dysrhythmia ++	Short bursts of monomorphic delta waves, often intermixed with frontal sharp transients	50–100 µV	1–3 Hz	Frontal

+++ abundant
++ common
+/– may or may not be present
AS = active sleep, QS = quiet sleep.

separated by prolonged periods of relatively flat tracing called inter-burst intervals (IBIs). With brain maturation, the number and duration of IBIs and the amplitudes of bursts decrease (see Table 5.1). By term-equivalent age, background activity is continuous while awake and during active sleep, whereas during quiet sleep, high-amplitude bursts persist and alternate with periods of relatively lower amplitude activity, a pattern named "tracé alternant" (Figure 5.7).

Specific physiological features appear and disappear at expected ages during brain maturation (see Table 5.2). In preterm EEGs, characteristic features include high-amplitude slow delta waves, delta brushes, and sharply contoured theta bursts. In term infants, characteristic normal EEG features are frontal sharp transients (also called "encoches frontales") and slow anterior dysrhythmia (Figure 5.8). These are all normal and should not be mistaken for epileptiform activity.

Amplitude-Integrated EEG (aEEG)

The main parameters of aEEG – continuity, amplitude and cyclic variation – change according to gestational age [7, 8] (Table 5.3).

The term "continuity" is somewhat ambiguous because it can relate both to the corresponding cEEG and to a specific set of parameters in aEEG. In aEEG, continuity is assessed through the upper and lower margins of the activity band. In the Hellstrom-Westas classification, the aEEG tracing is considered continuous when the lower margin amplitude stays above 5 µV and the upper margin amplitude is at least 10 µV [9]. Notably, while an upper margin of 10 µV is sufficient to categorize an aEEG as continuous using the Hellstrom-Westas system, typically upper margin amplitudes in healthy neonates are higher, often 30–50 µV. A discontinuous aEEG is characterized by lower margin amplitude below 5 µV, while upper margin remains above 10 µV (and often higher) (Figure 5.9). The discontinuous aEEG pattern in preterm infants correlates with the "tracé discontinu" pattern seen on cEEG. In contrast, a burst suppression pattern on aEEG shows an absence of variability, as well as a very low (typically <3 µV) lower margin amplitude (Figure 5.10). In parallel with EEG, aEEG becomes gradually more continuous with age; this is reflected by the lower margin of the aEEG activity band raising with increasing conceptional age. In alternative aEEG grading systems, continuity may be measured

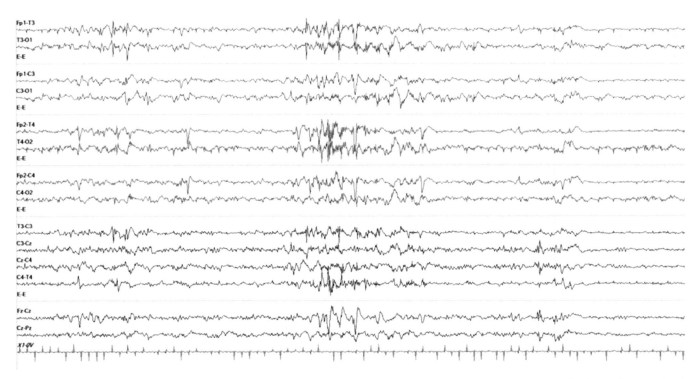

Figure 5.7 Tracé alternant in a term neonate. Display is set at 60 seconds per screen to best visualize the subtle alternating pattern of higher and lower amplitude activity.

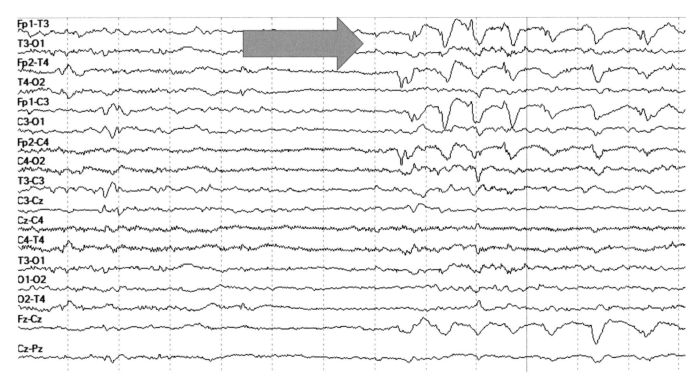

Figure 5.8 EEG from a 39-weeks gestational age infant, on day 4 after birth, after receiving therapeutic hypothermia for suspected hypoxic-ischemic encephalopathy (HIE). The EEG includes normal frontal sharp transients in the bilateral frontal channels, along with anterior dysrhythmia [arrow]. These are normal features in a term neonate.

differently. For example, in the Burdjalov classification approach to aEEG, the term "continuity" refers to the density of the aEEG band itself [10].

Amplitude – In healthy term neonates, the mean amplitude of the upper margin is between 10 and 30 μV with rare bursts of activity greater than 50 μV [11]. Presence of more frequent bursts before 30 weeks gestational age are normal. In

Table 5.3 Age-related patterns on aEEG in healthy preterm and full-term neonates

Conceptional age	Predominant background pattern	Lower margin typical amplitude (µV)	Upper margin typical amplitude (µV)	Sleep–wake cycling
24–27 weeks	Discontinuous with sparse intermixed high-amplitude "bursts"	2–5	12–40	Immature[#]
28–31 weeks	Discontinuous	2–5	10–30	Immature[#]
32–35 weeks	Borderline continuous while awake Discontinuous in quiet sleep	3–6	10–30	Mature[*]
36–37 weeks	Continuous while awake Discontinuous in quiet sleep	5–10	15–30	Mature[*]
38–40 weeks	Continuous	5–15	15–40	Mature[*]

[#] Only some developed cyclic variation in the lower amplitude.
[*] Clearly identifiable sinusoidal variations between discontinuous and more continuous background activity, cycle duration >20 min.

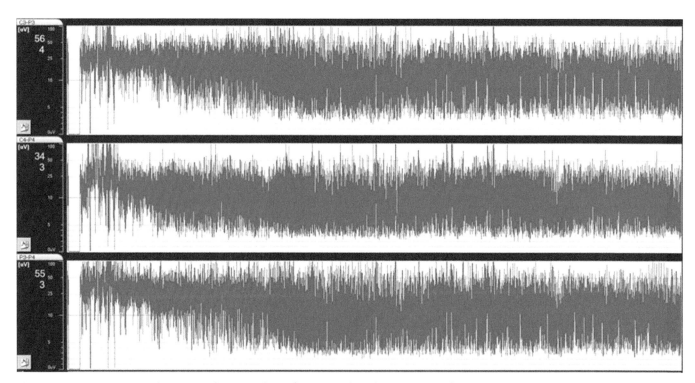

Figure 5.9 Discontinuous aEEG from a 38-week gestational age infant initiating hypothermia treatment for hypoxic-ischemic encephalopathy. Six hours of aEEG is displayed. While the initial segment features higher amplitudes, the majority is characterized by a lower margin below 5 µV with an upper margin above 10 µV.

premature infants, the number of bursts is inversely correlated with conceptional age.

Sleep–Wake Cycling – Cyclic variation of aEEG background activity may be detected even in premature infants. Neurologically normal preterm infants exhibit at least two different patterns of aEEG activity, corresponding to awake and asleep. The presence of cyclical variation of aEEG activity is useful for prediction of good outcome in preterm infants [11]. From as early as 30 weeks conceptional age, quiet sleep periods are clearly discernable in the aEEG as periods that

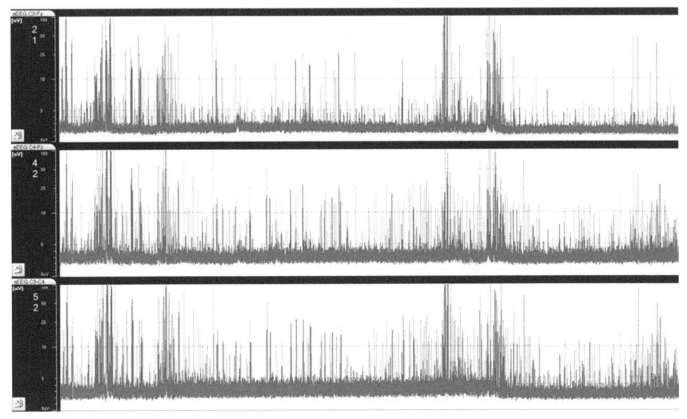

Figure 5.10 Burst suppression on aEEG. aEEG from a 5-day-old term neonate with multiple anomalies, following bowel perforation and sepsis. Note activity band predominantly below 3 µV with very brief high-amplitude bursts rising above.

have increased bandwidth. At term, the aEEG pattern in quiet sleep reflects the "tracé alternant" pattern seen on cEEG. The presence of discernable sleep–wake cycling before 30 weeks conceptional age is less well established. Cyclic variations in the most premature infants might suggest immature sleep–wake cycling. At the same time, variability in EEG background at these ages may be observed without consistent concordance with sleep or wake behavioral changes [12, 13].

Age-Specific Aspects

24–27 Weeks Conceptional Age

cEEG

"Tracé discontinu" describes an EEG background characterized by IBIs having duration often greater than 30 seconds in very preterm neonates, separated by high-amplitude bursts of varying duration. Tracé discontinu may be present as early as 27 weeks conceptional age (Figure 5.11). Variability is present and characterized by variable duration of IBIs.

Behaviorally, periods of rest alternate with period of motor activity, albeit with low correlation between behavior and EEG. Tactile stimulation provokes few EEG changes (low reactivity).

Specific EEG features at this age are bursts of high-amplitude delta waves (0.3–1 Hz, >500 µV) mixed with diffuse or temporal sharp theta bursts (200 µV).

aEEG

Two variations of a discontinuous pattern can be identified. A low-voltage discontinuous pattern is present in the most premature newborns, with minimum amplitudes <3µV, higher amplitudes typically ranging from 15 to 30 µV, and high-amplitude bursts infrequent. A higher voltage discontinuous pattern may also be seen, with higher minimum amplitudes of 3–5 µV, typical higher amplitudes ranging from 20 to 40 µV, and rare bursts >100µV.

28–31 Weeks Conceptional Age

cEEG

Active wakefulness, active sleep, and quiet sleep are now established with early sleep–wake cycling present and good concordance of behavioral state with specific EEG features. Discontinuity is marked, particularly during quiet sleep, with IBIs of duration up to 35 seconds and longer bursts of activity present, at times lasting up to 160 seconds. In bursts, theta waves are predominant (especially in the temporal regions), and delta brushes appear. Their number increases with age and will be maximal around 33 weeks conceptional age. Tactile stimulation causes increased continuity and a reduction of amplitude.

aEEG

From approximately 30 weeks gestational age, aEEG background activity becomes continuous (lower margin >5 µV)

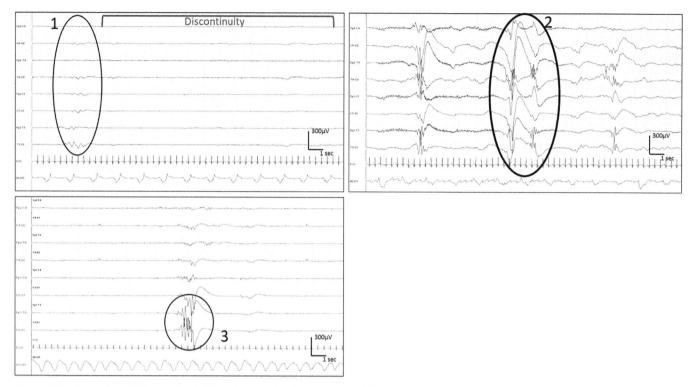

Figure 5.11 Conventional EEG recording in 26 week conceptional age premature infant.
1. Period of approximately 16 seconds of discontinuity with a low-amplitude burst of activity.
2. High-amplitude biphasic delta wave (>700 μV), with superimposed theta activity, predominantly distributed in occipital area.
3. Burst of theta waves associated with a high-amplitude slow wave, in left temporal area.
Longitudinal montage, 0.57 Hz–70 Hz bandwidth, notch filter (50 Hz), ECG: electrocardiogram, RESP: thoracic respiratory movements

during wakefulness and active sleep but stays discontinuous in quiet sleep.

32–35 Weeks Conceptional Age

cEEG

During wakefulness and active sleep, the EEG tracing is nearly continuous. During quiet sleep, the background activity remains discontinuous, with IBI durations around 15–20 seconds at 32 weeks conceptional age, 10 seconds at 34 weeks conceptional age, and less than 10 seconds at 35 weeks conceptional age (Figure 5.12). Reactivity to tactile stimulation is consistent during active sleep, manifesting as reduction of amplitude, but is more difficult to elicit during quiet sleep. This period is marked by an abundance of delta brushes and a decline of temporal activity with a progressive reduction of amplitudes. Immature frontal sharp transients begin to appear at 34 weeks conceptional age, frequently appearing smooth, incomplete, and asymmetrical at this age.

aEEG

The tracing is continuous, with a lower margin above 5 μV. The bandwidth narrows as compared to younger ages, and now fluctuates with sleep–wake cycles.

36–37 Weeks Conceptional Age

cEEG

The EEG tracing is continuous with mixed frequency activity of medium amplitude, sometimes called "activité moyenne." This pattern is present during wakefulness and active sleep, whereas quiet sleep is characterized by the tracé alternant pattern of amplitudes that, while always greater than 25 μV, alternate between higher and lower voltages. Frontal transient sharp waves (encoches frontales) and slow anterior dysrhythmia may be present and constitute an important marker of normal brain maturation in neonates approaching term age. Delta brushes gradually fade away during this period. Theta or alpha waves with low amplitudes are observed in the central and temporal areas in active sleep.

aEEG

The aEEG is similar to that of term neonates, with continuity and established sleep–wake cycling.

Term Infants: 38–42 Weeks Conceptional Age

cEEG

During wakefulness and active sleep, EEG is characterized by the activité moyenne pattern, containing mixed frequencies. In

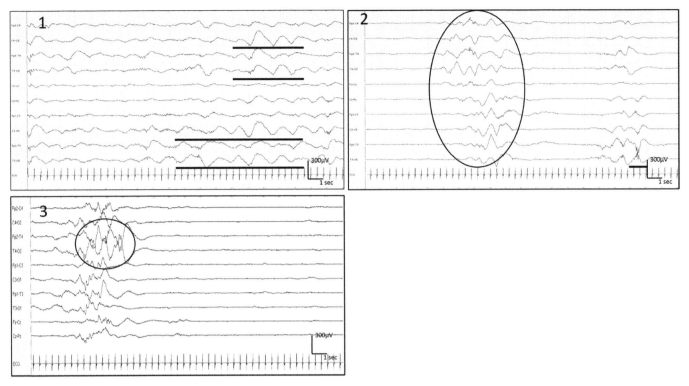

Figure 5.12 Conventional EEG recording in 32 week conceptional age premature infant.
1. Quiet wakefulness, continuous tracing with bursts of delta brushes observed on bilateral occipital areas [underline].
2. Quiet sleep, discontinuous tracing (IBI = 4 seconds) with bursts of activity composed of delta brushes [circle] and low amplitude theta waves in left temporal area [underline].
3. Quiet sleep, discontinuous tracing (IBI = 13 seconds) with bursts of theta waves in the right temporal area.
Longitudinal montage, 0.57 Hz–70 Hz bandwidth, notch filter (50 Hz), ECG: electrocardiogram.

quiet sleep, tracé alternant appears at 37–38 weeks conceptional age and disappears after 44 weeks conceptional age. EEG reactivity (e.g., to arousal) typically manifests as attenuation of background activity, which it is important not to mistake for abnormal discontinuity. Frontal sharp transients and slow anterior dysrhythmia are frequent and remain an important marker of normal brain maturation at this age (Figures 5.13 and 5.14). Delta brushes are rare at this age.

aEEG

Normal term infant aEEG is characterized by continuous tracing with mature sleep–wake cycling. Regular sinusoidal variations of amplitude appear with a cycle 20 minutes. The broader bandwidth corresponds to quiet sleep (tracé alternant) and the narrower bandwidth corresponds to continuous activity during wakefulness and active sleep. The sleep–wake cycling is also easy to identify with DSA (see Figure 5.13).

Infants and Children

Overview

In infants and children, normal EEG shows a mixture of waveforms and frequencies that evolve with age and behavioral state. With maturation, background activity frequencies increase and overall amplitudes decrease. Also, with increasing age there is less inter-subject variability; normal EEG largely approximates adult EEG from 10 years of age onward (Table 5.4).

During wakefulness, a posterior dominant rhythm is recognizable during eye closure from 3 months of age. This initially has a frequency of around 5 Hz, progressively increasing to around 7 Hz by 2 years, around 9 Hz by 7 years, and around 10 Hz by 15 years. The amplitude varies from 30 to 100 μV. Theta and delta waves are abundant. The total quantity of theta progressively increases to reach a peak at 5 years of age and then declines with subsequent age [14, 15]. Delta slow waves are the prominent frequency during the first year of life, followed by theta waves as the main frequency between 2 and 5 years of age. Overabundance of focal or diffuse delta waves is nonspecific marker of brain dysfunction.

During drowsiness, rhythmic diffuse patterns appear at 3 to 5 Hz during the first year of age, increasing in frequency to 4 to 6 Hz by age 5 (Figure 5.15). They are sometimes mixed with high-voltage (as high as 350 μV) bisynchronous 3 to 5 Hz bursts, called hypnagogic hypersynchrony. These are very common between ages 3 and 5 years. The superimposition of these waves may create sharp aspects that should not be confused with generalized spike-waves. These normal drowsy bursts disappear with deeper sleep, in contrast to abnormal spike-wave complexes, which either persist or increase in sleep.

During non-REM sleep, vertex waves, spindles and K complexes are physiological features. They are good markers of normality. Vertex waves are generally high-voltage diphasic sharp waves of maximal amplitude at the central electrodes (Cz, C3, and C4), lasting up to 200 msec. They begin to appear

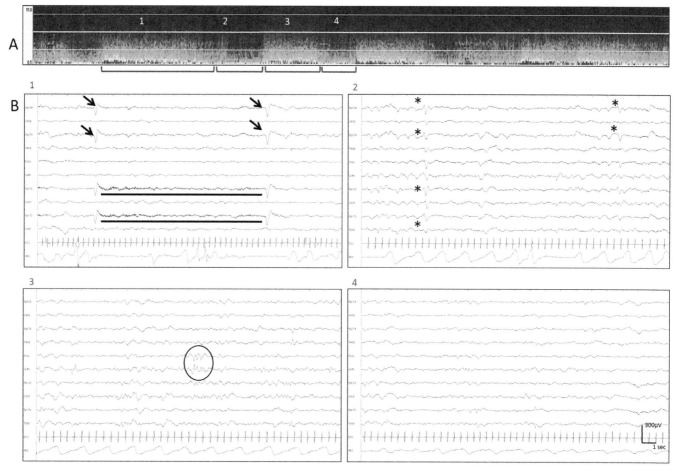

Figure 5.13 Conventional EEG recording in a full-term infant with accompanying DSA.
A. Density spectral array (DSA): display of activity over time on the x-axis (12 hours) with y-axis showing frequencies between 0.5 and 17 Hz. Color scale: from the blue color for the less predominant frequencies to red for dominant frequencies. Cyclic variation seen on DSA correlates with cEEG for (1) wakefulness, (2) active sleep, (3) quiet sleep, and (4) active sleep.
B.
1. Wakefulness: continuous tracing with low amplitude polyfrequency activity ("activité moyenne") with muscular artifacts [underline] and ocular movements [arrows] in frontal channels during wakefulness.
2. Active sleep (AS): continuous tracing with slightly higher amplitudes than later active sleep, frontal transient sharp waves [*] ("encoches frontales"), irregular respirations.
3. Quiet sleep (QS): "tracé alternant" with theta rhythms in central area (Cz) [circle], regular cardiac and respiratory frequency.
4. Active sleep (AS): with a typical "activité moyenne" pattern.
Longitudinal montage, 0.57 Hz–70 Hz bandwidth, notch filter (50 Hz), ECG: electrocardiogram, RESP: thoracic respiratory movements

at around 3 months of age. Their occurrence increases until 3 to 4 years. They may occur in short sequences of repetitive runs that are normal (Figure 5.15). Spindles are rhythmic runs of 12 to 14 Hz waves localized over frontal and central regions, less often seen diffusely. They are a marker of non-REM sleep. They may be present as early as at term-equivalent age and are abundant by age 3 months, though sometimes are asynchronous. Their length and quantity decline with age (Figure 5.15). K complexes are high-amplitude (>100 µV), broad (>200 ms), diphasic transient features and are often associated with sleep spindles. They are maximal at the midline.

During slow wave sleep the dominant frequency is high-amplitude delta. High-voltage rhythmic patterns may be observed at the time of transition between non-REM and REM sleep. They sometimes may mimic a seizure but their occurrence just before a sleep state change helps to distinguish them as a normal feature.

During REM sleep, the EEG has some similarities with the patterns observed during wakefulness. This has given it the name of "paradoxical sleep." Theta waves are the dominant frequency. Eye movements and lack of muscle movements are helpful in distinguishing REM sleep from wakefulness if video or behavioral correlation is not available.

During the first few months, arousal consists of attenuation of voltage. Isolated diphasic slow waves and diffuse theta rhythmic waves appear during arousal from the end of the first year of age. This persists until 4 to 5 years of age and is similar to patterns observed during drowsiness. Between 5 and 7 years, arousal gradually attains a pattern on EEG similar to that seen in adults: a rapid conversion from sleep to awake EEG within 1 to 2 seconds. When arousal occurs during deep, non-REM sleep, a brief delta/theta burst may appear.

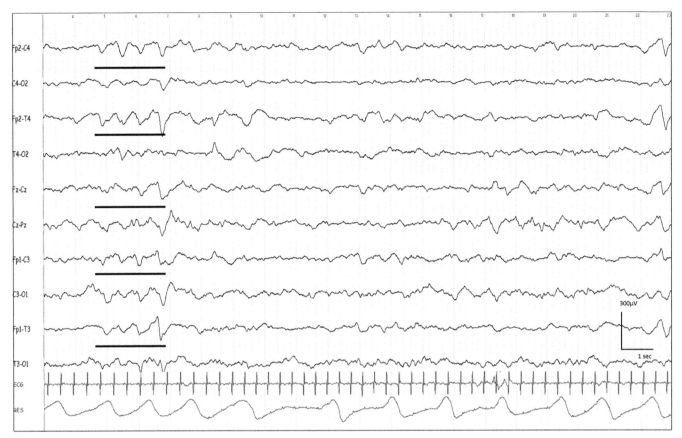

Figure 5.14 Conventional EEG recording in a full-term infant.
Continuous tracing in active sleep with slow anterior dysrhythmia in frontal areas [underline]. Longitudinal montage, 0.57 Hz–70 Hz bandwidth, notch filter (50 Hz), ECG: electrocardiogram, RESP: thoracic respiratory movements.

Table 5.4 Age-related specific EEG features in infants 1 month to children 15 years old

Age	Wakefulness	Sleep onset	NREM stage 1–2	NREM stage 3–4	REM
1 to 24 months	Mixed frequency, <75 µV, emergence of posterior dominant rhythm from 4 Hz (3 months) to 7 Hz (24 months)	Active/REM sleep onset disappears by 2 to 3 months post-term Diffuse high-amplitude 3–5 Hz activity	Mixed frequencies, spindles appear by 1–3 months post-term. Asynchronous spindles possible up to 6 months post-term. K complexes appear by 6 months post-term	Slow wave activity of high amplitude (up to 400 µV) present by 6 months post-term	Theta waves usually preceded by burst of very high-amplitude delta activity at REM onset
2 to 5 years	Posterior dominant rhythm 7–8 Hz intermixed with theta	Hypnagogic hypersynchrony: diffuse bisynchronous sinusoidal rhythmic up to 300 µv waves	K complexes in repetitive runs Typical vertex sharp waves by 16 months post-term	Slow wave activity	
5 to 10 years	Posterior dominant rhythm 9–10 Hz, intermixed 5–8 Hz decreasing with increasing age	Slowing of posterior dominant rhythm frequency Rhythmic anterior theta activity	Vertex sharp waves Represents 55% of total sleep time	Represents 30% of total sleep time	Low amplitude mixed frequency activity Represents 25% of total sleep time
10 years and older	Posterior dominant rhythm 9–10 Hz	Slowing of posterior dominant rhythm frequency	Diffuse low amplitude 4–7 Hz Spindles Represents 50% of total sleep time	Represents 25% of total sleep time	Represents 15% of total sleep time

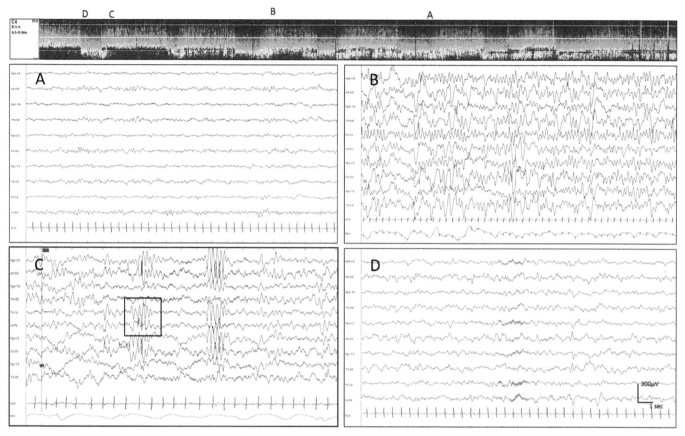

Figure 5.15 Conventional EEG recording in a 2-year-old child.
Top. Density spectral array (DSA) display of activity over time on the x-axis (12 hours) with y-axis showing frequencies between 0.5 and 17 Hz. Color scale: from the blue color for the less predominant frequencies and red for dominant frequencies.
A. Quiet wakefulness.
B. Hypnagogic physiological hypersynchrony in sleep onset.
C. Physiological theta burst in central areas in non-REM sleep (stage 1).
D. Symmetric spindles in non-REM sleep in central areas.
Longitudinal montage, 0.57 Hz–70 Hz bandwidth, notch filter (50 Hz), ECG: electrocardiogram, RESP: thoracic respiratory movements

QEEG

There are no normative data on QEEG background in infants and children. However, continuity, amplitude, asymmetry, and sleep–wake cycling can still be used to assess the appropriateness of the EEG background and monitor recovery after a neurological insult [16].

Age-Specific Aspects

From 1 Month to 2 Years

While awake, dominant rhythms are high-amplitude (up to 75 µV) theta waves, with frequencies from 4 Hz increasing to 6–7 Hz by 2 years of age. These are located in centro-occipital regions in early infancy, then become occipital and are notably interrupted by eye opening from 3 months of age onward. Delta and abundant theta activity is mixed with the posterior dominant rhythm during the second year.

During the first 3 months of age, infants fall asleep directly into active sleep (equivalent of REM sleep in adults). Synchronous theta waves in drowsiness and transition to sleep appear around 6 months of age with rhythmic 3–4 Hz waves, 100 to 250 µV (hypersynchrony).

In sleep, the typical neonatal tracé alternant pattern disappears around the end of the first month, replaced by a continuous, slow wave pattern with approximately 1 Hz, 100 µV, delta waves. Sleep spindles are present as early as term and always by 3 months corrected age. Sleep spindles have a duration up to 10 seconds each, and are typically asynchronous during infancy, becoming synchronous by age 2 years. Vertex waves appear around 6 months. They may constitute trains of vertex sharp waves during the second year. In non-REM deeper sleep there is a predominance of high-amplitude delta waves with a more pronounced occipital location after 1 year of age. In REM sleep, there are low amplitude diffuse theta diffuse or delta waves.

Arousal appears similar to drowsiness in this age group.

From 2 to 5 Years

In wakefulness, the posterior dominant rhythm progressively contains higher frequencies with age, by 5 years consisting largely of alpha activity with some persistent theta and delta waves (see Figure 5.15).

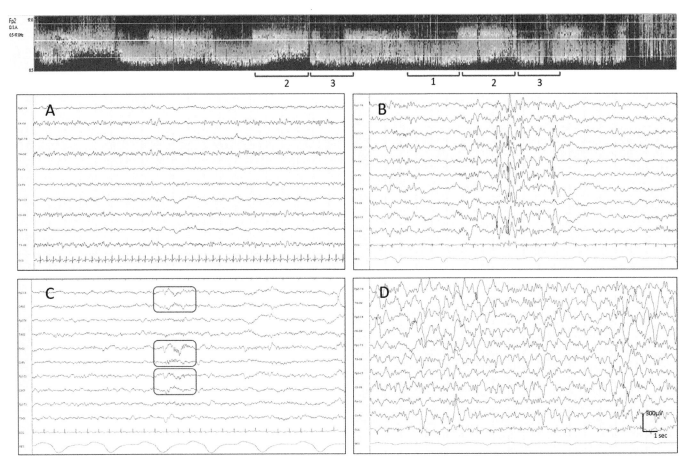

Figure 5.16 Conventional EEG recording in a 5-year-old child.
Top. Density spectral array (DSA): display of activity over time on the x-axis (12 hours) with y-axis showing frequencies between 0.5 and 17 Hz. Color scale: from the blue color for the less frequent predominant frequencies and red for dominant frequencies. Cyclic variation allows identification of quiet wakefulness (1), non-REM sleep (2), and REM sleep (3).
A. Quiet wakefulness.
B. K complex and vertex sharp waves.
C. Non-REM sleep (stage 2), spindles in central areas [circle].
D. Non-REM sleep (stage 3).
Longitudinal montage, 0.57 Hz–70 Hz bandwidth, notch filter (50 Hz), ECG: electrocardiogram, RESP: thoracic respiratory movements

Drowsiness is characterized by the hypersynchronous pattern less commonly with increasing age, but may be seen in normal EEG until 13 years of age. In drowsiness, theta waves with a sharp aspect appear and should not be confused for an abnormal pattern.

In sleep, vertex sharp waves are frequently seen intermixed with K complexes, having a maximum at the vertex.

Arousal patterns are nonspecific at this age.

From 5 to 10 Years

In wakefulness, by around 10 years of age the posterior dominant rhythm is alpha (10–11 Hz) of high amplitude (as high as 100 μV at 8–9 years, then decreasing with age) (Figure 5.16).

In sleep, spindles are shorter (1 to 2 seconds) and are located centrally but with spreading in frontal regions. During REM sleep, low amplitude theta and alpha rhythms are predominant.

At this age, arousal consists of a transition from sleep to awake that is rapid.

From 10 Years to Adulthood

Wakefulness is characterized by an alpha frequency (10–12 Hz), posterior dominant rhythm of low amplitude (Figure 5.17).

In drowsiness, the alpha rhythm gradually becomes slower, less prominent, and fragmented. Central or frontocentral theta activity, beta activity, and some occipital sharp transients appear. Hypnagogic hypersynchrony may persist.

During non-REM light sleep activity is slow with theta and then delta predominance. There are spindles, vertex waves and K complexes of high amplitude (>100 μV) and duration (>200 ms), with a diphasic aspect, and often associated with sleep spindles. During non-REM deep sleep polymorphic delta activity is prominent, of high amplitude (>75 μV) with few sleep spindles and K

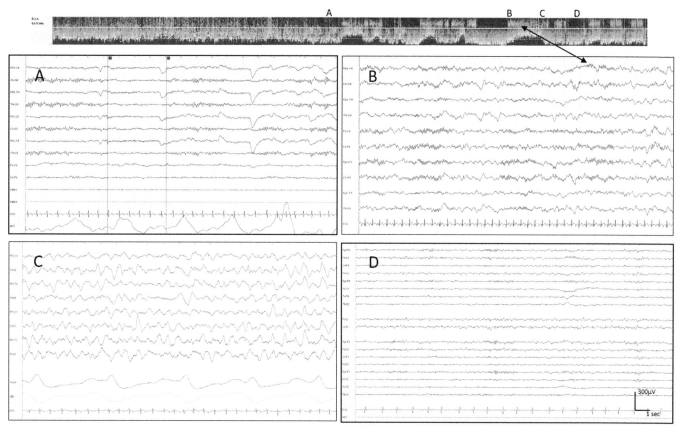

Figure 5.17 Conventional EEG recording in a 10-year-old child.
Top. Density spectral array (DSA): display of activity over time on the x-axis (12 hours) with y-axis showing frequencies between 0.5 and 17 Hz. Color scale: from the blue color for the less frequent predominant frequencies and red for dominant frequencies.
A. Quiet wakefulness with reactivity to eye opening and closure [vertical lines].
B. Non-REM sleep (stage 2), with spindles in central areas [arrow].
C. Non-REM sleep (stage 3).
D. REM sleep.
Longitudinal montage, 0.57 Hz–70 Hz bandwidth, notch filter (50 Hz), ECG: electrocardiogram, RESP: thoracic respiratory movements

complexes. During REM sleep EEG rhythms are desynchronized with theta and beta waves of low amplitude. REM sleep is characterized by presence of rapid eye movements observed on video and/or recorded as eye movement artifact in the frontal channels.

Physiological and Environmental Artifacts

Artifacts are superimposed features on the background activity that do not reflect brain activity. They can have different origins: technical, environmental, or physiological. They can be sustained or brief, transient or repetitive. Recognition of artifact is highly important for EEG interpretation.

Physiological Artifacts

Physiological artifacts are those noncerebral signals that appear on EEG that have origin in other body parts.

Muscular contractions may cause intermittent or sustained artifact, characterized by a frequency greater than 50 Hz (Figure 5.18). While EEG software may have filters designed

to reduce muscle artifact, it cannot be completely removed by additional EEG filters. Moreover, filtering may modify EEG morphology, making patterns more difficult to recognize as artifact.

Movement artifact may result from spontaneous patient movement, or from handling (e.g., rocking or patient care) (Figure 5.19). Movement artifact may appear on EEG as slow waves at the frequency of the movements, or abrupt and irregular. These artifacts can be prolonged, more or less regular and sometimes quite rhythmic; thus, they can closely mimic the EEG appearance of seizures. The use of an EMG electrode to document muscle activity or time-locked video can both be invaluable to clarify that movement is the source of the EEG activity.

Ocular artifact occurs as the result of eye movements, typically manifesting as frontal slow waves (Figure 5.20). These artifacts can be identified by bedside observation, video or dedicated electro-oculogram channels. Eye movement artifacts can be useful for identifying behavioral states, notably active sleep in preterm neonates and REM sleep in children.

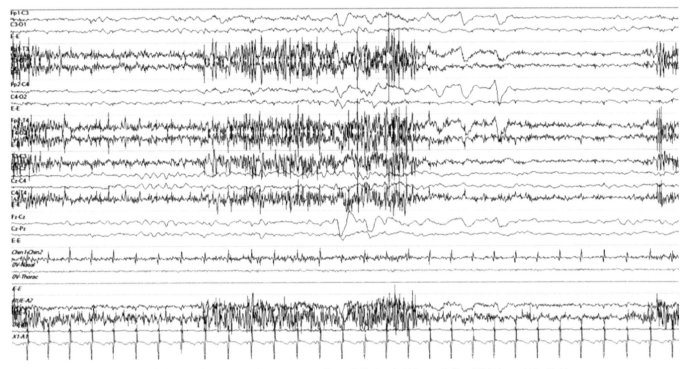

Figure 5.18 Muscle artifact in a full-term infant. Neonatal montage, 0.57 Hz to 70 Hz bandwidth, notch filter (60 Hz), sensitivity 7 μV.

Common in ICU tracings are cardiac and respiratory artifacts (Figures 5.21 and 5.22). Cardiac pulse or respiratory movements can be recorded on EEG tracing and sometimes imitate ictal discharges because they are rhythmic, stereotyped, and may evolve over time. The simultaneous recording of ECG and at least one respiratory sensor with cEEG allows one to distinguished many of these artifacts. Similarly, these typically appear at a frequency equal to the heart rate or respiratory rate.

Hiccup artifacts occur isolated or in series, often with a repetitive aspect (Figure 5.23). They may occur simultaneously on the respiratory channel and on EEG derivations as the head has subtle movement.

Sucking artifacts are rhythmic and composed of fast rhythms of muscular origin inconsistently superimposed on slow waves (theta-delta) (Figure 5.24). They are often recorded in temporal areas and can be prolonged, and more or less regular in rhythm. They may be of varying amplitude.

Electrodermogram artifact (sometimes called "sweat artifact") is characterized by slow drifts on the baseline (less than 0.5 Hz) with superimposed physiological activity (Figure 5.25).

Technical and Environmental Artifacts

Patting is a common environmental artifact seen in neonatal EEG (Figure 5.26). Because patting typically is rhyth-mic, evolves in frequency and/or amplitude, and then stops after seconds or minutes, it is a common seizure mimic. Patting is most easily identified if there is accompanying video, though may also be recognized by simultaneous movement seen in non-cerebral (EKG, respiratory, or EMG) channels.

"Line noise," electrical artifacts, is characterized by a superimposed frequency coming from the power supply (50 Hz in Europe, 60 Hz in the United States) (Figure 5.27). This added noise is traditionally reduced by filtering with a "notch" filter centered on the alternating current frequency. Similar artifacts may be present when EEG recording equipment or the patient comes into contact with other medical devices or even personal devices such as mobile phones, tablets, or laptop computers.

Artifactual asymmetry in amplitude should be considered when there is asymmetry solely in amplitude between the two hemispheres, without asymmetry in frequency content. Any asymmetry should be interpreted with caution on a bipolar montage because it could simply be due to asymmetric inter-electrode distances or asymmetric scalp edema, such as cephalohematoma. Therefore, confirmation of the amplitude asymmetry using a referential montage is required.

Electrode artifacts can be of various types, including spiky waves with an abrupt initial phase inconsistently

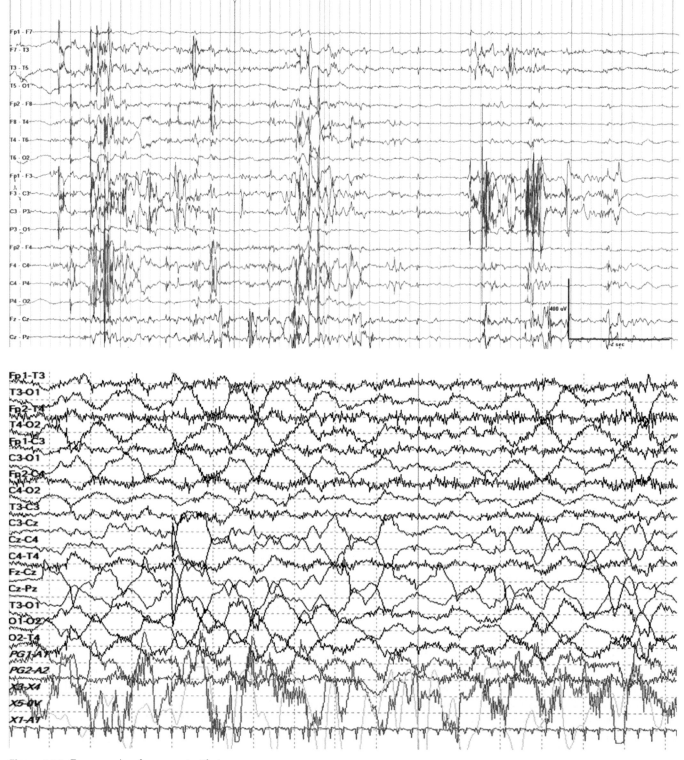

Figure 5.19 Two examples of movement artifact.
Top. EEG from a 3-year-old following cardiac arrest. Brief, abrupt artifact is seen where patient is moved during care.
Bottom. EEG from a term neonate monitored for spells of eye movements. Slow, semi-rhythmic waves reflect rocking movement.

followed by a slow wave, occurring transiently or in repeat sequences with regular intervals of a few seconds (Figure 5.28). These should resolve with adjustment of the electrode.

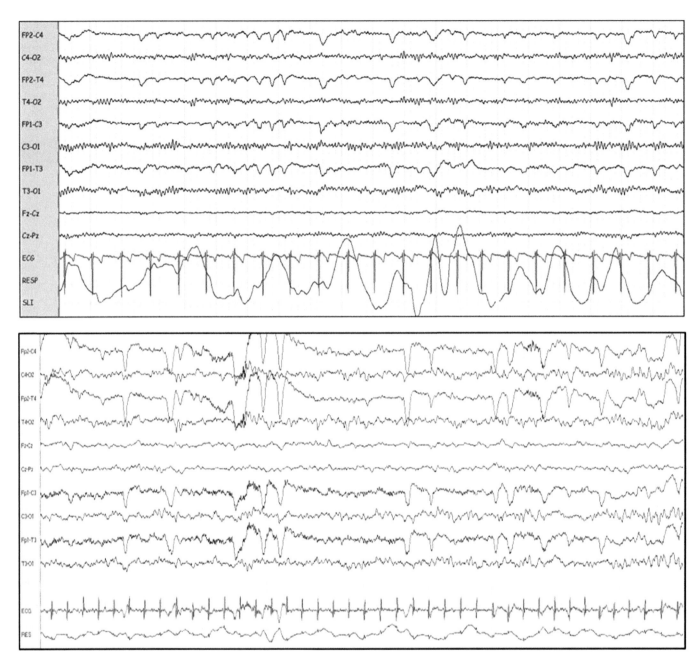

Figure 5.20 Examples of ocular artifact.
A. Ocular artifact appearing as theta activity in the frontal channels in a 10-year-old boy.
B. Ocular artifact appearing as theta frequency sharply contoured activity in the frontal channels in a 3-year-old girl. High pass filter 0.5 Hz, low pass filter: 70 Hz, notch filter 50 Hz. Gain of amplitude μV/mm.

Artifacts on QEEG

Artifacts are especially important to keep in mind when brain monitoring is performed via QEEG. False normal aEEG may be observed due to elevation of the overall amplitude by high-voltage electrocardiographic, high-frequency ventilation or muscular artifacts. This may occur in as many as 15% of cases in encephalopathic, ventilated newborns receiving hypothermia [17] with flat trace on raw EEG [18]. Brief or intermittent elevation of the lower margin may also occur with nursing cares such as patting. This pattern may be mistaken for seizures.

In order to reduce the potential for artifact, it is essential to record and to check raw EEG data at the beginning of a recording and whenever there is a sudden change in appearance of the QEEG trace. While QEEG can be a very helpful tool for bedside neuromonitoring, specific education of bedside caregivers on proper interpretation is essential. When suspected abnormalities are identified on QEEG, if possible, critical management decisions should be deferred until review of both QEEG and cEEG by skilled personnel.

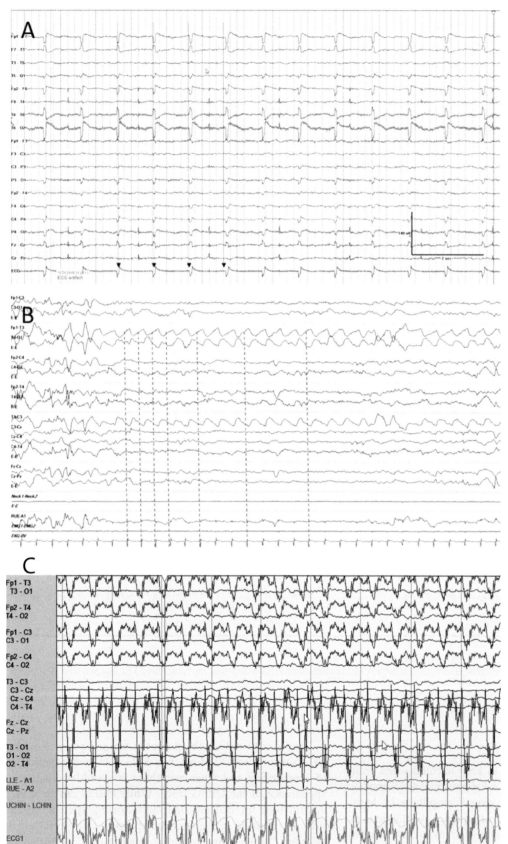

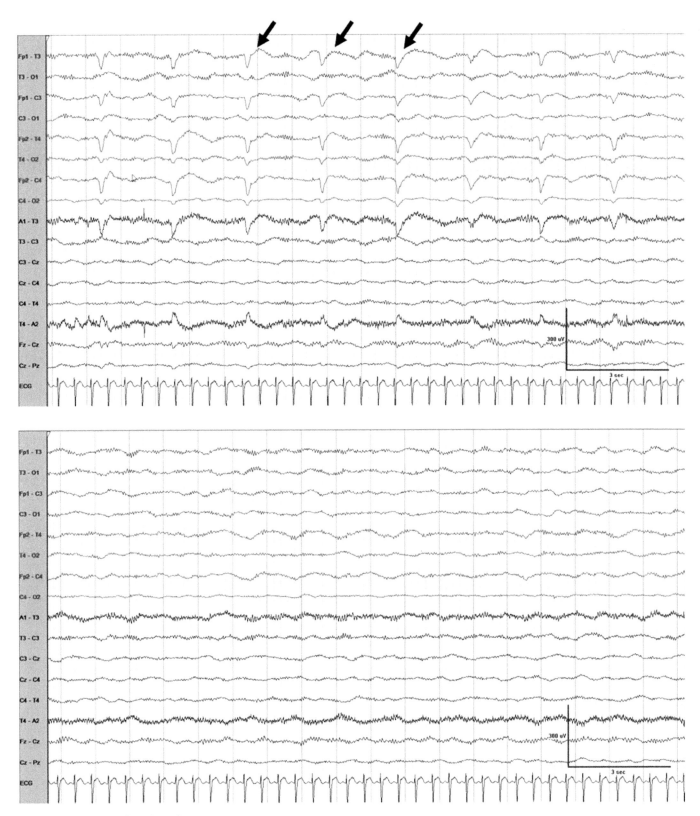

Figure 5.22 Example of droplet artifact.
Top: Artifact resembling periodic discharges [arrow] caused by droplets in ventilation circuit.
Top: Same patient with artifact resolved after suction of tubing.

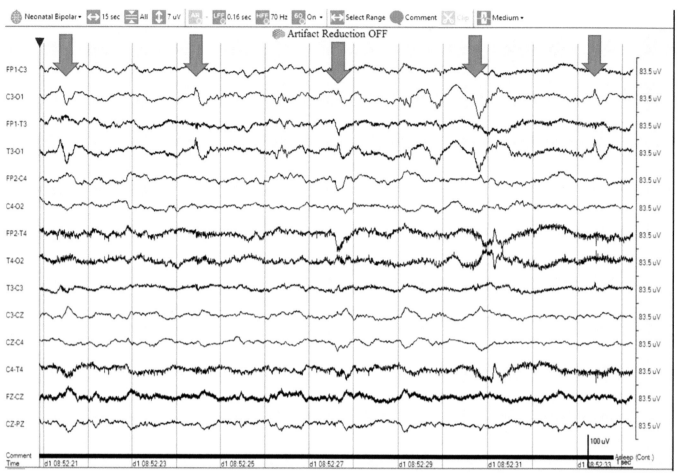

Figure 5.23 Hiccup artifact in a term neonate. Abrupt, repetitive artifact at O1 (arrows) corresponded to hiccups seen on video.

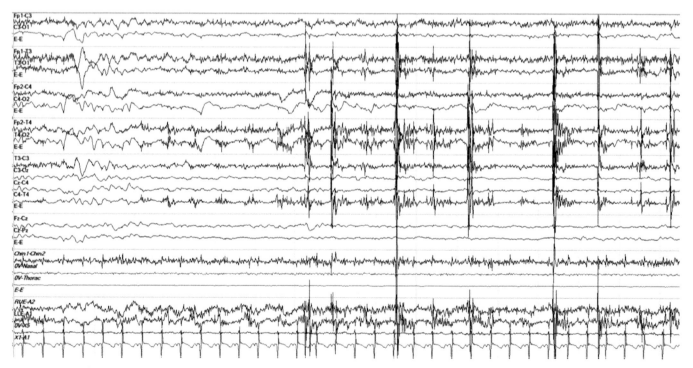

Figure 5.24 Sucking in a 35 week neonate. In this example, artifact is maximal in the temporal channels, and while initially, low amplitude is very high amplitude in the second half of the tracing.

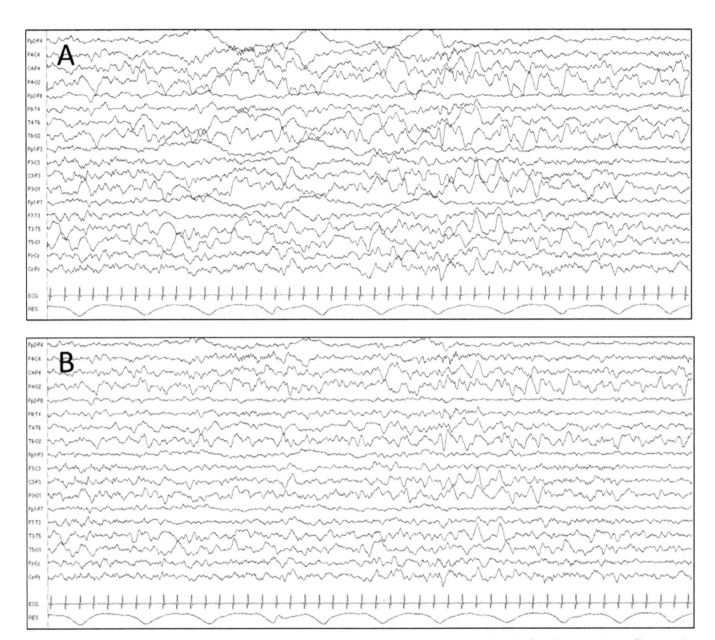

Figure 5.25 Sweat artifact in a 2-year-old child. (A) Sweat artifact appears as very slow delta waves predominantly in the frontal regions. High pass filter 0.5 Hz, low pass filter 70 Hz, notch filter 50 Hz. Gain of amplitude 15 μV/mm. (B) Sweat artifacts are less visible after adjusting the high pass filter to 1.6 Hz.

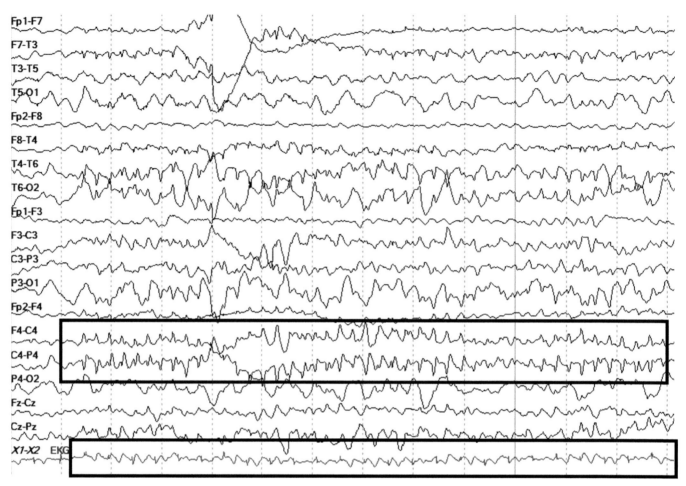

Figure 5.26 Patting artifact. While rhythmic and sharply contoured, this patting artifact does not have a plausible physiologic field, and can also be seen in the EKG channel.

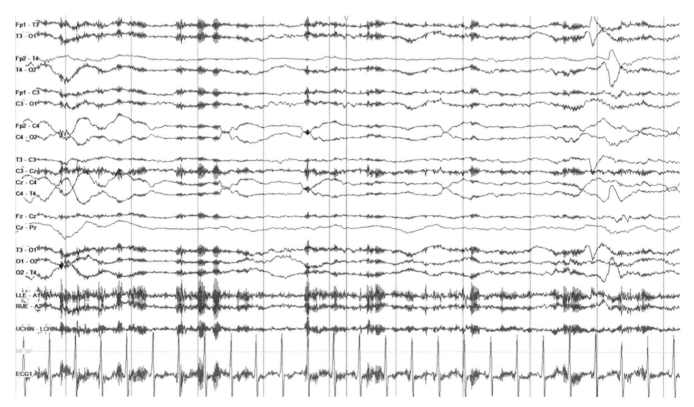

Figure 5.27 Neonatal EEG showing electrical artifact. Neonatal montage, 1Hz–70 Hz bandwidth, notch filter (60 Hz), Sensitivity 10 μV. High frequency artifact appears across all channels intermittently, in this case as other electrical equipment came near the EEG recording device.

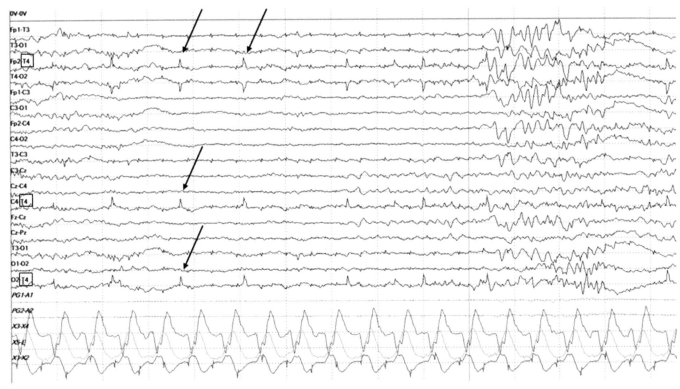

Figure 5.28   Electrode artifact. Five-day-old male born at 36 weeks with prenatal diagnosis of Ebstein's anomaly and hydrops. EEG following bradycardic arrest postdelivery, recorded while patient on VA-ECMO. Electrode artifact ("pop") [arrow] is evident at T4. There is also lower amplitude ECG artifact at T3. Sensitivity 5 µV, 15 seconds per page, HF 70 Hz Tc 0.1s.

References

1. Stewart CP, Otsubo H, Ochi A, et al. Seizure identification in the ICU using quantitative EEG displays. *Neurology.* 2010 Oct;**75**(17):1501–8.

2. Shellhaas RA, Chang T, Tsuchida T, et al. The American Clinical Neurophysiology Society's Guideline on continuous electroencephalography monitoring in neonates. *J Clin Neurophysiol.* 2011 Dec;**28**(6):611–17.

3. Lamblin MD, de Villepin-Touzery A. EEG in the neonatal unit. *Neurophysiol Clin.* 2015 Mar;**45**(1):87–95.

4. Seltzer LE, Swartz M, Kwon JM, et al. Intraoperative electroencephalography predicts postoperative seizures in infants with congenital heart disease. *Pediatr Neurol.* 2014 Apr;**50**(4):313–7.

5. Curzi-Dascalova L, Figueroa JM, Eiselt M, et al. Sleep state organization in premature infants of less than 35 weeks' gestational age. *Pediatr Res.* 1993 Nov;**34**(5):624–8.

6. André M, Lamblin M-D, d'Allest AM, et al. Electroencephalography in premature and full-term infants. Developmental features and glossary. *Neurophysiol Clin.* 2010 May;**40**(2):59–124.

7. Zhang D, Liu Y, Hou X, et al. Reference values for amplitude-integrated EEGs in infants from preterm to 3.5 months of age. *Pediatrics.* 2011 May; **127**(5):e1280–7.

8. Vesoulis ZA, Paul RA, Mitchell TJ, et al. Normative amplitude-integrated EEG measures in preterm infants. *J Perinatol.* 2015 Jun;**35**(6):428–33.

9. Hellstrom-Westas L, Rosen I, de Vries LS, Greisen G. Amplitude-integrated EEG classification and interpretation in preterm and term infants. *NeoReviews.* 2006; 7(2):e76–87.

10. Burdjalov VF, Baumgart S, Spitzer AR. Cerebral function monitoring: a new scoring system for the evaluation of brain maturation in neonates. *Pediatrics.* 2003 Oct;**112**(4):855–61.

11. Hellstrom-Westas L. Continuous electroencephalography monitoring of the preterm infant. *Clin Perinatol.* 2006 Sept;**33**(3):633–647.

12. Selton D, Andre M, Hascoët JM. Normal EEG in very premature infants: reference criteria. *Clin Neurophysiol.* 2000 Dec;**111**(12):2116–24.

13. Vecchierini M-F, André M, d'Allest AM. Normal EEG of premature infants born between 24 and 30 weeks gestational age: terminology, definitions and maturation aspects. *Neurophysiol Clin.* 2007 Nov;**37**(5):311–23.

14. Corbin HP, Bickford RG. Studies of the electroencephalogram of normal children: comparison of viscal and automatic frequency analyses. *Electroencephalogr Clin Neurophysiol.* 1955 Feb;**7**(1):15–28.

15. Hagne I. Development of the EEG in health infants during the first year of life, illustrated by frequency analysis. *Electroencephalogr Clin Neurophysiol.* 1968 Jan;**24**(1):88.

16. Oh SH, Park KN, Kim YM, et al. The prognostic value of continuous amplitude-integrated electroencephalogram applied immediately after return of spontaneous circulation in therapeutic hypothermia-treated cardiac arrest patients. *Resuscitation.* 2013 Feb;**84**(2):200–5.

17. Marics G, Csekő A, Vásárhelyi B, et al. Prevalence and etiology of false normal aEEG recordings in neonatal hypoxic-ischaemic encephalopathy. *BMC Pediatr.* 2013;**13**:194.

18. Hagmann CF, Robertson NJ, Azzopardi D. Artifacts on electroencephalograms may influence the amplitude-integrated EEG classification: a qualitative analysis in neonatal encephalopathy. *Pediatrics.* 2006 Dec;**118**(6):2552–4.

Abnormal EEG in the Intensive Care Unit

Jessica Carpenter and Tammy Tsuchida

Chapter 6

Key Points

- Identification of EEG background patterns can aid in evaluation of encephalopathy across the age span.
- Certain EEG abnormalities indicate recent injury or risk for seizures.
- EEG is essential for seizure diagnosis and distinction from other paroxysmal patterns.
- Quantitative EEG trends facilitate quick recognition of changes in background patterns over time.

Introduction

While EEG in the intensive care unit (ICU) is often associated with seizure detection, it may be useful for the detection of a variety of abnormalities. Focal abnormalities on EEG can indicate a localized process such as ischemia, hemorrhage, or mass lesion. Diffuse background abnormalities can be helpful in predicting neurodevelopmental outcome for neonates with acute injury. Other patterns can indicate high risk for seizures or even suggest a particular epilepsy diagnosis [1]. Recognition of acute changes in EEG background could prompt changes in clinical management, such as when focal slowing is noted in a patient at risk for focal hypoperfusion and thus prompts adjustments to increase cerebral perfusion pressure. Significant diffuse EEG background deterioration can similarly alert the clinician to impending herniation. In all cases, recognition of the abnormal EEG or QEEG findings is the essential first step. This chapter will describe a variety of common EEG abnormalities seen in neonates and children in the ICU and provide an overview of their clinical correlates.

Background Abnormalities

Neonates

Neonatal EEG background patterns that have received the most study are for the full-term neonate. The background pattern can be characterized by features of continuity and amplitude. When assessing for continuity there is a continuum ranging from continuous or appropriately discontinuous, to excessively discontinuous, to burst suppressed. Unlike the normal discontinuous patterns of tracé discontinu and tracé alternant, an abnormally discontinuous EEG has an inter-burst interval (IBI) that is longer than expected for postmenstrual age (PMA) (Table 6.1). Neonates can have an excessively discontinuous EEG due to a variety of CNS insults, including hypoxia-ischemia, meningoencephalitis, hyperammonemia, and many others. Abnormally discontinuous

Table 6.1 Normal inter-burst interval (IBI) duration values displayed according to postmenstrual age (PMA)

Postmenstrual age	Maximum inter-burst interval
<30 weeks	35 seconds
30–33 weeks	20 seconds
34–36 weeks	10 seconds
37–40 weeks	6 seconds

Adapted from: Tsuchida TN, Wusthoff CJ, Shellhaas RA, et al. American clinical neurophysiology society standardized EEG terminology and categorization for the description of continuous EEG monitoring in neonates: report of the ACNS critical care monitoring committee. *J Clin Neurophysiol.* 2013 Apr;30(2):161–73.

patterns can be distinguished from the normal discontinuous patterns seen in preterm neonates by the presence of abnormal waveforms within the bursts of activity in the abnormally discontinuous trace, such as excessive delta slow waves, or sharp wave discharges. An assessment of the degree of discontinuity can be clinically informative. For example, the length of IBI has been shown to correlate with ammonia level in neonates with citrullinemia [2] (Figure 6.1).

Another feature to characterize in potentially abnormal EEG is whether state changes are present. A state change is defined as at least one sustained minute in each of more than one state, with each demonstrating distinctly different EEG patterns (discontinuity, amplitudes, and frequencies). For EEGs that are abnormal due to the absence of active or quiet sleep features, the presence or absence of a state change is an additional useful descriptor, as absence of state changes is even more worrisome than absence of normal sleep architecture with preserved state changes.

Burst suppression is the most severely abnormal discontinuous pattern (Figure 6.2). Unlike the excessively discontinuous EEG, the burst suppression pattern has no normal features. By definition, in burst suppression the amplitude of the IBI must be below 5 μV peak-to-peak (pp) and the bursts contain no normal activity. The burst suppression background also contains no variability or reactivity (Table 6.2). When an EEG contains state changes alternating between excessive discontinuity and a pattern that otherwise appears to be burst suppression, it overall should be described as excessively discontinuous, as burst suppression is a background pattern lacking state changes.

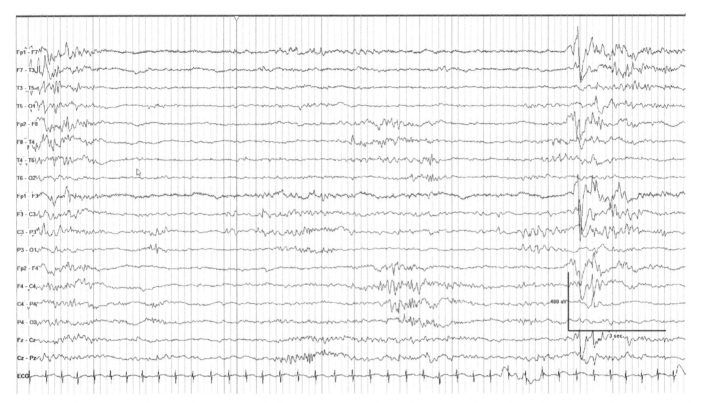

Figure 6.1 EEG from a 3-week-old term infant with mild citrullinemia, presenting with several days' history of worsening respiratory status and decreased level of consciousness (LOC) despite normal serum ammonia levels. EEG demonstrates dysmature pattern with excessive discontinuity for age and marked asynchrony of bursts.

Amplitude is also an important descriptor and is conventionally broken down into four categories based on patterns that are predictive of neurodevelopmental outcome in full-term infants [3]. In normal background, voltages should be 25 μV pp or greater in all behavioral states (awake, active sleep, quiet sleep). Low-voltage suppressed is defined as activity with amplitude between 2 and 10 μV pp in a tracing that is also invariant and unreactive with no normal background features. Electrocerebral inactivity (ECI) is defined as the absence of any activity with amplitude ≥2 μV pp, when reviewed at a sensitivity of 2 μV/mm and in an EEG recording acquired utilizing special technical parameters. These requirements include use of a full set of scalp electrodes, impedances under 10,000 Ω but over 100 Ω, and demonstration during the recording of the integrity of the recording system [4]. If the study is not performed using specific ECI technical parameters but nonetheless lacks apparent activity ≥2 μV pp, it would be described as possibly consistent with ECI but not meeting technical recording criteria to determine ECI. EEG to assess for ECI can be an ancillary study in the diagnosis of brain death in children; in cases of brain death, it is essential the EEG is recording in accordance with specific technical parameters to declare ECI [4, 5]. It is also important to recognize that brain death is a clinical determination and cannot be made based on the presence of ECI on EEG alone.

An intermediate neonatal amplitude category is a pattern with some normal features, but also with voltages continuously less than 25 μV but ≥10 μV pp. This background pattern has

been defined by the American Clinical Neurophysiology Society (ACNS) guideline as borderline low voltage; it is of uncertain significance [3].

For neonates with seizures or hypoxia-ischemia, EEG backgrounds that are low-voltage suppressed, burst suppression, or inactive are strongly associated with subsequent long-term neurological impairment [6–10]. It is important to use strict definitions for these background patterns because of their importance in predicting outcome [3]. For example, among neonates described as having "burst suppression" on EEG, but where the EEG shows variability and IBI amplitudes > 5 μV, only a minority have a poor neurological outcome [11]. Similarly, if the EEG is reactive, few neonates have an adverse neurological outcome [12]. It is additionally important to consider that immediately after an acute hypoxic-ischemic injury, neonates can have a very abnormal, even inactive, EEG that can later improve over hours to days. For this reason, EEG is most accurate for prognosis when it is assessed following an interval of at least 24 hours after an insult [10, 13, 14]. Likewise, as compared to single EEGs, the prognostic value of EEG background improves significantly when assessed over time with continuous or serial EEGs [15–19].

While amplitude abnormalities can indicate a poor prognosis, one must be certain that the low amplitude is due to abnormal brain activity and not due to other factors, such as soft tissue edema and/or neuroactive medications [20, 21]. To avoid misinterpreting increased distance between the electrode and brain as a low-amplitude recording, sensitivity

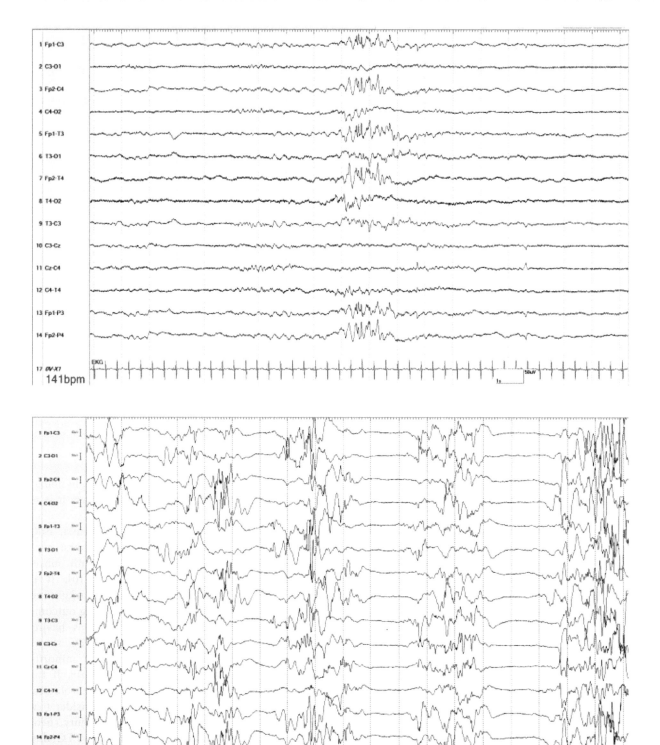

Figure 6.2 A discontinuous neonatal EEG contrasted with a burst suppression pattern. Top: This EEG from a 1-day-old full-term infant with hypoxic-ischemic injury is excessively discontinuous. IBIs are greater than 6 seconds in duration, and activity in the IBI has amplitudes >5 μV. Bottom: This EEG from a full-term infant with early infantile epileptic encephalopathy due to an *ARX* mutation shows burst suppression. The IBIs have amplitudes <5 μV, activity has no normal features, and the pattern is invariant.

settings can be decreased – if normal waveforms and frequencies appear, the low amplitude is not due to decreased brain activity but is instead due to scalp edema or intracranial fluid.

While there is some literature indicating that select background patterns have equivalent prognostic significance in preterm and full-term neonates, the majority of research on preterm EEG considers different prognostic

Table 6.2 Characterization of neonatal background continuity

	Normal discontinuity	Abnormal discontinuity	
		Excessive discontinuity	Burst suppression
Normal activity	+	+/−	−
Normal IBI duration for age	+	−	−
IBI voltage	<25–50 µV pp	<25 µV pp	<5 µV pp
Variability	+	+	−
Reactivity	+	+	−

pp, peak-to-peak.

markers and/or finds different prognostic value in features than when they are seen in term neonatal EEG. For example, in preterm neonates, an EEG with inactive or burst suppression pattern is associated with death or long-term disability [17, 22]. Most studies use IBI duration, dysmaturity, disorganization, positive Rolandic sharp waves, seizures, and sleep–wake cycling to predict outcomes [23–27]. Dysmaturity is typically defined as a 2 week or greater difference between EEG patterns and postmenstrual age (PMA) (Figure 6.3). Disorganization indicates a background with distorted delta waves, abnormal sharp waves, and abnormal delta brushes (cogwheel shaped or beta is high amplitude and/or more spiky).

Similar to the full-term infant, timing and serial EEGs improve prognostic accuracy. A normal EEG shortly after an acute event is more often associated with normal outcomes than an EEG obtained weeks later [28]. If the background pattern changes within a day from burst suppression or inactive to a nearly normal pattern, the prognosis improves [28]. One study combined severity of background abnormalities with persistence of the pattern and found a graded association between EEG severity on serial EEGs and neurodevelopmental outcomes at 2 years of age [27].

Neonatal background patterns can also be help identify neonates at risk for seizures. Seizures are less likely with a normal background and are more likely with runs of epileptiform discharges [29–32]. In addition, background patterns that are excessively discontinuous without state changes, burst suppression or inactive more likely to be associated with seizures [33].

Infants and Children

The significance of EEG background patterns in infants outside the neonatal period and in older children is less well studied. Findings from adult and neonatal studies are often applied to older children, as it is likely there is overlap in the significance of specific background patterns.

There are several pediatric studies on the role of EEG in predicting outcome after anoxia or cardiac arrest. A normal background confidently predicts a favorable neurological outcome [34]. Conversely, three background patterns are consistently associated with poor neurological outcome or death: burst suppression, low amplitude or suppressed EEG background, and lack of reactivity [34–41]. These patterns also have prognostic value in encephalopathy from other acute insults, such as encephalitis, or in infants with surgery for congenital heart defects, though literature for these populations is limited.

Abnormal background patterns can be difficult to interpret in a variety of circumstances. A burst suppression pattern is not universally predictive of poor outcome, particularly if due to a reversible etiology (i.e., pharmacological, intoxication, metabolic) [42–44]. A low-voltage, slow, nonreactive background may not predict poor outcome if seen in the setting of high doses of sedating or anesthetic medication. Finally, rhythmic coma patterns are likely to have a different prognostic value in children than they do in adults. In one study, there was no difference in etiology or outcome between theta, alpha, and beta coma patterns in children. Like other background patterns, outcome is more favorable when reactivity is present [45].

There are a few studies that suggest the time at which the EEG is obtained affects prognostic accuracy. For example, a normal or slow background within 12 hours of return of spontaneous circulation is more often associated with good outcomes than an EEG with the same patterns obtained later [34].

There has been some variability in definitions of these background patterns but the studies above and the ACNS terminology utilize the following criteria: **Discontinuity** is defined as a background with intervals of attenuation (>10 µV but <50% of background voltage) or suppression (<10 µV), present in 10%–49% of the background (Figure 6.4). When the intervals of suppression make up <50% of the background, the pattern is described as **burst suppression** (Figure 6.5). The **suppression** background is a pattern with activity persistently <10 µV (Figure 6.6). **Reactivity** has been defined as a change in background amplitude or frequency with stimulation [41].

Another potentially useful standardized characterization of the EEG background was adopted by the Pediatric Critical

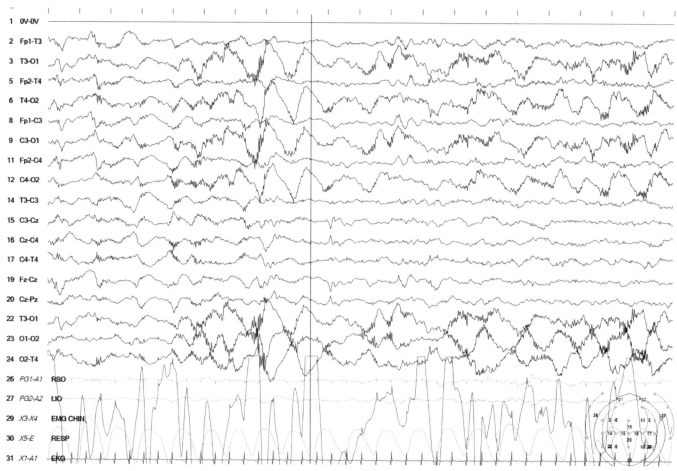

Figure 6.3 EEG from a 1-day-old neonate born at 37 weeks 1 day via emergency caesarean section following gestation notable for preeclampsia. Initial concern for hypoxic-ischemic encephalopathy prompted therapeutic hypothermia. EEG appears dysmature, with excessive delta brushes for postmenstrual age, and absence of features typically seen in term neonatal EEG, such as encoche frontales. (Modified 10–20 neonatal montage, 7 μV, 20 sec/page.)

Care EEG Group (PCCEG) in 2013 [46]. In a large multicenter study, background patterns from EEGs obtained in the pediatric intensive care unit (PICU) and cardiac intensive care unit (CICU) were grouped into normal-sleep, slow-disorganized, discontinuous, burst suppression, and attenuated-featureless (Figure 6.7). The slow-disorganized pattern is seen in abundance in the PICU and CVICU settings and includes a broad range of backgrounds (Figure 6.8). With this categorization, increased risk for electrographic seizures was seen with any background abnormality on the initial EEG [46].

Multiple studies suggest the EEG background is best used to provide prognostic information when combined with other assessments such as clinical exam, neuroimaging and evoked potentials [47, 48].

Seizures and Interictal Abnormalities

Seizures

The recent increased use of EEG monitoring has led to increased awareness of nonconvulsive seizures in critically ill patients. Seizures may be electroclinical, where a clinical seizure is coupled with a simultaneous EEG correlate. Seizures may alternately be electrographic-only, where an EEG seizure occurs without a clear clinical correlate. In the ICU, seizures are more commonly electrographic-only, especially after administration of anti-seizure medications [49, 50]. By definition, an electrographic seizure is an abnormal, paroxysmal, encephalographic event that differs from background activity and *evolves* in frequency, morphology, amplitude, or spatial distribution on EEG with a duration of at least 10 seconds [3, 51]. It should be noted that while the neonatal literature has historically considered clinical seizures without EEG confirmation, more recent studies focus primarily on neonates with electrographic and electroclinical seizures [52–54]. Individual seizures are distinguished when there is at least 10 seconds between events. Electrographic seizures can be identified by evolving sharply contoured activity (Figure 6.9) or a more subtle buildup of rhythmic activity, often delta or theta frequency (Figure 6.10). Identifying a physiological field is an important step in distinguishing a seizure from rhythmic artifact. A physiological field manifests as activity in anatomically adjacent regions, while artifact often has synchronous activity in distant regions. In the ICU, studies are often reviewed at faster paper speed (e.g., 20 seconds per page vs. the standard 10

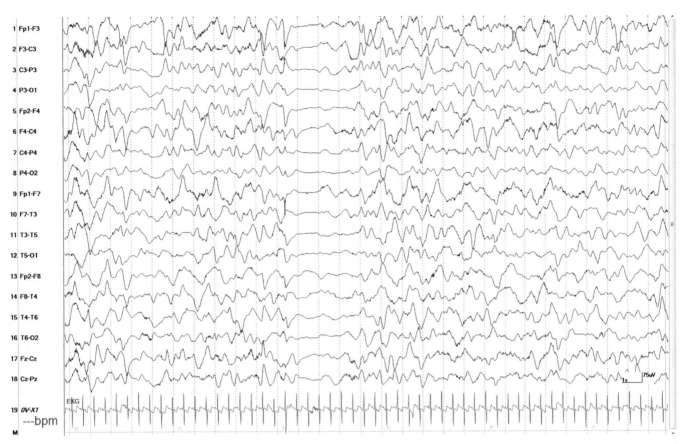

Figure 6.4 Discontinuous EEG with intervals of attenuation or suppression present in 10%–49% of the background. (Standard 10–20 montage, 15 µV, 30 sec/page.)

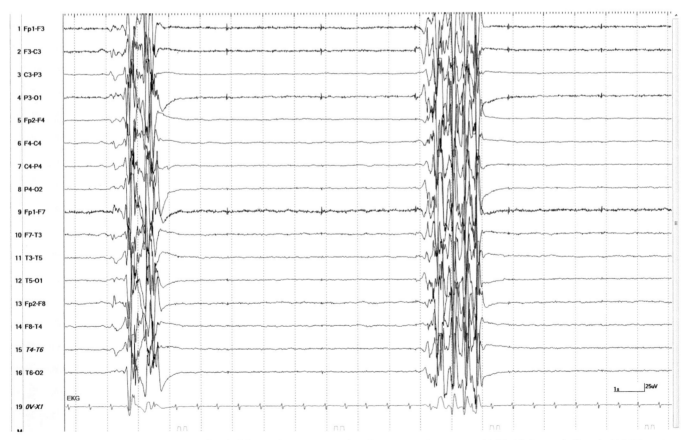

Figure 6.5 EEG recording from a 13-year-old female following bupropion overdose. Burst suppression pattern with IBI of 8–9 seconds. (Standard 10–20 montage, 5 µV, 20 sec/page.)

Jessica Carpenter and Tammy Tsuchida

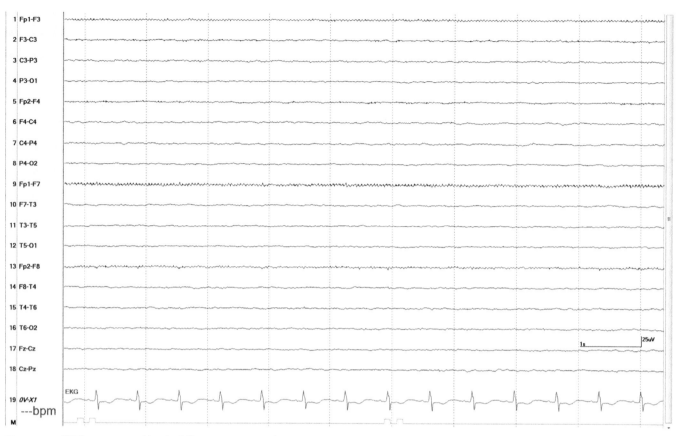

Figure 6.6   EEG from a 4-year-old male. Diffuse suppression with activity persistently <10 μV. (Standard 10–20 montage, 5 μV, 10 sec/page.)

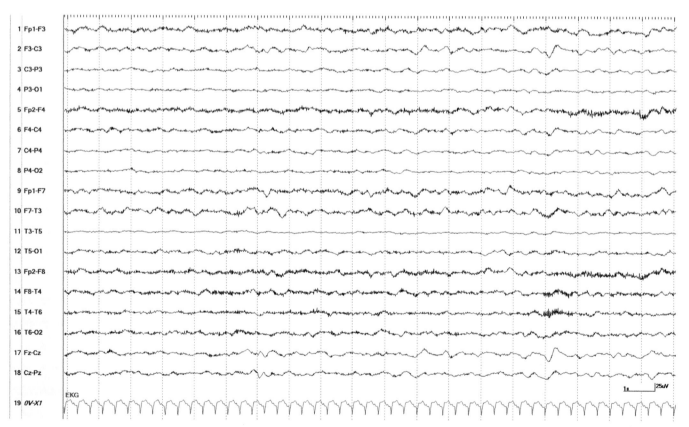

Figure 6.7   EEG from a 20-month-old male. Attenuated featureless background. (Standard 10–20 montage, 5 μV, 20 sec/page.)

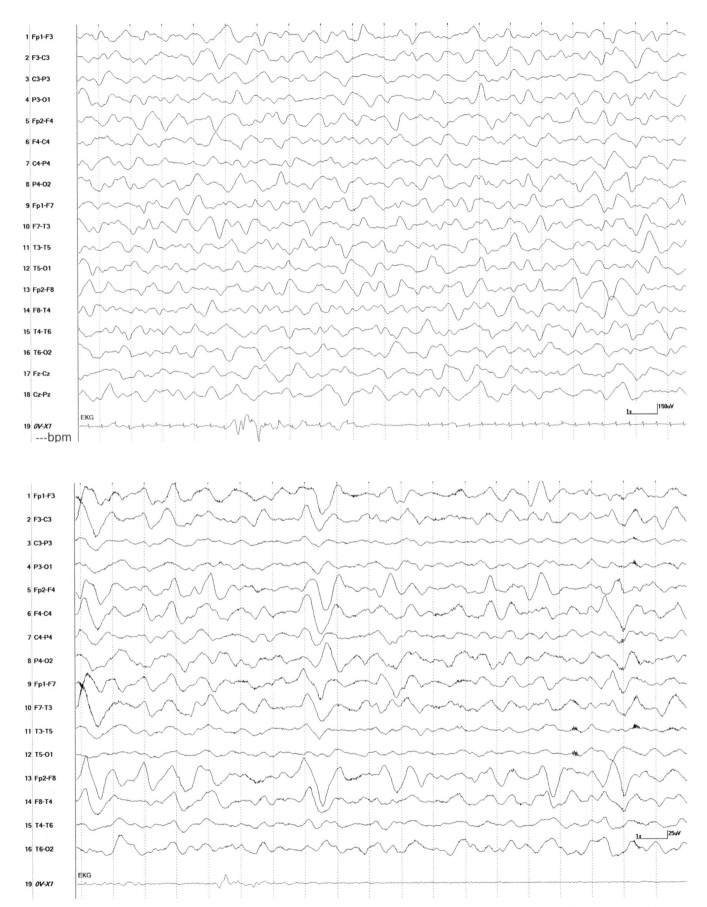

Figure 6.8 Two examples of slow-disorganized background. Top: EEG from a 13-month-old female. 30 μV, 20 sec/page. Bottom: EEG from a 13-year-old female. (Standard 10–20 montage, 5 μV, 20 sec/page.)

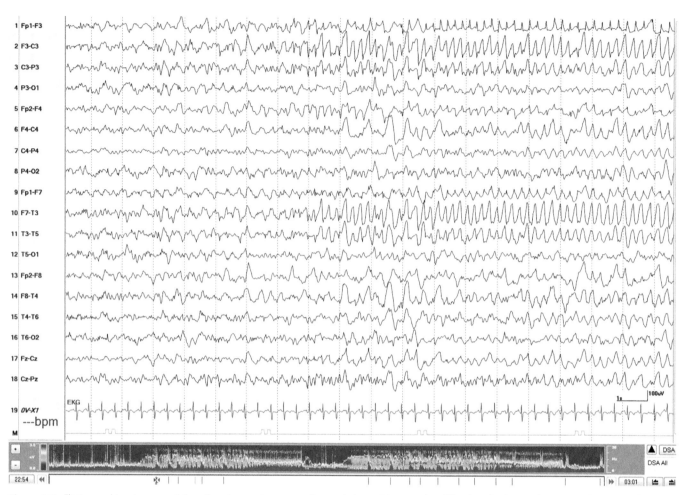

Figure 6.9 Electrographic seizure consisting of an abnormal, paroxysmal, encephalographic event that differs from background activity and evolves in frequency, morphology, voltage, and spatial distribution. The seizure arises in the left central and temporal channels with subsequent spread to surrounding regions. It is also visible on DSA at the bottom of the screen, with the pink marker indicating the corresponding segment on DSA. (Standard 10–20 montage, 20 μV, 20 sec/page.)

seconds per page) to facilitate identification of seizures with slow evolution, and to facilitate the distinction between periodic discharges and the evolving discharges required for a seizure (Figure 6.10). Seizure identification is typically easier after the first few seizures are identified within a recording, as seizure morphology remains similar throughout a recording. Among patients who receive sedatives, paralytics and anti-seizure medications, seizures are more commonly electrographic-only. It is also worth noting the appearance of seizures can change after the administration of seizure medications, making them more subtle and difficult to recognize [20] (Figure 6.11).

Continuous EEG monitoring (cEEG) provides the highest yield when there is video and audio accompaniment. Video review can help not only with documentation of clinical signs of seizures but also to distinguish rhythmic or periodic cerebral activity from EEG artifact. It should be noted that the video can miss subtle motor movements and/or vital sign changes that may be visible to a bedside observer. Family members and bedside caregivers should be encouraged to document clinical events of concern, and feedback should be provided as to whether these events are or are not confirmed to be electrographic seizures.

Status epilepticus is typically defined as a seizure of 30 minutes' duration, or multiple seizures occurring over 30 minutes without an intervening return to baseline. In 2012, the Neurocritical Care Society (NCS) proposed modifying the operational definition of clinical status epilepticus to convulsions lasting longer than 5 minutes [55]. Adoption and widespread use of this definition are slowly increasing but it is not yet universally accepted. With the increase of digital EEG and continuous monitoring, a definition of electrographic status was needed. Currently, the definition of status epilepticus by EEG is single or recurrent electrographic seizures with total summed duration composing more than 50% (30 minutes) of an arbitrary 1 hour epoch. With newer studies suggesting worse outcomes in patients with a maximum hourly seizure burden of as little as 12 minutes, the electrographic definition of status epilepticus likely underestimates the cut off for clinically a significant seizure burden [56, 57].

Electrographic status epilepticus can sometimes be difficult to identify. Early in status epilepticus with generalized tonic-clonic seizures, seizures are distinct on EEG but as the status epilepticus continues, the seizures merge and may appear more like waxing and waning frequencies of epileptiform discharges

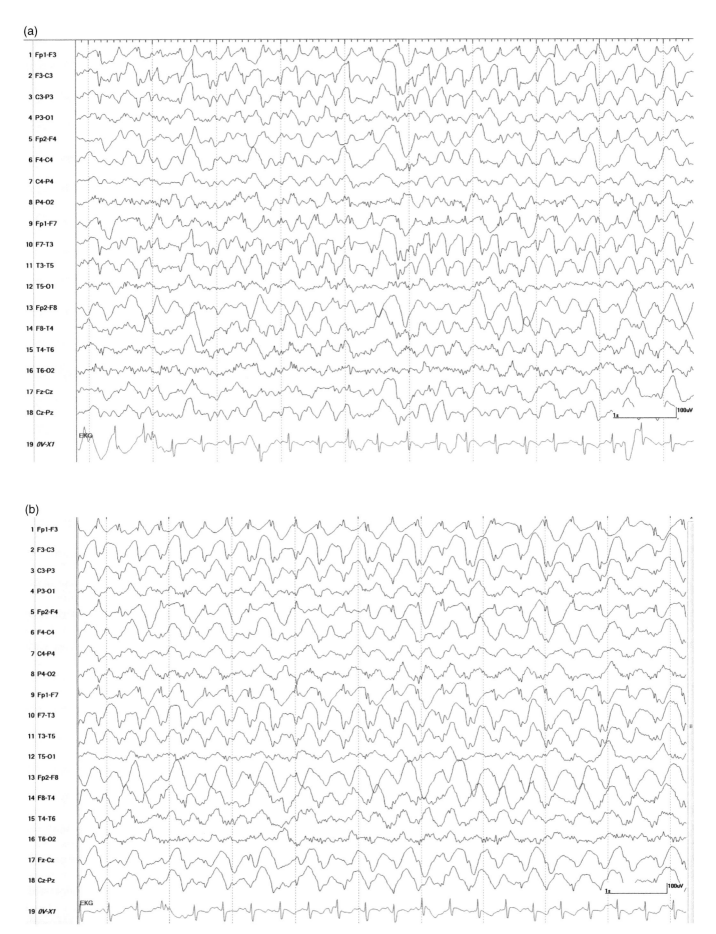

Figure 6.10 EEG from a 13-month-old female. Electrographic seizure composed of evolving rhythmic delta. Comparison of (a) and (b) with (c) demonstrates how adjustment of display parameters may facilitate recognition of slower evolving rhythms. (a) and (b) are a continuation of the same seizure, displayed with a standard 10–20 montage, sensitivity of 20 μV, and at 10 seconds per page/screen. (c) The same seizure at a faster paper speed, with subtle evolution more easily appreciated (20 seconds per page/screen).

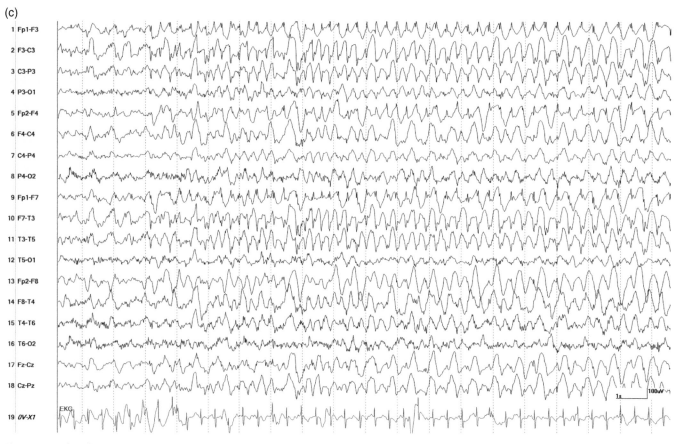

(c)

Figure 6.10 (cont.)

rather than a seizure. As status epilepticus continues, the activity may evolve to have the appearance of rhythmic discharges and there may be no associated clinical change. Even later in status epilepticus, there may be periods of flattening of the EEG and finally the EEG pattern may evolve to periodic discharges [58]. When a patient with encephalopathy is found to have any of these patterns, one should consider whether these patterns are reflective of electrographic status epilepticus and thus potentially responsive to administration of seizure medications.

Interictal Epileptiform Discharges

Interictal epileptiform discharges are transient waveforms that stand out from the surrounding background activity. Like a seizure, the presence of a physiological field makes it more likely that the discharges are due to abnormal brain activity rather than artifact. Neonatal interictal epileptiform discharges are defined slightly differently from those of children and adults. Spikes have a duration of <100 milliseconds for neonates, rather than <70 milliseconds as in children and adults. Sharp waves are 100–200 milliseconds in duration in neonates and 70–200 milliseconds in children.

A key distinction is that while typically any epileptiform discharge is considered abnormal in children, some sharp discharges occur often in normal neonates, particularly in quiet sleep. For this reason, quantification of sharp waves to determine whether they are normal or excessive should only be performed during wakefulness or active sleep in neonates, and never during quiet sleep. Neonatal sharp wave discharges are more likely to be abnormal if they are excessive in number, if unifocal, if occurring in runs (≥3 in a row), or they occur in the less typical frontal, vertex, or occipital locations (Figure 6.12). Epileptiform discharges are typically negative in polarity and thus adjacent channels have waveforms that point toward each other. In contrast, positive sharp waves point away from each other and are often due to artifact in children. In a neonate, epileptiform discharges at the vertex with spread to the Rolandic regions are characteristic of, but not exclusive to, abnormal brain activity resulting from white matter injury and are called positive Rolandic sharp waves (Figure 6.13) [29, 59].

Brief Rhythmic Discharges

Another pattern seen in neonates is brief rhythmic discharges (BRDs) (Figure 6.14). This transient pattern has the same features as a seizure, but lasts less than 10 seconds [3]. The presence of BRDs should raise very high suspicion for seizures, as they are most often (but not exclusively) seen in neonates who also have seizures. The significance of BRDs without seizures is uncertain, though at least one study reports neonates with isolated BRDs had similar adverse outcomes as neonates with seizures [60].

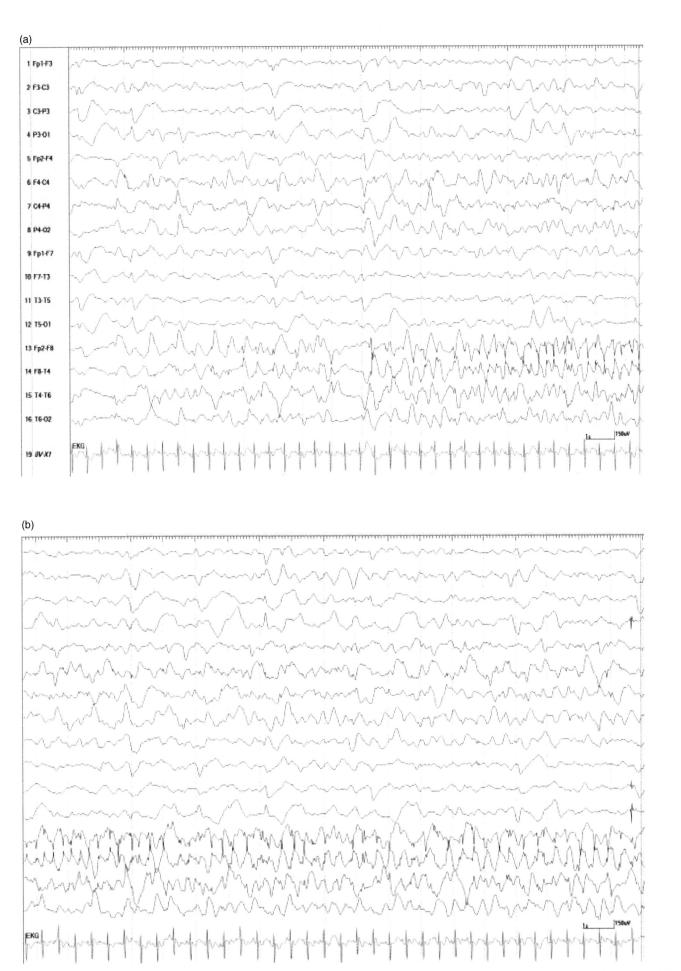

Figure 6.11 Evolution of a seizure before and after medication administration. (a) and (b) Electrographic seizure (standard 10–20 montage, 20 μV, 20 sec/page). (c) and (d) Electrographic seizure in the same patient after seizure medication administered. Note the change in amplitude and morphology, with evolution less apparent.

(c)

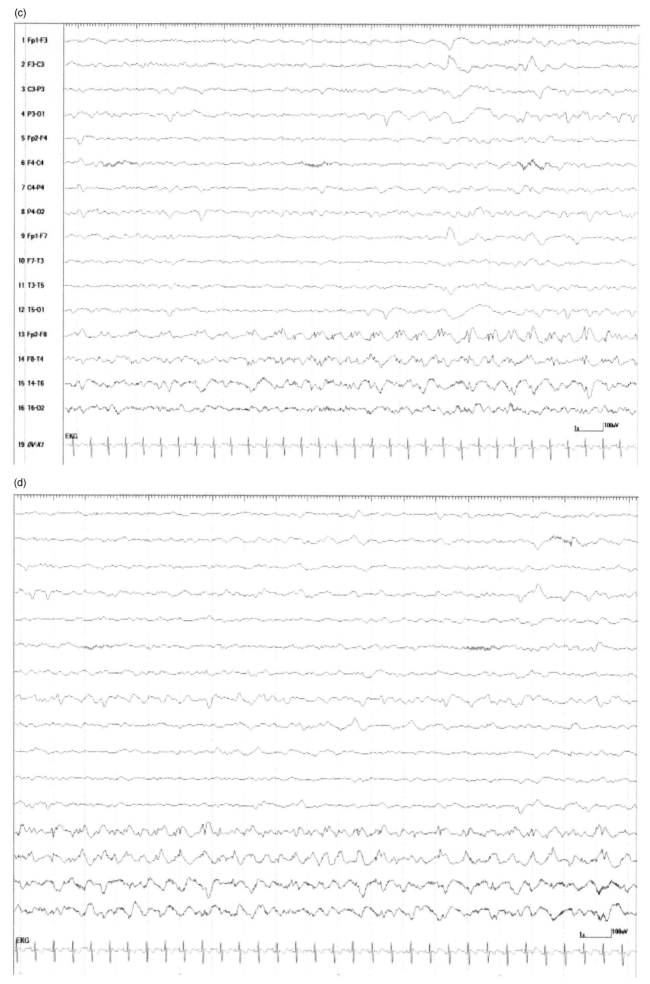

(d)

Figure 6.11   (cont.)

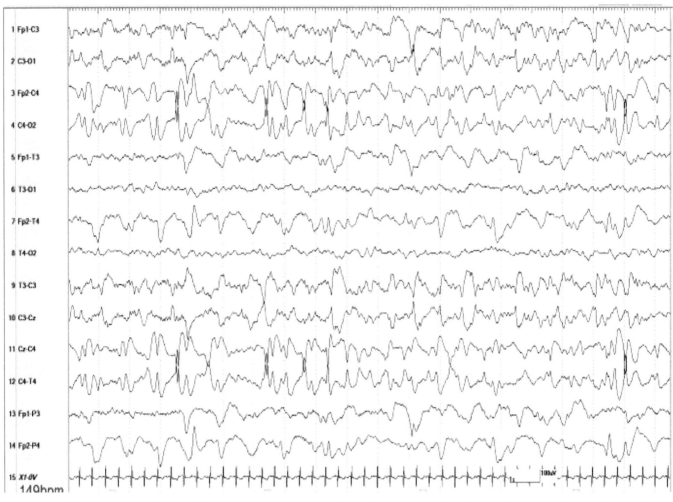

Figure 6.12 Full-term neonate with cerebral dysgenesis and runs of spike and wave discharges (negative polarity) at the right central region. The waveforms at channels 3 and 4 and 11 and 12 point toward each other, indicating a negative polarity. (Modified 10–20 neonatal montage, 20 μV, 20 sec/page.)

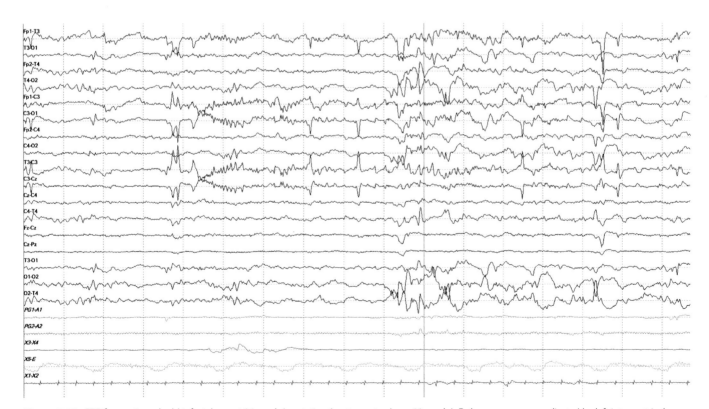

Figure 6.13 EEG from a 6-week-old infant, born at 26 weeks' gestation (postmenstrual age 32 weeks). Early course was complicated by left intraventricular hemorrhage. EEG shows positive sharp waves at C3 extending to T3. (Modified 10–20 neonatal montage, 7 μV, 20 sec/page.)

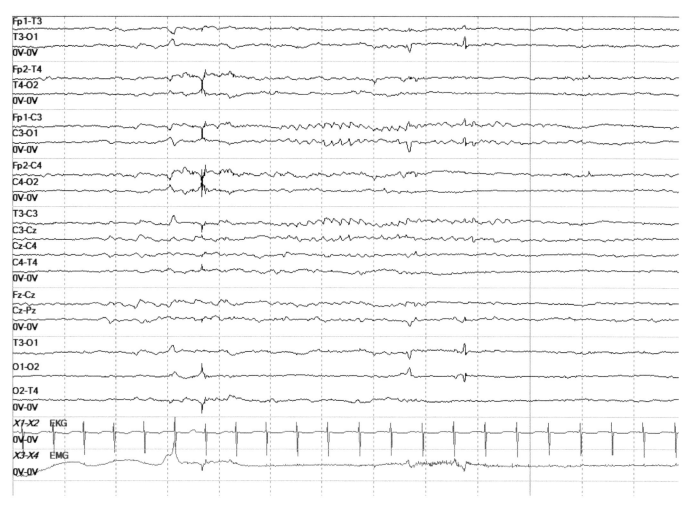

Figure 6.14 EEG from the first day of life in a neonate born at 35 weeks, presenting with hypoxic-ischemic encephalopathy due to placental abruption. EEG shows brief rhythmic discharges at C3: while these are paroxysmal and evolving, they are not sustained long enough to constitute seizure. This patient did have seizures at other points in the recording. (Modified 10–20 neonatal montage, 7 μV, 15 sec/page.)

In older infants and children, interictal epileptiform discharges, periodic discharges, and rhythmic delta activity are all associated with an increased risk for seizures [50].

Quantitative EEG

With the increased use of digital EEG monitoring has come a variety of quantitative EEG (QEEG) tools that can be used to increase the efficiency of EEG screening by neurophysiologists. QEEG can also be used as a bedside tool for clinicians for real time identification of background changes and potential seizures. The QEEG format or trend that is most extensively used in the ICU is the amplitude-integrated EEG (aEEG), which is widely used in neonates.

Amplitude-Integrated EEG (aEEG)

Amplitude-integrated EEG (aEEG) was originally developed to evaluate depth of anesthesia in adults, but was subsequently embraced by neonatologists as a bedside tool to monitor brain function and detect seizures (marketed as a CFM: cerebral function monitor). The aEEG

graphically displays EEG amplitude on a linear scale from 0 to 10 microvolts (to emphasize lower voltages), and a logarithmic scale from 10 to 100 microvolts. The aEEG can be displayed continuously at the bedside, and is intended for real time review and interpretation, to allow clinicians to detect significant background changes or seizures. While not as widely used in the PICU as in the NICU, the principles are the same for neonates and older children.

Two main systems guide the interpretation of aEEG to predict outcomes after hypoxic-ischemic injury in term neonates (Table 6.3). The voltage characterization system is simpler, using three categories solely based on the predominant voltage of the activity band. The pattern classification system incorporates voltage and pattern recognition and has five categories. While requiring more user expertise, the pattern classification system has a higher specificity and positive predictive value than the voltage classification system for predicting a poor outcome in term neonates. Both systems have similar ability to predict a good outcome in term neonates.

Comparing these two systems, both consider a persistently low-voltage aEEG to be the most severe abnormality, with the

Table 6.3 Comparison of two neonatal aEEG classification systems

	Voltage system		Pattern system		
Category	Lower margin	Upper margin	Lower margin	Upper margin	Category
Normal	>5 µV	>10 µV	5 to 10 µV	10 to 50 µV	Continuous normal voltage (CNV)
Moderately abnormal	≤5 µV	>10 µV	<5 µV	>10 µV	Discontinuous normal voltage (DNV)
			0–2 µV invariant	>25 µV	Burst suppression (BS)
Suppressed	<5 µV invariant	<10 µV invariant	≤5 µV	≤5 µV	Low voltage (LV)
			<5 µV	<5 µV	Inactive, flat trace (FT)

voltage system using a criteria of <10 µV for the upper margin and the pattern system using around 5 µV or less. The pattern system further divides the most severe abnormalities into low-voltage (LV) or inactive, flat trace (FT). The LV and FT patterns have similar upper and lower margin values, resulting in a low-voltage, narrow band of activity (bandwidth) (Figure 6.15). The systems are also similar in their characterization of normal aEEG, where a lower margin of >5 µV and upper margin of >10 µV is used for both "normal voltage" and "continuous normal voltage" (CNV) patterns. The systems diverge with the voltage system moderately abnormal voltage category. Moderately abnormal voltage aEEG background is associated overall with abnormal outcomes. However, this category has upper and lower margin voltages that are the same as the pattern system category of discontinuous normal voltage (DNV), which is associated with good outcomes. At the same time, some moderately abnormal voltage tracings with the same amplitude criteria correspond to the pattern of burst suppression (BS), which is associated with poor outcomes (see Table 6.3). In the pattern system, the BS lower margin value of 0–2 µV is much lower than DNV, and, unlike DNV, tends not to vary over hours. In addition, the BS upper margin of >25 µV is much higher than the DNV pattern. The larger difference between the upper and lower margin values can result in a wider BS bandwidth than DNV. When both have a very wide bandwidth, the variation over hours in amplitude of the DNV lower margin helps distinguish DNV from BS. The two patterns are also distinguishable since the BS longer inter-burst intervals result in spaces in between the bursts that give the appearance of the teeth on a comb (Figure 6.15). Regardless of the classification system used, at least two channels (C3, P3, C4, P4) are needed to detect unilateral abnormalities [61].

Superimposed upon aEEG background patterns are sleep–wake cycles. Normal sleep–wake cycling results in regularly alternating changes of amplitude and bandwidth. Sleep–wake cycles are not used for classifying aEEG in the voltage system. In comparison, the pattern classification system characterizes varying degrees of sleep–wake cycling. Normal sleep–wake cycling alternates between CNV and DNV, corresponding to awake or active sleep and quiet sleep, respectively. Immature

sleep–wake cycling has some fluctuation, but poor cyclic variation of the lower margin amplitude (Figure 6.16). It is helpful to recognize that there are some terms used with different meanings when describing aEEG as compared to when describing full EEG. For example, an aEEG tracing might meet criteria for the descriptor "burst suppression" if baseline amplitudes are low and individual bursts rise sharply above on the activity band, even as the corresponding full EEG might not meet all the criteria for true burst suppression if there is reactivity or variability. Normal and severely abnormal patterns are more likely to have the same appearance on aEEG and EEG [62–65]. Moderately abnormal amplitude and burst suppression patterns on aEEG do not correlate as well with raw EEG. Similar to full array EEG, the prognostic value of aEEG improves when assessed over multiple time points [66, 67].

The above systems only apply to term neonates; other aEEG classification systems are used for characterizing patterns in premature neonates. All take into account the expected increase in continuous activity with increasing postmenstrual age (PMA) [68–70]. In addition, all characterize the increase in minimum amplitude (lower margin on aEEG) with increasing postmenstrual age. Because the premature infant has very low amplitude-inter-burst interval activity and long inter-burst intervals, the aEEG in a normal preterm neonate can look somewhat similar to the BS pattern in a full-term neonate (Figure 6.17). Currently there is no single system utilized for predicting outcomes based on aEEG in preterm neonates.

Amplitude-integrated EEG is used widely for seizure detection. The two channel aEEG (typically including channels C3-P3 and C4-P4), when combined with review of the source EEG tracing, detects up to three-quarters of neonates having seizures [71]. Single channel aEEG using central or parietal electrodes can detect 12–54% of individual seizures [31, 72]. Frontally placed aEEG electrodes, while easily placed and visible, have lower rates of seizure detection and should be avoided [73]. While aEEG cannot identify all seizures, the evidence suggests that 57%–100% of neonates with seizures will have at least one seizure detectable on aEEG [31, 62, 64, 71]. The exact sensitivity for seizure detection in a given patient

(a)

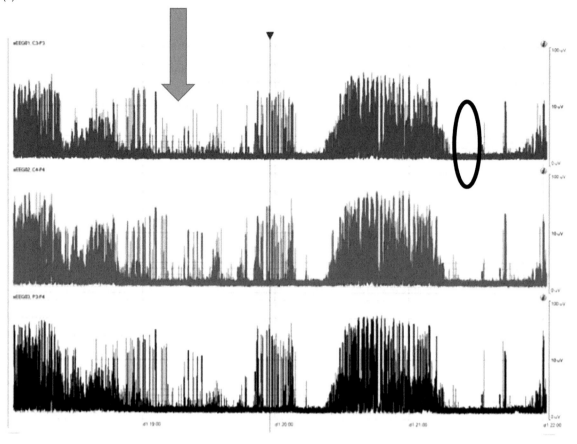

(b)

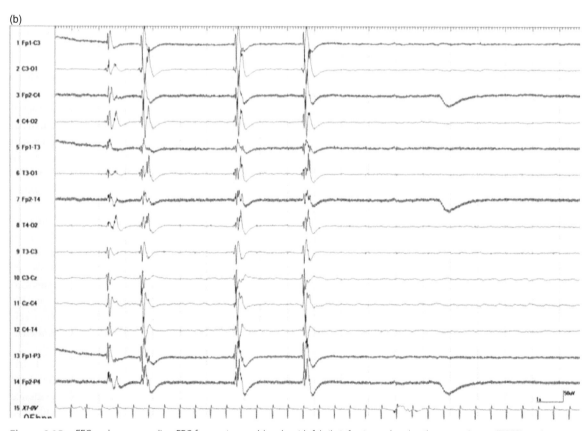

Figure 6.15   aEEG and corresponding EEG from a 4-year-old male with febrile infection–related epilepsy syndrome (FIRES), undergoing pentobarbital-induced pharmacological coma. (a) aEEG shows alternating burst suppression pattern [arrow], with voltages at baseline 0–2 μV interspersed with upward deflections of 15–25 μV, having the appearance of teeth of a comb. Brief segments of aEEG show flat trace pattern [circle], with amplitudes entirely under 5 μV for both the upper and lower margins. The vertical line indicates where the corresponding EEG is sampled. (b) The corresponding EEG, showing burst suppression. (Double distance electrodes, 7 μV, 20 sec/page.)

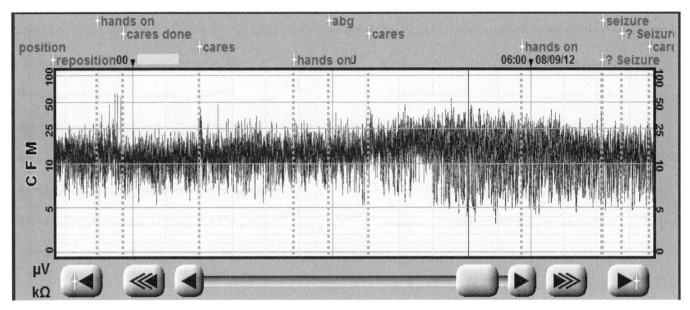

Figure 6.16 Immature sleep–wake cycling. aEEG shows bandwidth with initially narrower bandwidth in the first half of the display, then a wider bandwidth. However, the typical features of normal sleep–wake cycling, such as a sinusoidal pattern, are not established.

depends in part on user experience, and in part on seizure characteristics. Shorter seizures are less likely to appear on aEEG, and seizures outside the central or parietal regions may not be detectable on aEEG.

In any age group, seizures can be identified on aEEG by elevation in the lower margin of the activity band, often accompanied by elevation in the upper margin giving an arch-like appearance. This occurs because seizures result in an abrupt increase in overall amplitude (Figure 6.18). Stretching out the aEEG display to show fewer hours per screen (e.g., 1 or 2 hours rather than 4–8 hours per screen) may increase the sensitivity of seizure detection [72]. Seizures most likely to be missed on aEEG include those that are less than 30 seconds in duration, those that are focal, and those with the amplitude is less than twice that of the background activity (Figure 6.19) [31, 64, 71, 72]. Review of the corresponding EEG tracing is essential when assessing for possible seizures on aEEG, because artifact can mimic seizures on aEEG [62, 71, 72, 74, 75]. For example, muscle artifact in full-term infants can mimic seizures [74]. While the source is unclear, preterm infants also can have artifact that mimics seizures [76].

Other QEEG Techniques

Quantitative EEG does not yet have as widespread use by intensivists in the PICU and CVICU as does aEEG in the NICU, though this is changing. Color Density Spectral Array

(CDSA) and aEEG are regularly used by neurophysiologists in older infants and children for seizure detection. Likewise, QEEG adoption by intensivists is increasing as continuous EEG monitoring becomes more prevalent [77–79]. There is evidence that non-neurophysiologists in the PICU can successfully use CDSA to detect seizures [80]. Adult ICU studies also suggest that aEEG may also be useful for seizure detection by both neurophysiologists and non-neurophysiologists [81–83]. Similar to neonates, these modalities can be useful for assessing dynamic background changes and allow for quick assessment of a physiological state (Figure 6.20).

Conclusion

EEG has many uses in the ICU setting; identification of abnormal patterns is useful across ages and diagnoses. Background patterns are useful for prognostication and can also direct clinical decisions. Certain EEG abnormalities can alert the clinician to a new cerebral injury or to risk for seizures. EEG is essential for seizure detection in ICU patients. Quantitative EEG trends are used most often to assist with seizure detection, but also facilitate a quick summary of changes in background patterns that could be clinically significant. The combined use of EEG and quantitative EEG can be an important tool in managing ICU patients with cerebral dysfunction.

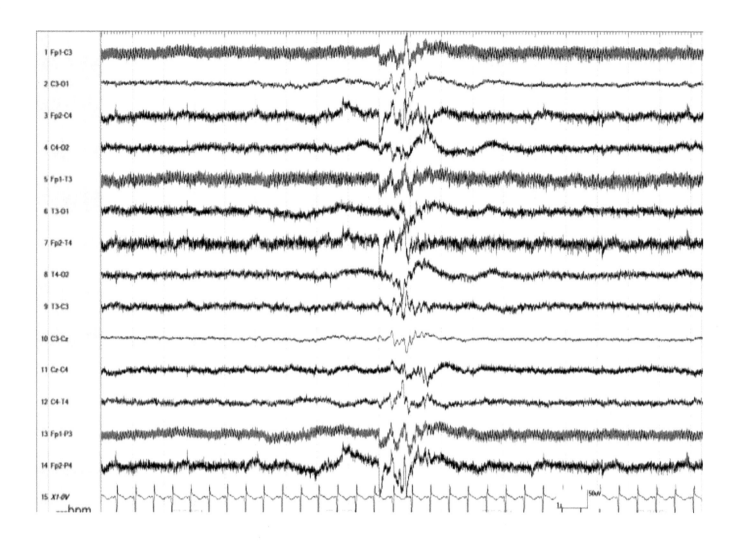

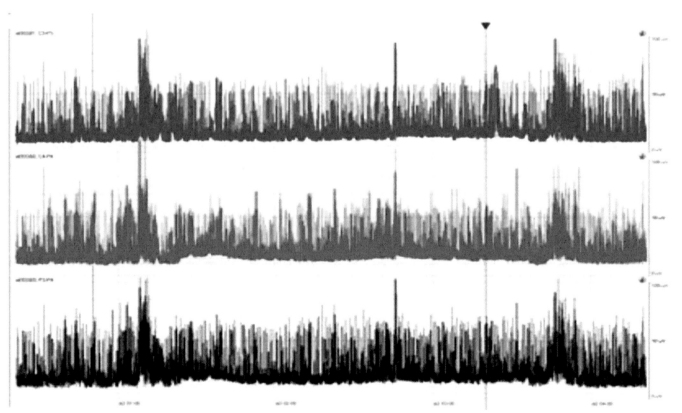

Figure 6.17 EEG and corresponding aEEG from a 35-week postmenstrual age (PMA) twin with aortic coarctation, during hypothermia therapy for hypoxic-ischemic encephalopathy. Top: The EEG is excessively discontinuous. Bottom: The aEEG has a somewhat comb-like appearance because the IBI duration on EEG is longer, up to 15 seconds. However, the aEEG pattern is DNV and not BS because the lower margin varies between 2 and 5 µV, unlike the invariant 0–2 µV lower margin of the BS.

(a)

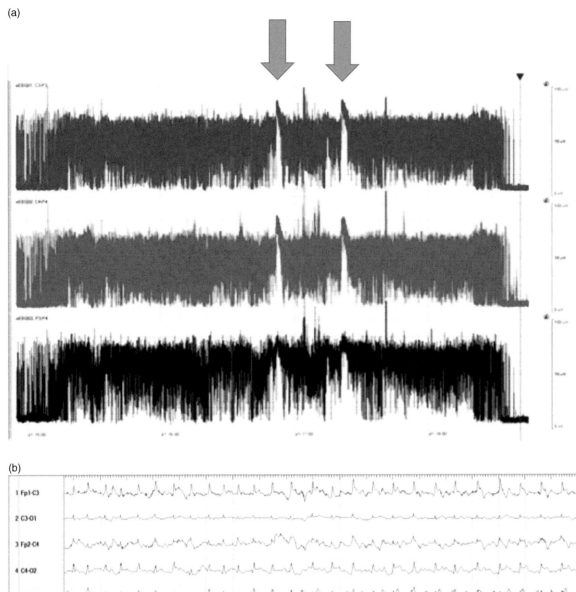

(b)

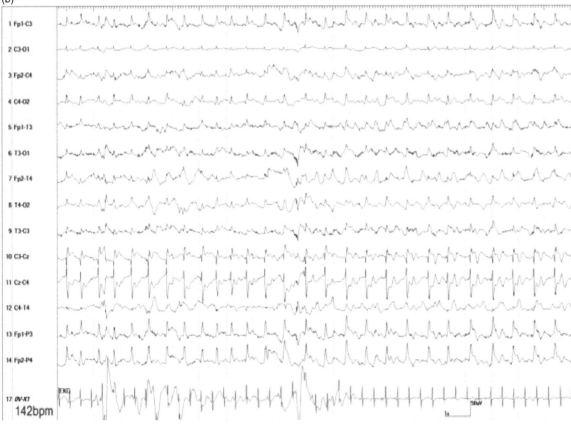

FIGURE 6.18   aEEG and EEG from a term-born neonate with hypoxic-ischemic encephalopathy. (a) aEEG demonstrates two seizures [arrows] over a 4-hour interval. Note the elevation of the lower margin of the activity band. (b) Corresponding EEG shows generalized seizure. (c) Later in aEEG recording, seizures are frequent, with multiple arc-shaped elevations of the lower margin, each representing individual seizures for this patient.

Jessica Carpenter and Tammy Tsuchida

(c)

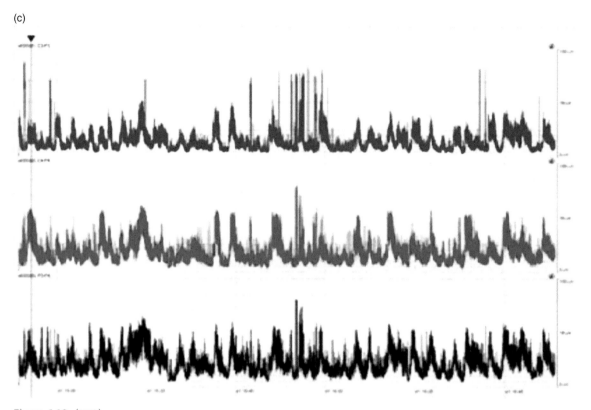

Figure 6.18 (cont.)

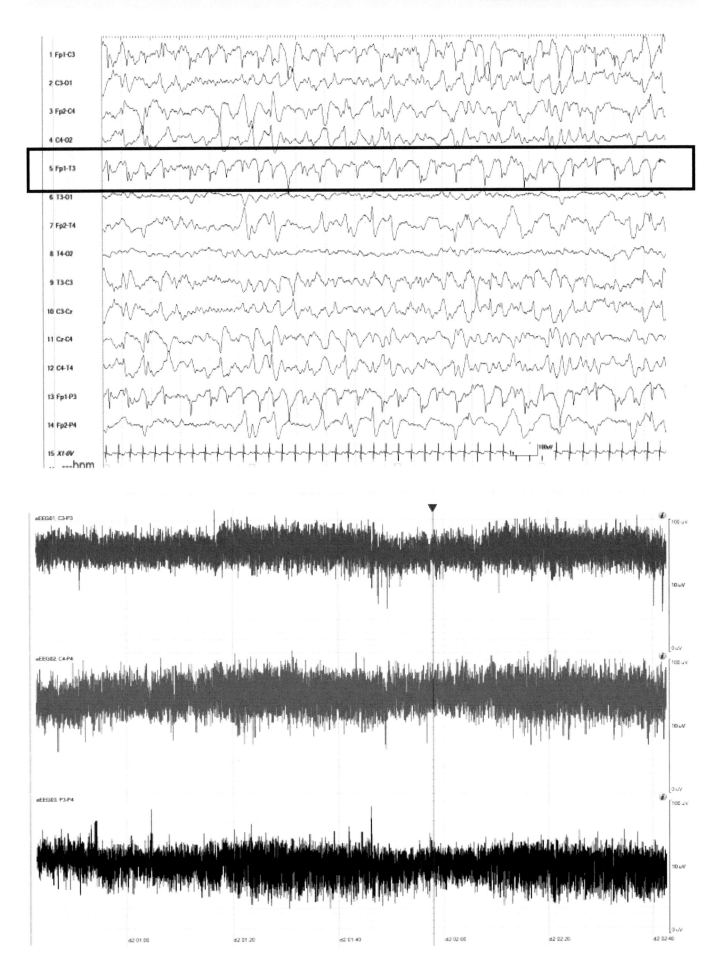

Figure 6.19 Term-born neonate with hypoxic-ischemic encephalopathy. Top: Left frontal seizures visible on full EEG [rectangle] Bottom: are not visible on corresponding aEEG.

(a)

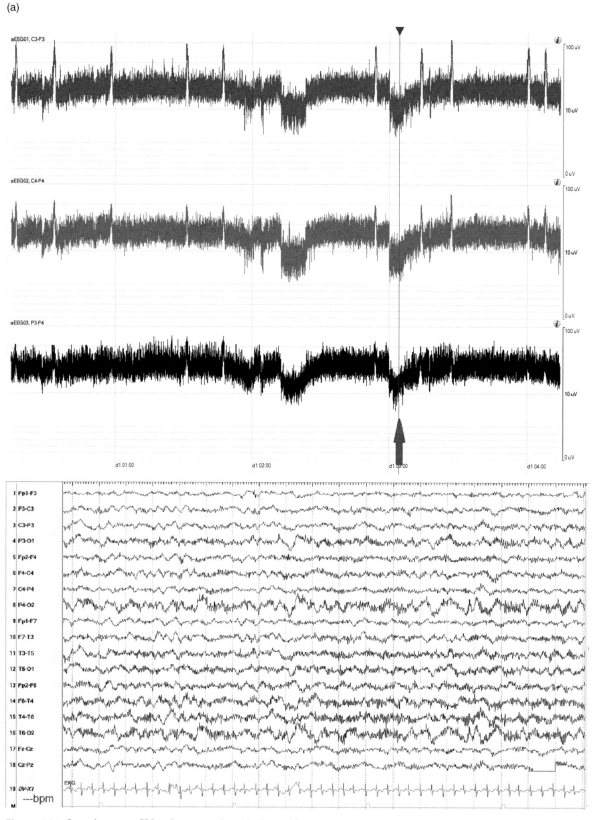

Figure 6.20 State changes on EEG and corresponding aEEG [arrows] from a 2-year-old female with tuberous sclerosis. (a) Wakefulness has overall lower amplitude activity and a narrower bandwidth on corresponding aEEG [arrow]. (b) Sleep is characterized by higher amplitude activity on EEG and corresponding aEEG [arrow]. (All EEG standard 10–20 montage, 7 μV, 20 sec/page.)

(b)

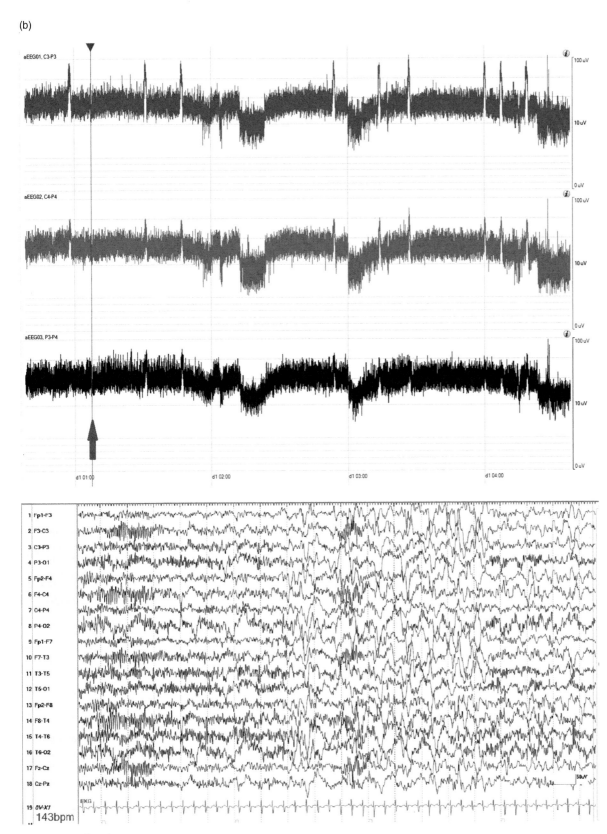

Figure 6.20 (cont.)

References

1. Hussain E, Nordli D. EEG patterns in acute pediatric encephalopathies. *J Clin Neurophysiol*. 2013 Oct;30(5):539–44.

2. Clancy RR, Chung HJ. EEG changes during recovery from acute severe neonatal citrullinemia. *Electroencephalogr Clin Neurophysiol*. 1991 Mar;78(3):222–7.

3. Tsuchida TN, Wusthoff CJ, Shellhaas RA, et al.; American Clinical Neurophysiology Society Critical Care Monitoring Committee. American Clinical Neurophysiology Society standardized EEG terminology and categorization for the description of continuous EEG monitoring in neonates: report of the American Clinical Neurophysiology Society critical care monitoring committee. *J Clin Neurophysiol*. 2013 Apr;30(2):161–73.

4. Stecker MM, Sabau D, Sullivan L, et al. American Clinical Neurophysiology Society Guideline 6: minimum technical standards for EEG recording in suspected cerebral death. *J Clin Neurophysiol*. 2016 Aug;33(4):324–7.

5. Nakagawa TA, Ashwal S, Mathur M, et al. clinical report-guidelines for the determination of brain death in infants and children: an update of the 1987 task force recommendations. *Pediatrics* 2011;128:e730–e40.

6. Rose AL, Lombroso CT. A study of clinical, pathological, and electroencephalographic features in 137 full-term babies with a long-term follow-up. *Pediatrics*. 1970 Mar;45(3):404–25.

7. Monod N, Pajot N, Guidasci S. The neonatal EEG: statistical studies and prognostic value in full-term and preterm babies. *Electroencephalogr Clin Neurophysiol*. May 1972;32(5):529–44.

8. Watanabe K, Miyazaki S, Hara K, Hakamada S. Behavioral state cycles, background EEGs and prognosis of newborns with perinatal hypoxia. *Electroencephalogr Clin Neurophysiol*. 1980;49(5–6):618–25.

9. Holmes G, Rowe J, Hafford J, et al. Prognostic value of the electroencephalogram in neonatal asphyxia. *Electroencephalogr Clin Neurophysiol*. 1982 Jan;53(1):60–72.

10. Pezzani C, Radvanyi-Bouvet MF, Relier JP, Monod N. Neonatal electroencephalography during the first twenty-four hours of life in full-term newborn infants. *Neuropediatrics*. Feb 1986;17(1):11–18.

11. Sinclair DB, Campbell M, Byrne P, Prasertsom W, Robertson CM. EEG and long-term outcome of term infants with neonatal hypoxic-ischemic encephalopathy. *Clin Neurophysiol*. 1999 Apr;110(4):655–9.

12. Holmes GL, Rowe J, Hafford J. Significance of reactive burst suppression following asphyxia in full term infants. *Clin Electroencephalogr*. 1983 Jul;14(3):138–41.

13. Hamelin S, Delnard N, Cneude F, Debillon T, Vercueil L. Influence of hypothermia on the prognostic value of early EEG in full-term neonates with hypoxic ischemic encephalopathy. *Neurophysiol Clin*. 2011 Feb;41(1):19–27.

14. Nash KB, Bonifacio SL, Glass HC, et al. Video-EEG monitoring in newborns with hypoxic-ischemic encephalopathy treated with hypothermia. *Neurology*. 2011 Feb 8;76(6):556–62.

15. Sarnat HB, Sarnat MS. Neonatal encephalopathy following fetal distress. A clinical and electroencephalographic study. *Arch Neurol*. 1976 Oct;33(10):696–705.

16. Takeuchi T, Watanabe K. The EEG evolution and neurological prognosis of neonates with perinatal hypoxia [corrected]. *Brain Dev*. 1989;11(2):115–20.

17. Holmes GL, Lombroso CT. Prognostic value of background patterns in the neonatal EEG. *J Clin Neurophysiol*. Jul 1993;10(3):323–52.

18. Pressler RM, Boylan GB, Morton M, Binnie CD, Rennie JM. Early serial EEG in hypoxic ischaemic encephalopathy. *Clin Neurophysiol*. Jan 2001;112(1):31–7.

19. Murray DM, Boylan GB, Ryan CA, Connolly S. Early EEG findings in hypoxic-ischemic encephalopathy predict outcomes at 2 years. *Pediatrics*. Sep 2009;124(3):e459–467.

20. Mathieson SR, Livingstone V, Low E, et al. Phenobarbital reduces EEG amplitude and propagation of neonatal seizures but does not alter performance of automated seizure detection. *Clin Neurophysiol*. 2016 Oct;127(10):3343–50.

21. Obeid R, Tsuchida TN. Treatment Effects on Neonatal EEG. *J Clin Neurophysiol*. 2016 Oct;33(5):376–81.

22. Tharp BR, Cukier F, Monod N. The prognostic value of the electroencephalogram in premature infants. *Electroencephalogr Clin Neurophysiol*. Mar 1981;51(3):219–36.

23. Hayashi-Kurahashi N, Kidokoro H, Kubota T, et al. EEG for predicting early neurodevelopment in preterm infants: an observational cohort study. *Pediatrics*. 2012 Oct;130(4):e891–7.

24. Le Bihannic A, Beauvais K, Busnel A, de Barace C, Furby A. Prognostic value of EEG in very premature newborns. *Arch Dis Child Fetal Neonatal Ed*. 2012 Mar;97(2):F106–9.

25. Selton D, Andre M, Debruille C, Deforge H, Hascoët JM. Cognitive outcome at 5 years in very premature children without severe early cerebral abnormalities. Relationships with EEG at 6 weeks after birth. *Neurophysiol Clin*. 2013 Dec;43(5–6):289–97.

26. Nunes ML, Khan RL, Gomes Filho I, Booij L, da Costa JC. Maturational changes of neonatal electroencephalogram: a comparison between intra uterine and extra uterine development. *Clin Neurophysiol*. 2014 Jun;125(6):1121–8.

27. Périvier M, Rozé JC, Gascoin G, et al. Neonatal EEG and neurodevelopmental outcome in preterm infants born before 32 weeks. *Arch Dis Child Fetal Neonatal Ed*. 2016 May;101(3):F253–9.

28. Wusthoff CJ, Bonifacio SB, Van Meurs KP. The use of EEG and aEEG in assessing the term and preterm brain. In Stevenson DK, Benitz WE, Sunshine P, Hintz SR and Druzin M, editors. *Fetal and Neonatal Brain Injury*, 5th ed. New York: Cambridge University Press; 2018.

29. Clancy RR, Tharp BR. Positive Rolandic sharp waves in the electroencephalograms of premature neonates with intraventricular hemorrhage. *Electroencephalogr Clin Neurophysiol*. 1984 May;57(5):395–404.

30. Laroia N, Guillet R, Burchfiel J, McBride MC. EEG background as predictor of electrographic seizures in high-risk neonates. *Epilepsia*. 1998;39(5):545–51.

31. Shellhaas RA, Clancy RR. Characterization of neonatal seizures by conventional and single channel EEG. *Clin Neurophysiol*. 2007;118:2156–61.

32. Pisani F, Copioli C, Di Gioia C, Turco E, Sisti L. Neonatal seizures: relation of ictal video-electroencephalography (EEG) findings with

neurodevelopmental outcome. *J Child Neurol.* 2008 Apr;**23**(4):394–8.

33. Glass HC, Wusthoff CJ, Shellhaas RA, et al. Risk factors for EEG seizures in neonates treated with hypothermia: a multicenter cohort study. *Neurology.* 2014 Apr 8;**82**(14):1239–44.

34. Ostendorf AP, Hartman ME, Friess SH. Early electroencephalographic findings correlate with neurologic outcome in children following cardiac arrest. *Pediatr Crit Care Med.* 2016 Jul;**17**(7):667–76.

35. Pampiglione G, Harden A. Prognostic value of neurophysiological studies in the first hours following resuscitation: a review of 120 children after cardiac arrest. *Electroencephalogr Clin Neurophysiol.* 1968 Jul;**25**(1):91.

36. Tasker RC, Boyd S, Harden A, Matthew DJ. Monitoring in non-traumatic coma. Part II: Electroencephalography. *Arch Dis Child.* 1988 Aug;**63**(8):895–9.

37. Mandel R, Martinot A, Delepoulle F, et al. Prediction of outcome after hypoxic-ischemic encephalopathy: a prospective clinical and electrophysiologic study. *J Pediatr.* 2002 Jul;**141**(1):45–50.

38. Ramachandrannair R, Sharma R, Weiss SK, Cortez MA. Reactive EEG patterns in pediatric coma. *Pediatr Neurol.* 2005a Nov;**33**(5):345–9.

39. Nishisaki A, Sullivan J, 3rd, Steger B, et al. Retrospective analysis of the prognostic value of electroencephalography patterns obtained in pediatric in-hospital cardiac arrest survivors during three years. *Pediatr Crit Care Med.* 2007 Jan;**8**(1):10–7.

40. Topjian AA, Sánchez SM, Shults J, et al. Early electroencephalographic background features predict outcomes in children resuscitated from cardiac arrest. *Pediatr Crit Care Med.* 2016 Jun;**17**(6):547–57.

41. Hirsch LJ, LaRoche SM, Gaspard N, et al. American Clinical Neurophysiology Society's Standardized Critical Care EEG Terminology: 2012 version. *J Clin Neurophysiol.* 2013 Feb;**30**(1):1–27.

42. Lowenstein DH, Aminoff MJ, Simon RP. Barbiturate anesthesia in the treatment of status epilepticus: clinical experience with 14 patients. *Neurology.* 1988 Mar;**38**(3):395–400.

43. Davidson AJ, Sale SM, Wong C, et al. The electroencephalograph during anesthesia and emergence in infants and children. *Paediatr Anaesth.* 2008 Jan;**18**(1):60–70.

44. Mundi JP, Betancourt J, Ezziddin O, et al. Dilated and unreactive pupils and burst-suppression on electroencephalography due to bupropion overdose. *J Intensive Care Med.* 2012 Nov-Dec;**27**(6):384–8.

45. Ramachandrannair R, Sharma R, Weiss SK, Otsubo H, Cortez MA. A reappraisal of rhythmic coma patterns in children. *Can J Neurol Sci.* 2005b Nov;**32**(4):518–23.

46. Abend NS, Arndt DH, Carpenter JL, et al. Electrographic seizures in pediatric ICU patients: cohort study of risk factors and mortality. *Neurology.* 2013 Jul 23;**81**(4):383–91.

47. Mewasingh LD, Christophe C, Fonteyne C, et al. Predictive value of electrophysiology in children with hypoxic coma. *Pediatr Neurol.* 2003 Mar;**28**(3):178–83.

48. Abend NS, Licht DJ. Predicting outcome in children with hypoxic ischemic encephalopathy. *Pediatr Crit Care Med.* 2008 Jan;**9**(1):32–9.

49. Shellhaas RA, Chang T, Tsuchida TN, et al. American Clinical Neurophysiology Society's guideline on continuous EEG monitoring in neonates. *J Clin Neurophysiol.* 2011;**28**(6):611–17.

50. Herman ST, Abend NS, Bleck TP, et al.; Critical Care Continuous EEG Task Force of the American Clinical Neurophysiology Society. Consensus statement on continuous EEG in critically ill adults and children, part I: indications. *J Clin Neurophysiol.* 2015 Apr;**32**(2):87–95.

51. Young GB, Jordan KG, Doig GS. An assessment of nonconvulsive seizures in the intensive care unit using continuous EEG monitoring: an investigation of variables associated with mortality. *Neurology.* 1996 Jul;**47**(1):83–9.

52. Holden KR, Mellits ED, Freeman JM. Neonatal seizures. I. Correlation of prenatal and perinatal events with outcomes. *Pediatrics.* 1982 Aug;**70**(2):165–76.

53. Legido A, Clancy RR, Berman PH. Neurologic outcome after electroencephalographically proven neonatal seizures. *Pediatrics.* 1991 Sep;**88**(3):583–96.

54. Boylan GB, Pressler RM, Rennie JM, et al. Outcome of electroclinical, electrographic, and clinical seizures in the newborn infant. *Dev Med Child Neurol.* 1999 Dec;**41**(12):819–25.

55. Brophy GM, Bell R, Claassen J, et al.; Neurocritical Care Society Status Epilepticus Guideline Writing Committee. Guidelines for the evaluation and management of status epilepticus. *Neurocrit Care.* 2012 Aug;**17**(1):3–23.

56. Payne ET, Zhao XY, Frndova H, et al. Seizure burden is independently associated with short term outcome in critically ill children. *Brain.* 2014 May;**137**(Pt 5):1429–38.

57. Kharoshankaya L, Stevenson NJ, Livingstone V, et al. Seizure burden and neurodevelopmental outcome in neonates with hypoxic-ischemic encephalopathy. *Dev Med Child Neurol.* 2016 Dec;**58**(12):1242–8.

58. Treiman DM, Walton NY, Kendrick C. A progressive sequence of electroencephalographic changes during generalized convulsive status epilepticus. *Epilepsy Res.* 1990 Jan-Feb;**5**(1):49–60.

59. Novotny EJ, Jr., Tharp BR, Coen RW, et al. Positive Rolandic sharp waves in the EEG of the premature infant. *Neurology* 1987;**37**:1481–6.

60. Oliveira AJ, Nunes ML, Haertel LM, Reis FM, da Costa JC. Duration of rhythmic EEG patterns in neonates: new evidence for clinical and prognostic significance of brief rhythmic discharges. *Clin Neurophysiol.* 2000 Sep;**111**(9):1646–53.

61. van Rooij LG, de Vries LS, van Huffelen AC, Toet MC. Additional value of two-channel amplitude integrated EEG recording in full-term infants with unilateral brain injury. *Arch Dis Child Fetal Neonatal Ed.* 2010 May;**95**(3):F160–8.

62. Hellström-Westas L. Comparison between tape-recorded and amplitude-integrated EEG monitoring in sick newborn infants. *Acta Paediatr.* 1992 Oct;**81**(10):812–19.

63. al Naqeeb N, Edwards AD, Cowan FM, Azzopardi D. Assessment of neonatal encephalopathy by amplitude-integrated electroencephalography. *Pediatrics.* 1999 Jun;**103**(6 Pt 1):1263–71.

64. Toet MC, van der Meij W, de Vries LS, Uiterwaal CS, van Huffelen KC. Comparison between simultaneously recorded amplitude integrated

electroencephalogram (cerebral function monitor) and standard electroencephalogram in neonates. *Pediatrics*. 2002 May;**109** (5):772–9.

65. Clancy RR, Dicker L, Cho S, et al. Agreement between long-term neonatal background classification by conventional and amplitude-integrated EEG. *J Clin Neurophysiol*. 2011 Feb;**28** (1):1–9.

66. Hallberg B, Grossmann K, Bartocci M, Blennow M. The prognostic value of early aEEG in asphyxiated infants undergoing systemic hypothermia treatment. *Acta Paediatr*. 2010 Apr;**99** (4):531–6.

67. Thoresen M, Hellström-Westas L, Liu X, de Vries LS. Effect of hypothermia on amplitude-integrated electroencephalogram in infants with asphyxia. *Pediatrics*. 2010 Jul;**126**(1): e131–9.

68. Burdjalov VF, Baumgart S, Spitzer AR. Cerebral function monitoring: a new scoring system for the evaluation of brain maturation in neonates. *Pediatrics*. 2003 Oct;**112**(4):855–61.

69. Olischar M, Klebermass K, Kuhle S, et al. Reference values for amplitude-integrated electroencephalographic activity in preterm infants younger than 30 weeks' gestational age. *Pediatrics*. 2004 Jan;**113**(1 Pt 1):e61–6.

70. Hellström-Westas L. Continuous electroencephalography monitoring of the preterm infant. *Clin Perinatol*. 2006 Sep;**33**(3):633–47, vi.

71. Shah DK, Mackay MT, Lavery S, et al. Accuracy of bedside electroencephalographic monitoring in comparison with simultaneous continuous conventional electroencephalography for seizure detection in term infants. *Pediatrics*. 2008 Jun;**121**(6):1146–54.

72. Rennie JM, Chorley G, Boylan GB, et al. Pressler R, Nguyen Y, Hooper R. Non-expert use of the cerebral function monitor for neonatal seizure detection. *Arch Dis Child Fetal Neonatal Ed*. 2004 Jan;**89**(1):F37–40.

73. Wusthoff CJ, Shellhaas RA, Clancy RR. Limitations of single-channel EEG on the forehead for neonatal seizure detection. *J Perinatol*. 2009 Mar;**29** (3):237–42.

74. de Vries NK, Ter Horst HJ, Bos AF. The added value of simultaneous EEG and amplitude-integrated EEG recordings in three newborn infants. *Neonatology*. 2007;**91**(3):212–16.

75. Evans E, Koh S, Lerner J, Sankar R, Garg M. Accuracy of amplitude integrated EEG in a neonatal cohort. *Arch Dis Child Fetal Neonatal Ed*. 2010 May;**95**(3):F169–73.

76. Suk D, Krauss AN, Engel M, Perlman JM. Amplitude-integrated electroencephalography in the NICU: frequent artifacts in premature infants may limit its utility as a monitoring device. *Pediatrics*. 2009 Feb;**123**(2): e328–32.

77. Stewart CP, Otsubo H, Ochi A, et al. Seizure identification in the ICU using quantitative EEG displays. *Neurology*. 2010 Oct 26;**75**(17):1501–8.

78. Akman CI, Micic V, Thompson A, Riviello JJ, Jr. Seizure detection using digital trend analysis: factors affecting utility. *Epilepsy Res*. 2011 Jan;**93**(1): 66–72.

79. Pensirikul AD, Beslow LA, Kessler SK, et al. Density spectral array for seizure identification in critically ill children. *J Clin Neurophysiol*. 2013 Aug;**30** (4):371–5.

80. Topjian AA, Fry M, Jawad AF, et al. Detection of electrographic seizures by critical care providers using color density spectral array after cardiac arrest is feasible. *Pediatr Crit Care Med*. 2015 Jun;**16**(5):461–7.

81. Dericioglu N, Yetim E, Bas DF, et al. Non-expert use of quantitative EEG displays for seizure identification in the adult neuro-intensive care unit. *Epilepsy Res*. 2015 Jan; **109**:48–56.

82. Swisher CB, White CR, Mace BE, et al. Diagnostic accuracy of electrographic seizure detection by neurophysiologists and non-neurophysiologists in the adult ICU using a panel of quantitative EEG trends. *J Clin Neurophysiol*. 2015 Aug;**32**(4):324–30.

83. Haider HA, Esteller R, Hahn CD, et al.; Critical Care EEG Monitoring Research Consortium. Sensitivity of quantitative EEG for seizure identification in the intensive care unit. *Neurology*. 2016 Aug 30;**87** (9):935–44.

Neonatal Encephalopathy

Geraldine B. Boylan and Deirdre M. Murray

Illustrative Cases

Case 2 Neonatal Hypoxic-Ischemic Encephalopathy

Case 5 Neonatal Birth Trauma

Key Points

- EEG is essential to grade the severity of neonatal encephalopathy, monitor response to anti-seizure therapy, and to predict outcome early in the neonatal period in infants with NE.
- EEG evolution and outcome prediction is altered by therapeutic hypothermia.
- Seizures are common in NE and seizure burden is altered by hypothermia.
- EEG and aEEG can assess severity of NE and predict outcome more accurately than clinical assessment alone.

Neonatal Encephalopathy

Clinical Presentation

Neonatal encephalopathy (NE) is the term used to describe persistent neurological dysfunction evident in the first few days after birth. The commonest cause of NE is hypoxia-ischemia, but a similar clinical presentation may occur in conditions such as sepsis, inborn errors of metabolism and epileptic encephalopathies [1]. In this chapter we will focus primarily on neonatal hypoxic-ischemic encephalopathy (HIE), which occurs following significant perinatal asphyxia and is the commonest cause of neonatal encephalopathy. The clinical presentation of HIE is that of a neonate, either term or preterm, who is unresponsive at birth, with low Apgar scores, requiring significant resuscitation in the first minutes of life. This presentation is usually associated with a mixed respiratory and metabolic acidosis, with pH < 7.10, increased base deficit, and an increased serum lactate. It is important to note that none of these biochemical markers can provide definitive diagnosis, and individually they have low positive predictive values for the development of HIE [2]. For the diagnosis of HIE, neonates must also develop an evolving encephalopathy with clinical, EEG and/or MRI abnormalities consistent with hypoxic-ischemic injury [3, 4]. All neonates should be screened for sepsis, and EEG monitoring will assist in ruling out persistent metabolic or epileptic encephalopathies. The severity of the subsequent encephalopathy predicts the risk of long-term disability. The commonest neurological assessment system, based

on the grading system proposed by Sarnat, categorizes severity of encephalopathy into one of three grades: mild, moderate, or severe. While the original Sarnat system was based on neurological status at 24 hours after birth, modified structured clinical assessment tools such as the Thompson score can be used to track the evolution of the encephalopathy over time [5, 6]. Assessment of neurological status and prediction of outcome is extremely difficult using clinical assessment alone; EEG monitoring can be very helpful.

Global Burden of Disease

The greatest burden of disease is in low- and middle-income countries. Worldwide, 10 million neonates will suffer perinatal respiratory depression, of which 1.15 million will develop clinical encephalopathy. In countries with low neonatal mortality rates (NMR) (<5) the incidence of neonatal encephalopathy is 1.6 per 1000 births. This rises to 12.1 per 1000 deliveries in countries with high NMR (>15) [7]. It is estimated that 23% of neonatal deaths worldwide can be attributed to asphyxia. This equates to nearly 1 million neonatal deaths per year. In countries with high NMR, the death rate is 8 times that of countries with low NMRs [8].

EEG/aEEG Use in NE

Electroencephalography (EEG) is extremely useful in NE. Neonates with a significant encephalopathy may be very sick and unable to tolerate long periods of handling; EEG may provide information about neurological function even when a clinical examination is limited. Because of the smaller head size in neonates as compared to adults and older children, a reduced number of EEG recording electrodes is typically used for neonatal monitoring, as is detailed in guidelines such as those by the American Clinical Neurophysiology Society [9]. The acquisition of other physiological signals including electrocardiogram (ECG) and respiratory movement patterns are recommended when monitoring neonates with encephalopathy. Eye movement (electrooculogram) and surface electromyography (EMG) can also be very useful. We have found simultaneous video monitoring to be invaluable during neonatal EEG monitoring to help identify subtle clinical seizure manifestations and distinguish artifacts [10, 11].

Neonatal EEG is advancing with improvements in sensor and digital technology. Recordings can now continue for several days due to increased digital storage capacity on most EEG

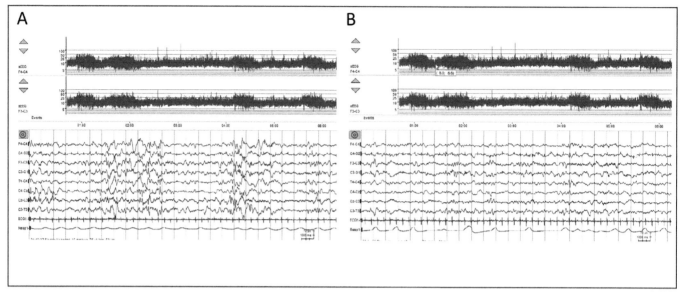

Figure 7.1 aEEG (top) and multichannel EEG from a healthy term baby. The aEEG is a compressed signal displaying 5 hours of aEEG activity and well-developed sleep cycles. The EEG (bottom) shows 25-second snapshots during a quiet sleep period (A) and an active sleep period (B).

machines or through direct server storage. Algorithms are in development for automated assessment of background patterns and for the identification of seizures. Of utmost importance, remote access to review the network-connected cot-side EEG as it is recording is now possible at many hospitals. A number of manufacturers have developed neonatal specific EEG sensors/electrodes to facilitate neonatal EEG monitoring, making it more accessible for units that do not have 24-hour neurophysiology available [12]. However, multichannel EEG does require careful attention to electrode application to ensure low electrode impedance and a low artifact level. Artifact occurs frequently in neonates due to patient movement or displacement of the EEG electrodes or leads. Therefore, it is imperative that experienced neurophysiologists and neurologists, skilled in the visual analysis of newborn EEG and in the recognition of neonatal seizures and identification of artifacts, interpret the EEG of neonates with encephalopathy.

In addition to neurophysiologist review of full EEG recordings, rapid bedside screening is possible with the use of amplitude-integrated EEG (aEEG). The modern aEEG system provides two-channel EEG monitoring and displays both the aEEG trend and the raw EEG signals for each channel. These allow superior accuracy to the older machines that displayed a single aEEG channel only [13]. The aEEG is an algorithm that filters, rectifies, smooths, and plots the raw EEG signal on a semi-logarithmic scale. The aEEG tracing is then displayed in a time-compressed manner, so that many hours of recording can be displayed on a single screen (Figure 7.1). Though aEEG is most often interpreted by neonatologists and bedside caregivers, it does require training for accurate interpretation. Amplitude-integrated EEG is excellent for providing an overview of the EEG background activity, identifying sleep–wake cycles, and for identifying more widespread, prolonged, and recurrent seizures.

EEG Abnormalities and Evolution in NE/HIE

In contrast to the EEG of the healthy term newborn in the immediate postnatal period [14, 15], EEG patterns in newborns with HIE are characteristically abnormal, similar to those seen in animal models of HIE [16]. A normal EEG from a term newborn in the first 24 hours should display continuous mixed frequency activity in the 25–100 μV range, with well-developed cycles of sleep alternating with wakefulness (Figure 7.2). In HIE, the severity of the abnormalities seen will depend on the timing of the EEG and the severity of the initial insult. Immediately following significant hypoxia and/or ischemia, the EEG becomes suppressed. In mild HIE, the EEG amplitude recovers quickly. In many cases of mild HIE, by the time the EEG is recorded at 4–6 hours after birth, the EEG is continuous. However, in these milder cases, sleep–wake cycles are typically disrupted, the EEG may be of lower amplitude, and normal features (such as anterior slow waves) may be absent. Rapid recovery of the EEG is associated with a good prognosis [17]. In moderate HIE, the EEG may remain suppressed for a longer time after delivery (Figure 7.3). As recovery begins, bursts of EEG activity are seen, alternating with periods of EEG suppression, constituting a discontinuous pattern (Figure 7.4). During this period of EEG recovery, seizures often occur. The most common time for postnatal seizures to occur is 18–20 hours after birth, though seizures may occur earlier or later than this [18]. In severe HIE, the EEG may remain suppressed for much longer; in very severe cases the EEG may not recover (Figure 7.5). Early return of sleep–wake cycles is a good prognostic sign. Studies using early continuous EEG in neonates have allowed demonstration of this gradual recovery of EEG activity [19].

Many EEG grading systems have been reported in the literature, with varied timings and durations of recordings;

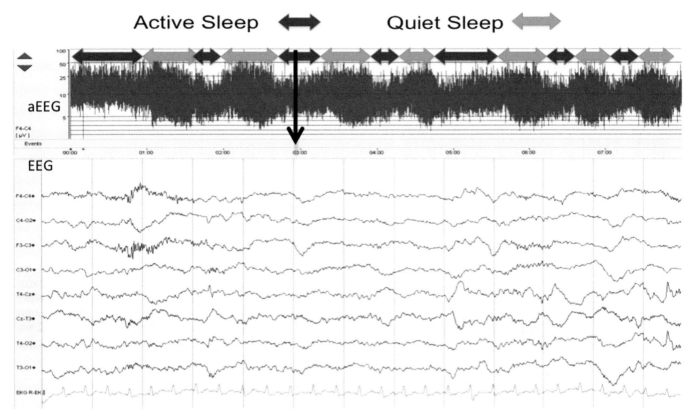

Figure 7.2 Showing relationship between aEEG and continuous multichannel EEG (cEEG) in a term neonate. The aEEG is a compressed trace which can display many hours of EEG on one screen (8 hours in this case). The black arrow demonstrates the point on the aEEG which corresponds to the raw cEEG tracing below. The cEEG shows the EEG on a second-by-second basis, allowing the observer to interrogate the frequency content of the signal and also symmetry and synchrony. The aEEG provides an overall summary of the EEG showing amplitude characteristics very well and also the presence or absence of sleep cycling.

however, very few have used early continuous EEG monitoring and related the background EEG pattern to outcome [20]. Using the grading system of Pressler displayed in Table 7.1 (a), EEG correlated well with neurodevelopmental outcome at 2 years in a non-cooled cohort of neonates with HIE [17, 19]. An alternative grading system by Holmes (Table 7.1[b]) has also been used to correlate EEG with MRI findings in a cohort of neonates who were cooled for HIE (Nash et al. 2011). It is clear that in both cooled and noncooled cohorts, the prognostic ability of individual grades depends greatly on the timing of the recording. Even a very low-voltage recording at 6 hours after birth may subsequently recover; if normalized by 24 hours, this can still be associated with a good prognosis. In contrast, a very low-voltage recording at 24 hours is almost universally associated with a poor outcome (death or severe motor disability). The prognostic utility of a moderately abnormal EEG varies considerably depending on the time it is recorded; it is only reliably predictive of a poor outcome if still present at 48 hours [19, 21]. For these reasons, is essential to begin EEG recording as soon as possible in neonates with HIE and to continue monitoring for at least 48 hours. This ensures that accurate information on the severity of the initial hypoxic-ischemic encephalopathy is available, that the evolution of the encephalopathy can be assessed, that the seizures can be identified quickly and treated promptly, and that useful

prognostic information is available in the immediate postnatal period.

aEEG Abnormalities in NE/HIE

Amplitude-integrated EEG is a commonly used method of EEG monitoring in the NICU, with modern systems generally displaying two aEEG channels and their associated raw EEG signals [22]. Two aEEG grading methods are commonly used for neonates. The amplitude method, described by al Naqeeb et al in 1999, is based exclusively on the upper and lower voltage of the aEEG band [23]. The pattern recognition method classifies the aEEG pattern into one of five grades based on recognition of patterns indicating continuity, amplitude, and bursts [24]. These grading systems are summarized in Table 7.2. The amplitude method is considered easier to interpret and requires less training as compared to the pattern-based method. However, it may provide less detailed information than pattern recognition, particularly by an expert eye [25]. The amplitude-based grading system was previously used as a method to assess for encephalopathy and thus determine eligibility for the largest randomized trial of therapeutic hypothermia for HIE [26]. However, as cooling has now become the standard of care in the developed world, aEEG's role in identifying those who will benefit from cooling has been questioned [27]. Continuous normal voltage (CNV) and Discontinuous

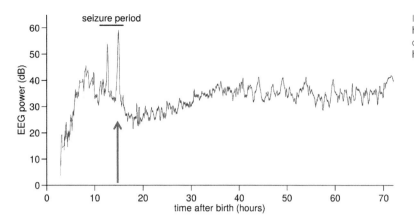

Figure 7.3 Typical recovery of EEG activity following moderate hypoxia ischemia during labor in a full-term infant. EEG monitoring commenced at 3 hours after birth and seizures emerged at 12 hours; they were treated with phenobarbitone [red arrow].

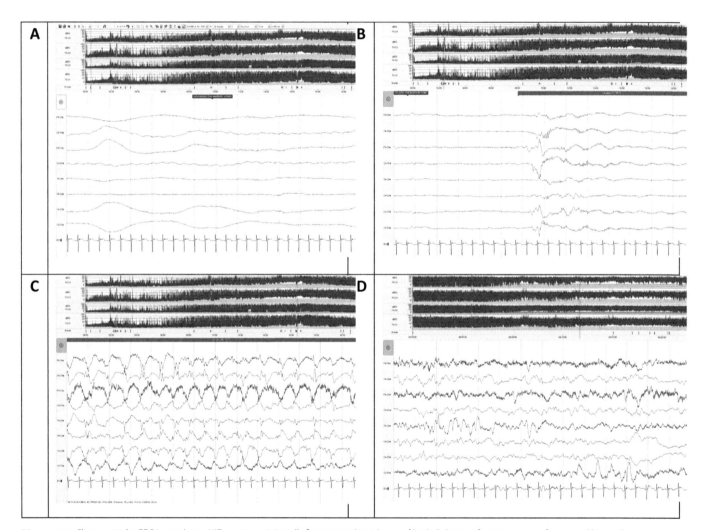

Figure 7.4 Changes in the EEG in moderate HIE over time. A. Initially flat trace within 6 hours of birth. B. Bursts of activity return after several hours. C. seizures appear at 12–24 hours. D. the EEG eventually becomes more continuous by 36 hours.

normal voltage (DNV) patterns are usually associated with a good outcome. Burst suppression patterns (BS), continuous low-voltage (CLV), and flat trace (FT) patterns are associated with a poor prognosis, though their reliability for prognosis again depends on the time of recording after birth.

While neither aEEG grading system includes information about sleep–wake cycling (SWC) as a specific criterion, the

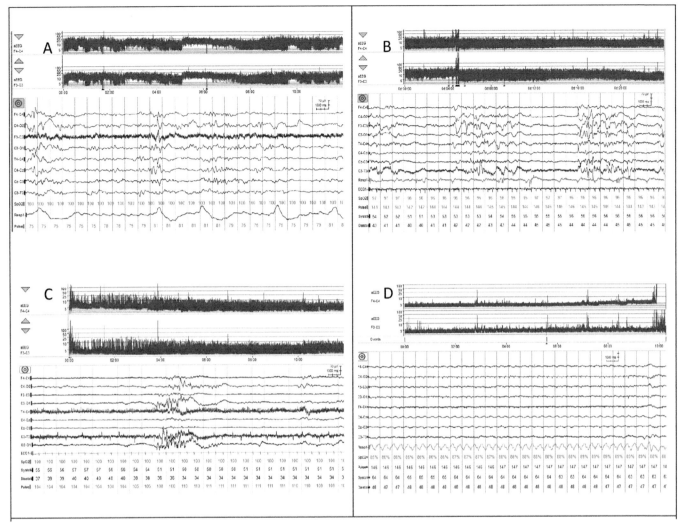

Figure 7.5 Picture A shows the neonatal EEG of a term neonate following a hypoxic-ischemic insult. EEG shows a mild-moderate pattern with reduced amplitude and disrupted sleep cycles in aEEG. A clear moderately abnormal EEG pattern is seen in B showing a discontinuous background pattern, note lower Border of aEEG is less than 5 μV. A severe pattern is seen in picture C, showing a low-voltage burst suppression pattern, both upper and lower borders of the aEEG are reduced <5 to <10 μV. In picture D, the EEG is completely suppressed and respiration artifact is evident, note the very reduced baseline on aEEG with overall amplitude less than 5 μV.

aEEG is extremely useful for the rapid visual recognition of SWC (Figure 7.2). A characteristic pattern of intermittent amplitude variation can be seen as the neonate alternates through periods of wakefulness, quiet sleep and active sleep [15]. The presence, or early return, of SWC following a hypoxic-ischemic insult is a good prognostic sign [28].

Both aEEG grading systems have been extensively reported and shown to correlate well with outcome in the pre-cooling era, where prognosis could be identified at 6 hours in 90% of neonates [29]. Prognostication using aEEG in the era of therapeutic hypothermia is more uncertain [30]. There can be considerable disagreement between individual grades of HIE on the multichannel EEG and aEEG [31]. Artifacts are also a problem during aEEG monitoring; certain artifacts (such as ventilator artifact) can elevate the amplitude of the aEEG baseline, making the aEEG difficult to grade (Figure 7.6) [32]. Visualization of the concurrent raw EEG signals is therefore essential to check for potentially misleading artifact. However,

aEEG may still provide useful information regarding the neurological status of neonates, and furthermore allows detection of subclinical seizures that would otherwise have gone undetected in the absence of monitoring [25]. Detailed outcome prediction in cooled and uncooled cohorts are discussed further below.

Use of EEG to Differentiate HIE from Other Causes of NE

Neonatal encephalopathy has a number of causes, not only hypoxia-ischemia. Clinical presentations of NE similar to that of HIE may occur with sepsis, stroke, inborn errors of metabolism, and epileptic encephalopathies. All may result in a neonate with a poor condition at birth, with a requirement for resuscitation and metabolic acidosis. However, other causes of NE can usually be ruled out by careful biochemical, microbiological, and genetic investigation. This process can take time.

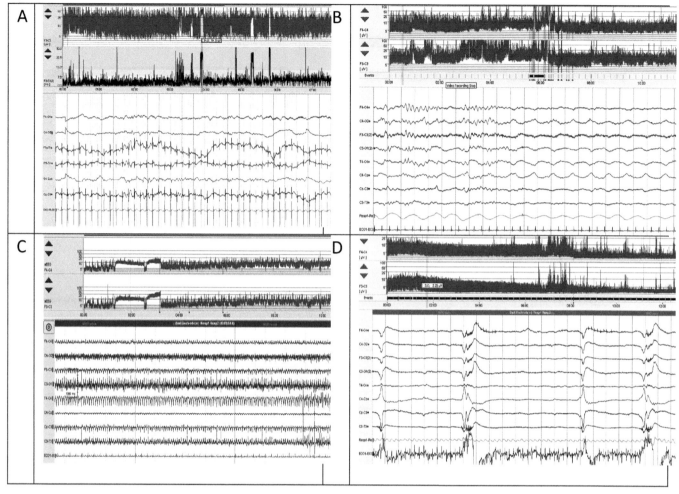

Figure 7.6 Examples of neonatal EEG and aEEG artifact
A. Intermittent ECG artifact causing an increase in the aEEG background. B. Respiration artifact on a severely suppressed background EEG pattern (note same frequency as respiratory channel). C. Clonus in a term baby with severe causing fast frequency movement artifact on the EEG and increasing the aEEG baseline. D. External mechanical artifact on all channels (note also on ECG channel) causing a slow high-voltage periodic artifact which has elevated the upper margin of the aEEG trace. When this artifact was eliminated, the baseline revealed a very suppressed background pattern.

Continuous multichannel EEG in the early postnatal period can be useful to help differentiate HIE and other causes of NE. In HIE, the evolving pattern described above is typically seen, except in those very severe cases where an isoelectric EEG is present that never recovers. Inborn errors of metabolism are characterized by a more static abnormal EEG pattern, which may worsen over time rather than recover. Seizure types and EEG/aEEG backgrounds patterns can be very different from those seen in HIE (Figure 7.7), which may help in diagnosis and differentiation [33]. In neonatal encephalopathies due to epileptic encephalopathy, such as early infantile epileptic encephalopathy or in early myoclonic encephalopathy, EEG patterns are very different from those seen in HIE. Epileptic encephalopathies feature EEGs characterized by high-voltage, often chaotic background activity interspersed with intractable seizures or a burst suppression pattern [34] (Figure 7.7). Neonates with other congenital disorders such as Zellweger syndrome or brain malformation disorders will also present in the neonatal period with encephalopathy; in these cases, the background EEG pattern is also very different to the patterns

seen in HIE (Figure 7.7). In summary, EEG can often help differentiate between different types of neonatal encephalopathy, particularly when HIE is included in the differential. It remains imperative that a good clinical history is obtained and a full neurological examination of the baby is performed. In addition to these, when the evolution of EEG background over the first hours and days does not fit the pattern typical of HIE, other etiologies for the encephalopathy should be considered.

Effects of Sedation and Other Neuroprotective Agents on EEG/aEEG Findings

Background EEG patterns may be significantly affected by the administration of sedative, analgesic, or anti-seizure medications. Most studies on the topic agree that medications, such as phenobarbital, benzodiazepines, and morphine, all affect the neonatal EEG and aEEG [35, 36], resulting in decreased amplitude and increased discontinuity. Notably, these effects tend to be more pronounced in neonates with already impaired

Table 7.1 Classification of EEG background activity: grading systems for early EEG findings reported by (a) Pressler et al[1] and (b) Holmes et al[2] that have been shown to correlate with long-term outcomes following neonatal hypoxic-ischemic encephalopathy

(a) Pressler System

Grade	Findings	Description
0	Normal EEG findings	Continuous background pattern with normal physiological features such as anterior slow waves
1	Normal/mild abnormalities	Continuous background pattern with slightly abnormal activity (e.g., mild asymmetry, mild voltage depression, or poorly defined SWC)
2	Moderate abnormalities	Discontinuous activity with IBI of <10 seconds, no clear SWC, or clear asymmetry or asynchrony
3	Major abnormalities	Discontinuous activity with IBI of 10–60 seconds, severe attenuation of background patterns, or no SWC
4	Inactive EEG findings	Background activity of <10 μV or severe discontinuity with IBI of >60 seconds

(b) Holmes System

Grade	Findings	Description
1	Normal pattern for gestational age	Transient periods of discontinuous activity occupying less than 50% of the recording, with presence of distinct state changes
2	Excessively discontinuous	Discontinuous activity occupying more than 50% of the recording and consisting of bursts of normal activity separated by abnormally long, inter-burst intervals of more than 6 seconds' duration, and amplitude between <25 and >5 μV, with poor state changes
3	Depressed and undifferentiated	Persistently low-voltage background activity with amplitude between 5 and 15 μV and without normal features
4	Burst suppression	Invariant and unreactive pattern of bursts of paroxysmal activity with mixed features but no age-appropriate activity lasting <10 seconds alternating with periods of marked voltage attenuation with amplitude <5 μV
5	Extremely low voltage	Invariant and unreactive pattern, with amplitude <5 μV or with no discernible cerebral activity.

IBI = Inter-burst interval; SWC = Sleep–wake cycling
[1] Pressler RM, Boylan GB, Morton M, et al. Early serial EEG in hypoxic ischaemic encephalopathy. *Clin Neurophysiol.* 2001 Jan;112(1):31–7. PubMed PMID: 11137658.
[2] Holmes GL, Lombroso CT. Prognostic value of background patterns in the neonatal EEG. *J Clin Neurophysiol.* 1993 Jul;10(3):323–52. Review. PubMed PMID: 8408599.

background EEG activity. Midazolam, in particular, may cause a significant decrease in background amplitude shortly after administration that may last for several hours [37]. Phenobarbital will cause electroclinical uncoupling leading to a reduction in the clinical manifestations of neonatal seizures, despite ongoing electrical seizures [38]. In addition, the characteristics of the electrographic seizures themselves change following PB administration [39]. Neuroprotective agents, such as Xenon, will also affect the background EEG and may have adjunct anticonvulsant effects [40].

Clinical and Electrographic Seizures in NE

Seizures are often the hallmark of neonatal encephalopathy but their clinical expression may be subtle or absent, making them difficult to detect without EEG monitoring [41]. When clinical signs do occur they may be misinterpreted, making under- and overestimation of seizures common based on clinical diagnosis alone [10, 42]. Until recently, treatment with phenobarbital was only shown to have a 50% success rate. It also may increase electroclinical uncoupling, thus leading to a reduction in associated clinical signs despite ongoing electrographic seizures [38, 43]. A recent study has shown a higher success rate with phenobarbital therapy which may be due to earlier initiation of treatment [44].

The characteristics of seizures in HIE are well described now in both cooled and noncooled cohorts. The characteristics of seizures in other causes of neonatal encephalopathy are less well reported [33].

Table 7.2 Most frequently used grading systems for visual analysis of amplitude-integrated EEG (aEEG)

Amplitude based			Pattern based	
Normal	Upper margin of band of aEEG activity > 10 µV and the lower margin > 5 µV		Continuous normal voltage (CNV)	
Moderate	Upper margin of band of aEEG activity > 10 µV and the lower margin ≤ 5 µV		Discontinuous normal voltage (DNV)	
Severe	Upper margin of band of aEEG activity <10 µV and the lower margin < 5 µV		Burst suppression (BS)	
			Continuous low-voltage (CLV)	
			Flat trace (FT)	

Timing of Seizures in HIE and Seizure Burden

Seizures are seen in term neonates with significant HIE, usually occurring within the first 24 hours after birth [18]. Seizures worsen hypoxic-ischemic injury in neonatal animal models; the same may be true for some neonates [45, 46]. Seizures occur in moderate and severe HIE and are often difficult to control (Figure 7.4). Very few studies were available to detail the evolution of electrographic seizure burden in neonates with HIE in the pre-therapeutic hypothermia era [18, 47]. Low et al. demonstrated that there was no significant difference in the median time of seizure onset between cooled and uncooled neonates in HIE; seizures started on average at 18 hours (IQR 12–22) after birth in normothermic neonates, as compared to 13 hours (IQR 11–22) in those receiving hypothermia [18]. In a cooled HIE population, Wusthoff and colleagues reported a later mean age of electrographic seizure onset at 35 hours; however, a large number of neonates had a seizure onset at less than 24 hours, with the latest seizure onset time being 95 hours [42]. Glass et al. reported a similar pattern, with a median age of seizure onset at 18 hours and the latest age of electrographic seizure onset was 62 hours [48]. Less often, seizures may begin, or recommence, during the rewarming phase. The wide range of seizure onset times in neonates with HIE who receive TH provides a challenge to providing adequate seizure surveillance in neonatal intensive care units where continuous EEG monitoring is not available. Lynch et al. examined the temporal distribution of seizures in neonates with HIE and found that seizures generally have a short period of high electrographic seizure burden near the time of seizure onset, followed by a longer period of low seizure burden [18].

In HIE, seizures can be multifocal in onset. They may or may not have spread to neighboring regions, and may even spread to involve the entire brain. This is in contrast with seizures in acute stroke, which typically have a single focus of onset, and to epileptic encephalopathies, as described below.

Total seizure burden is reduced in neonates receiving therapeutic hypothermia as compared to normothermic groups. This is particularly true in moderate HIE, with little difference in seizure burden among those cooled or not cooled for severe HIE [47, 49]. Although overall seizure burden is decreased with hypothermia, the number of neonates who have any seizures is

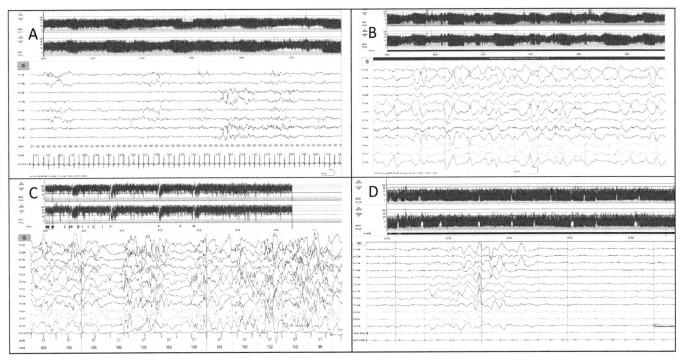

Figure 7.7 EEG background patterns in NE (other than HIE). A. Molybdenum cofactor deficiency showing gross asynchrony in the background pattern. B. Lissencephaly showing abnormal sleep cycles on aEEG (lower margin of aEEG less than 5 µV) and asynchronous high-voltage slow waves. C. Ohathara syndrome showing chaotic high-voltage burst suppression pattern. aEEG shows intermittent electrodecremental periods during sequential seizures. D. Zellweger syndrome showing a persistent burst suppression pattern with loss of higher frequency activity during the burst periods. The aEEG shows intermitted elevations of the baseline pattern during seizures.

relatively unchanged. Low et al. showed very similar rates of affected neonates in noncooled and cooled cohorts (52% and 48%, respectively) [47]. These reported rates are consistent with other studies using multichannel EEG [21, 42, 50]. In the more recent studies [21, 42], the recorded seizure burden was not quantified and a control cohort (noncooled) was not available for comparison; we are therefore unable to compare total seizure burden, which is suspected to have a greater effect on outcome than solely presence or absence of seizures.

Accurate quantification of seizure burden is difficult with aEEG alone, without full array EEG for confirmation. Artifacts are common with aEEG; some artifacts such as EKG or respiratory artifact can look like seizures. For this reason, suspected seizures on aEEG must be confirmed on the source, raw EEG channels at a minimum. In addition, inter-observer variability in aEEG interpretation is high; this is particularly true for novice users. Furthermore, seizure recognition is particularly unreliable with aEEG alone for focal and low amplitude seizures [51]. For all these reasons, while aEEG may be a useful screening tool for identifying whether a neonate is having any seizures, it has significant limitations in attempting to quantify seizure burden.

Status epilepticus, defined as 30 minutes or more of continuous or intermittent seizures within a 1-hour period [9], occurs in neonates with both moderate and severe HIE and occurs in approximately 23% of neonates undergoing

therapeutic hypothermia [42, 47]. In cooled cohorts, moderate and severe brain injury remains more common in neonates with status epilepticus than those without [21, 52]. Srinivasakumar et al. confirmed these findings and reported that 5 of 19 neonates with status epilepticus had severe brain injury on MRI [49]. Even during therapeutic hypothermia, seizures remain a risk factor for significant brain injury, particularly in neonates with status epilepticus.

Seizures in Other Causes of Neonatal Encephalopathy

Seizures are common in all types of neonatal encephalopathy, though the clinical presentation and electrographic characteristics may vary depending on the cause of the encephalopathy. There are no studies to date that describe in detail the characteristics of seizures in all causes of neonatal encephalopathy; some valuable information is available in a number of important case series. In early infantile epileptic encephalopathies (e.g., *KCNQ2* encephalopathy, *SCN2A* encephalopathy, Ohtahara syndrome), epileptic spasms and tonic seizures are common and the background EEG pattern shows persistent multifocal epileptiform activity or a burst suppression pattern [34, 53, 54]. In early myoclonic encephalopathies (EME), such as nonketotic hyperglycinemia, erratic myoclonia is common and the EEG background demonstrates a burst suppression pattern [55]. However, in EME, during burst suppression the bursts are short and there are long periods of suppression [34, 55]. These conditions are described in further detail in the chapter on neonatal epilepsies.

Prediction of Outcome in NE

Using the Sarnat score, neonates are graded as having mild, moderate, or severe encephalopathy depending on their clinical signs [5]. In most cohorts, the approximate breakdown tends to be mild (39%), moderate (39%), and severe (22%) [7]. Management and outcome vary significantly with grade of HIE. The overall death rate in neonatal encephalopathy of all grades is 9.9% in developed countries, but this rises to 30% among those who qualify for cooling and precipitously to 76.8% when considering severe encephalopathy alone [7, 56].

Prior to the cooling era, among neonates who survived beyond the neonatal period, approximately 26% had moderate or severe disability long term, with a further 14% surviving with mild impairment. Reported rates of cerebral palsy following neonatal encephalopathy vary but are generally 10%–13% among survivors of moderate to severe encephalopathy. Dyskinetic CP and spastic quadriplegia are the most common subtypes, with 80% of dyskinetic CP attributable to perinatal hypoxia-ischemia at term [57]. High rates of hearing loss (17%) and visual deficits (41%) also occur [58]. Therapeutic hypothermia improves the outlook for neonates with moderate to severe HIE, with increased likelihood of survival with normal IQ (RR=1.31) and improved survival without neurological abnormalities (RR=1.6) at follow-up at 6-7 years of life [59].

Many studies have shown that long-term cognitive and behavioral difficulties are frequent in surviving children without motor disability. Specific memory impairments correspond with reduced hippocampal volume on MRI [60]. Reduced attention, behavioral difficulties, and reduced school readiness have been reported [61, 62]. Marlow et al also demonstrated memory, attention/executive function impairments and lower educational achievement in children following moderate and severe HIE assessed at age 7 years [63]. Odd et al. have shown that infants with encephalopathy had lower working memory, reading accuracy, and comprehension scores and increased requirement for educational support (OR=6.24) between 8 and 11 years [64]. The outcome for children following mild HIE is less clear. Initial studies reported an outcome similar to non-HIE NICU survivors. However, more recently, a number of small long-term studies have shown increased rates of disability, both cognitive and behavioral [62]. Most large prospective studies of outcome following intervention have not included the mild HIE group, as they are not currently eligible for intervention, and so we have very little contemporaneous data on outcome after mild HIE. The longer children are followed, the more evident it becomes that survivors of NE often have significant long-term, non-motor, effects.

Prediction of Outcome Using EEG in Cooled and Noncooled Neonates

As above, the predictive ability of the EEG recording depends on several factors: timing of the EEG, whether the neonate is cooled or noncooled, administration of sedative medications. Bearing these factors in mind, the best available evidence for prediction of outcome using EEG is summarized in Table 7.3. Different grading systems and different outcome measures make direct comparison difficult; however, the prediction based on grade is similar whether cooled or uncooled. Best evidence suggests that, regardless of TH intervention, a normal EEG at 6 hours is very predictive of normal outcome. A normal EEG at 48 hours may be falsely reassuring if earlier EEG recordings are not available or have normalized. Definite prediction of poor outcome becomes reliable at 48 hours. If EEG is severe or inactive at 24–48 hours, abnormal outcome is seen in 90–100%. Moderate abnormalities are more difficult to interpret. If this pattern is seen at 6–24 hours, a neonate has a 40%–50% chance of an abnormal outcome. If seen at 48 hours or beyond, this risk increases to around 70% [19, 21].

Prediction of Outcome Using aEEG in Cooled and Noncooled Neonates

Prior to the introduction of therapeutic hypothermia, aEEG was repeatedly shown to have excellent predictive ability even as early as 3–6 hours following delivery. An aEEG graded as either burst suppression (BS), flat trace (FT) or continuous low-voltage (CLV) at 3 hours had a sensitivity and specificity for poor outcome of 0.85 and 0.77, respectively. At 6 hours, these patterns had a sensitivity and specificity of 0.91 and 0.86, respectively [29]. Similarly promising results were found using the amplitude based grading system when assessed within the first 12 hours after delivery; a moderately or severely depressed aEEG trace had a PPV of 85% and a NPV of 100% for the prediction of a poor outcome [23]. Similarly, the return of SWC was a good prognostic indicator in noncooled cohorts, with a return of SWC by 36 hours giving accurate outcome prediction in 82% of neonates [65].

Therapeutic hypothermia alters the evolution of aEEG and its early predictive ability. In 2009, very soon after the widespread introduction of therapeutic hypothermia, Hallberg et al. reported in a small cohort of 26 cooled neonates that BS/CLV/FT aEEG recordings at 6 hours had only a 32% PPV for abnormal outcome at 18–24 months. This increased to 60% at 24 hours, but confident prediction was not possible until 48 hours [66]. Further evidence regarding the impact of hypothermia on aEEG evolution and predictive value came from the direct comparison between cooled and noncooled neonates with HIE randomized within the selective head cooling trial [30]. In this study, the PPV of an abnormal trace at 6 hours for abnormal outcome was 84% in normothermic neonates, but only 54% in hypothermic neonates. In neonates treated with hypothermia, PPV did not increase to 90% until

Table 7.3 EEG grade and outcome based on timing of EEG recording

EEG findings	Predicted outcome based on timing of EEG recording*			
	6 hours	24 hours	48 hours	Beyond 48 hours
Normal amplitude continuous EEG induced hypothermia	100% normal/mild MRI	100% normal/mild MRI	93% normal/mild MRI	92% normal/mild MRI
Mild EEG normothermic	100% normal outcome at 2 years 75% intact survival at 5 years	100% normal outcome at 2 years 65% intact survival at 5 years	73% normal outcome at 2 years N/A at 5 years	N/A
Mild EEG Induced hypothermia	73% Normal/mild MRI findings	77% Normal/mild MRI findings	81% Normal/mild MRI findings	77% Normal/mild MRI findings
Moderate EEG normothermic	100% intact survival at 2 years 45% intact survival at 5 years	66% intact survival at 2 years 57% intact survival at 5 years	0% intact survival at 2 years N/A at 5 years	N/A
Moderate EEG abnormalities Induced hypothermia	50% Normal MRI	40% Normal MRI	29% Normal MRI	33% Normal MRI
Major/Severe EEG abnormalities normothermic	20% intact at 2 years 42.9% intact survival at 5 years	10% intact at 2 years 11% intact survival at 5 years	0–15% intact at 2 years 0% intact survival at 5 years	N/A
Severe depression, undifferentiated, burst suppression Induced hypothermia	29% Normal MRI	0% Normal MRI	0% Normal MRI	0% Normal MRI
Very low voltage Amplitude <5 µV normothermic	14% intact survival at 2 and 5 years	0% intact survival at 2 or 5 years	0% intact survival at 2 or 5 years	0% intact survival at 2 or 5 years
Very low voltage Amplitude <5 µV Induced hypothermia	43% Normal MRI	0% Normal MRI	0% Normal MRI	0% Normal MRI

* Note that for all infants the presence of seizures will worsen prognosis and in particular with a high seizure burden or status epilepticus. N/A = no available data. Grading system of Pressler et al. used for normothermic infants and Holmes et al. for hypothermic cohort.

24 hours, and 100% at 48 hours. Time to normal trace and return of SWC were both useful in prognostication. Similar results have been reported for neonates following whole body cooling, where the predictive ability of an early abnormal trace was reduced in the cooled arm of the trial [67].

Hence, we now have good evidence that very early aEEG is less useful for outcome prediction in cooled neonates, likely due to the variable effect of the therapeutic intervention. aEEG may identify encephalopathy requiring neuroprotective intervention, but not the neonate's response to that intervention. In summary, similar to EEG, a normal early aEEG trace is reassuring, but an abnormal trace does not reliably predict poor outcome in the first 48 hours after birth.

When Is the Best Time to Record and Interpret EEG and/or aEEG Findings in NE to Aid in Outcome Prediction?

Ideally, continuous EEG monitoring would be available to all neonates immediately following hypoxic-ischemic injury to allow accurate prognosis and rapid detection of seizures. However, this is not always possible; many centers have access to aEEG and/or intermittent EEG only. In those cases, the combination aEEG monitoring with an early EEG within the first 6-12 hours and a repeat EEG at 48 hours is likely to provide the most information. If normal and continuous activity with sleep–wake cycling is seen on aEEG by 6 hours, the prognosis is excellent. On the other hand, abnormalities seen at this stage, even if severe in nature, may improve rapidly. Continued abnormalities at 48 hours, especially if moderate or severe in nature are associated with significant long-term disability.

References

1. Douglas-Escobar M, Weiss MD. Hypoxic-ischemic encephalopathy: a review for the clinician. *JAMA Pediatr.* 2015;**169**(4):397–403.

2. Ferriero DM, Bonifacio SL. The search continues for the elusive biomarkers of neonatal brain injury. *J Pediatr.* 2014;**164**(3):438–40.

3. Rutherford M, Malamateniou C, McGuinness A, et al. Magnetic resonance imaging in hypoxic-ischaemic encephalopathy. *Early Hum Dev.* 2010;**86**(6):351–60.

4. Bonifacio SL, Glass HC, Vanderpluym J, et al. Perinatal events and early magnetic resonance imaging in therapeutic hypothermia. *J Pediatr.* 2011;**158**(3): 360–5.

5. Sarnat HB, Sarnat MS. Neonatal encephalopathy following fetal distress. A clinical and electroencephalographic study. *Arch Neurol.* 1976;**33**(10):696–705.

6. Thompson CM, Puterman AS, Linley LL, et al. The value of a scoring system for hypoxic ischaemic encephalopathy in predicting neurodevelopmental outcome. *Acta Paediatr.* 1997;**86**(7):757–61.

7. Lee AC, Kozuki N, Blencowe H, et al. Intrapartum-related neonatal encephalopathy incidence and impairment at regional and global levels for 2010 with trends from 1990. *Pediatr Res.* 2013;**74**(Suppl 1):50–72.

8. Lawn JE, Cousens S, Zupan J; the Lancet Neonatal Survival Steering Team. 4 million neonatal deaths: when? Where? Why? *Lancet.* 2005;**365**(9462):891–900.

9. Tsuchida TN, Wusthoff CJ, Shellhaas RA, et al.; American Clinical Neurophysiology Society Critical Care Monitoring. American Clinical Neurophysiology Society standardized EEG terminology and categorization for the description of continuous EEG monitoring in neonates: report of the American Clinical Neurophysiology Society critical care monitoring committee. *J Clin Neurophysiol.* 2013;**30**(2):161–73.

10. Murray DM, Boylan GB, Ali I. et al. Defining the gap between electrographic seizure burden, clinical expression and staff recognition of neonatal seizures. *Arch Dis Child Fetal Neonatal Ed.* 2008;**93**(3):F187–91.

11. Boylan GB. EEG monitoring in the neonatal intensive care unit: a critical juncture. *Clin Neurophysiol.* 2011;**122**(10):1905–7.

12. Herman ST, Abend NS, Bleck TP, et al.; E. E. G. T. F. o. t. A. C. N. S. Critical Care Continuous. Consensus statement on continuous EEG in critically ill adults and children, part I: indications. *J Clin Neurophysiol.* 2015;**32**(2):87–95.

13. El-Dib M, Chang T, Tsuchida TN, Clancy RR. Amplitude-integrated electroencephalography in neonates. *Pediatr Neurol.* 2009;**41**(5):315–26.

14. Korotchikova I, Connolly S, Ryan CA, et al. EEG in the healthy term newborn within 12 hours of birth. *Clin Neurophysiol.* 2009;**120**(6):1046–53.

15. Korotchikova I, Stevenson NJ, Livingstone V, Ryan CA, Boylan GB. Sleep-wake cycle of the healthy term newborn infant in the immediate postnatal period. *Clin Neurophysiol.* 2016;**127**(4):2095–101.

16. Gunn AJ, Thoresen M. Animal studies of neonatal hypothermic neuroprotection have translated well into practice. *Resuscitation.* 2015;**97**:88–90.

17. Pressler RM, Boylan GB, Morton M, Binnie CD, Rennie JM. Early serial EEG in hypoxic ischaemic encephalopathy. *Clin Neurophysiol.* 2001;**112**(1):31–7.

18. Lynch NE, Stevenson NJ, Livingstone V, et al. The temporal evolution of electrographic seizure burden in neonatal hypoxic ischemic encephalopathy. *Epilepsia.* 2012;**53**(3):549–57.

19. Murray DM, Boylan GB, Ryan CA, Connolly S. Early EEG findings in hypoxic-ischemic encephalopathy predict outcomes at 2 years. *Pediatrics.* 2009;**124**(3):e459–67.

20. Walsh BH, Murray DM, Boylan GB. The use of conventional EEG for the assessment of hypoxic ischaemic encephalopathy in the newborn: a review. *Clin Neurophysiol.* 2011;**122**(7):1284–94.

21. Nash KB, Bonifacio SL, Glass HC, et al. Video-EEG monitoring in newborns with hypoxic-ischemic encephalopathy treated with hypothermia. *Neurology.* 2011;**76**(6):556–62.

22. Boylan G, Burgoyne L, Moore C, O'Flaherty B, Rennie J. An international survey of EEG use in the neonatal intensive care unit. *Acta Paediatr.* 2010;**99**(8):1150–5.

23. al Naqeeb N, Edwards AD, Cowan FM, Azzopardi D. Assessment of neonatal encephalopathy by amplitude-integrated electroencephalography. *Pediatrics.* 1999;**103**(6 Pt 1):1263–71.

24. de Vries LS, Toet MC. How to assess the aEEG background. *J Pediatr.* 2009;**154**(4):625–6; author reply 626–7.

25. Hellstrom-Westas L. Monitoring brain function with aEEG in term asphyxiated infants before and during cooling. *Acta Paediatr.* 2013;**102**(7):678–9.

26. Azzopardi D, Brocklehurst P, Edwards D, et al. The TOBY Study. Whole body hypothermia for the treatment of perinatal asphyxial encephalopathy: a randomised controlled trial. *BMC Pediatr.* 2008;**8**:17.

27. Shankaran S, Pappas A, McDonald, SA, et al.; H. Eunice Kennedy Shriver National Institute of Child and N. Human Development Neonatal Research. Predictive value of an early amplitude integrated electroencephalogram and neurologic examination. *Pediatrics.* 2011;**128**(1):e112–20.

28. Cseko AJ, Bango M, Lakatos P, et al. Accuracy of amplitude-integrated electroencephalography in the prediction of neurodevelopmental outcome in asphyxiated infants receiving hypothermia treatment. *Acta Paediatr.* 2013;**102**(7):707–11.

29. Toet MC, Hellstrom-Westas L, Groenendaal F, Eken P, de Vries LS. Amplitude integrated EEG 3 and 6 hours after birth in full term neonates with hypoxic-ischaemic encephalopathy. *Arch Dis Child Fetal Neonatal Ed.* 1999;**81**(1):F19–23.

30. Thoresen M, Hellstrom-Westas L, Liu X, de Vries LS. Effect of hypothermia on amplitude-integrated electroencephalogram in infants with asphyxia. *Pediatrics.* 2010;**126**(1):e131–9.

31. Evans E, Koh S, Lerner J, Sankar R, Garg M. Accuracy of amplitude

integrated EEG in a neonatal cohort. *Arch Dis Child Fetal Neonatal Ed.* 2010;**95**(3):F169–73.

32. Marics G, Cseko A, Vasarhelyi B, et al. Prevalence and etiology of false normal aEEG recordings in neonatal hypoxic-ischaemic encephalopathy. *BMC Pediatr.* 2013;**13**:194.

33. Olischar M, Shany E, Aygun C, et al. Amplitude-integrated electroencephalography in newborns with inborn errors of metabolism. *Neonatology.* 2012;**102**(3):203–11.

34. Yamamoto H, Okumura A, Fukuda M. Epilepsies and epileptic syndromes starting in the neonatal period. *Brain Dev.* 2011;**33**(3):213–20.

35. Young GB, da Silva OP. Effects of morphine on the electroencephalograms of neonates: a prospective, observational study. *Clin Neurophysiol.* 2000;**111**(11):1955–60.

36. Shany E, Benzaquen O, Friger M, Richardson J, Golan A. Influence of antiepileptic drugs on amplitude-integrated electroencephalography. *Pediatr Neurol.* 2008;**39**(6):387–91.

37. Hellstrom-Westas L. Midazolam and amplitude-integrated EEG. *Acta Paediatr.* 2004;**93**(9):1153–4.

38. Scher MS, Alvin J, Gaus L, Minnigh B, Painter MJ. Uncoupling of EEG-clinical neonatal seizures after antiepileptic drug use. *Pediatr Neurol.* 2003;**28**(4):277–80.

39. Mathieson SR, Livingstone V, Low E, et al. Phenobarbital reduces EEG amplitude and propagation of neonatal seizures but does not alter performance of automated seizure detection. *Clin Neurophysiol.* 2016;**127**(10):3343–50.

40. Azzopardi D, Robertson NJ, Kapetanakis A, et al. Anticonvulsant effect of xenon on neonatal asphyxial seizures. *Arch Dis Child Fetal fNeonatal Ed.* 2013;**98**(5):F437–9.

41. Hellstrom-Westas L, Rosen I, Swenningsen NW. Silent seizures in sick infants in early life. Diagnosis by continuous cerebral function monitoring. *Acta Paediatr Scand.* 1985;**74**(5):741–8.

42. van Rooij LG, Hellstrom-Westas L, de Vries LS. Treatment of neonatal seizures. *Semin Fetal Neonatal Med.* 2013;**18**(4):209–15.

43. Wusthoff CJ, Dlugos DJ, Gutierrez-Colina A, et al. Electrographic seizures during therapeutic hypothermia for neonatal hypoxic-ischemic encephalopathy. *J Child Neurol.* 2011;**26**(6):724–8.

44. Sharpe C, Reiner GE, Davis SL, et al. Levetiracetam versus phenobarbital for neonatal seizures: a randomized controlled trial. *Pediatrics.* 2020;**145**(6):e20193182.

45. Wirrell EC, Armstrong EA, Osman LD, Yager JY. Prolonged seizures exacerbate perinatal hypoxic-ischemic brain damage. *Pediatr Res.* 2001;**50**(4):445–54.

46. Miller SP, Weiss J, Barnwell A, et al. Seizure-associated brain injury in term newborns with perinatal asphyxia. *Neurology.* 2002;**58**(4):542–8.

47. Low E, Boylan GB, Mathieson SR, et al. Cooling and seizure burden in term neonates: an observational study. *Arch Dis Child Fetal Neonatal Ed.* 2012;**97**(4):F267–72.

48. Glass HC, Wusthoff CJ, Shellhaas RA, et al. Risk factors for EEG seizures in neonates treated with hypothermia: A multicenter cohort study. *Neurology.* 2014;**82**(14):1239–44.

49. Srinivasakumar P, Zempel J, Wallendorf M, et al. Therapeutic hypothermia in neonatal hypoxic ischemic encephalopathy: electrographic seizures and magnetic resonance imaging evidence of injury. *J Pediatr.* 2013;**163**(2):465–70.

50. Rafay MF. , Cortez MA, de Veber GA, et al. Predictive value of clinical and EEG features in the diagnosis of stroke and hypoxic ischemic encephalopathy in neonates with seizures. *Stroke.* 2009;**40**(7):2402–7.

51. Shellhaas RA, Soaita AI, Clancy RR. Sensitivity of amplitude-integrated electroencephalography for neonatal seizure detection. *Pediatrics.* 2007;**120**(4):770–7.

52. Glass HC, Nash KB, Bonifacio SL, et al. Seizures and magnetic resonance imaging-detected brain injury in newborns cooled for hypoxic-ischemic encephalopathy. *J Pediatr.* 2011;**159**(5):731–5 e731.

53. Howell KB, McMahon JM, Carvill GL, et al. SCN2A encephalopathy: a major cause of epilepsy of infancy with migrating focal seizures. *Neurology.* 2015;**85**(11):958–66.

54. Pisano T, Numis AL, Heavin SB, et al. Early and effective treatment of KCNQ2 encephalopathy. *Epilepsia.* 2015;**56**(5):685–91.

55. Dulac O. Epileptic encephalopathy with suppression-bursts and nonketotic hyperglycinemia. *Handb Clin Neurol.* 2013;**113**:1785–97.

56. Azzopardi DV, Strohm B, Edwards AD, et al. Moderate hypothermia to treat perinatal asphyxial encephalopathy. *N Engl J Med.* 2009;**361**(14):1349–58.

57. Rennie JM, Hagmann CF, Robertson NJ. Outcome after intrapartum hypoxic ischaemia at term. *Semin Fetal Neonatal Med.* 2007;**12**(5):398–407.

58. Mercuri E, Anker S, Guzzetta A, et al. Visual function at school age in children with neonatal encephalopathy and low Apgar scores. *Arch Dis Child Fetal Neonatal Ed.* 2004;**89**(3):F258–62.

59. Azzopardi D, Strohm B, Marlow N, et al. Effects of hypothermia for perinatal asphyxia on childhood outcomes. *N Engl J Med.* 2014;**371**(2):140–9.

60. van Handel M, de Sonneville L, de Vries LS, Jongmans MJ, Swaab H. Specific memory impairment following neonatal encephalopathy in term-born children. *Dev Neuropsychol.* 2012;**37**(1):30–50.

61. de Haan M, Wyatt JS, Roth S, et al. Brain and cognitive-behavioural development after asphyxia at term birth. *Dev Sci.* 2006;**9**(4):350–8.

62. van Handel M, Swaab H, de Vries L, Jongmans MJ. Behavioral outcome in children with a history of neonatal encephalopathy following perinatal asphyxia. *J Pediatr Psychol.* 2010;**35**(3):286–95.

63. Marlow N, Rose AS, Rands CE, Draper E. S. Neuropsychological and educational problems at school age associated with neonatal encephalopathy. *Arch Dis Child Fetal Neonatal Ed.* 2005;**90**(5):F380–7.

64. Odd DE, Lewis G, Whitelaw A, Gunnell D. Resuscitation at birth and cognition at 8 years of age: a cohort study. *Lancet.* 2009;**373**(9675):1615–22.

65. Osredkar D, Toet MC, van Rooij LG, et al. Sleep-wake cycling on amplitude-integrated electroencephalography in term newborns with hypoxic-ischemic encephalopathy. *Pediatrics.* 2005;**115**(2):327–32.

66. Hallberg B, Grossmann K, Bartocci M, Blennow M. The prognostic value of early aEEG in asphyxiated infants undergoing systemic hypothermia treatment. *Acta Paediatr.* 2010;**99**(4):531–6.

67. Azzopardi D, TOBY Study Group. Predictive value of the amplitude integrated EEG in infants with hypoxic ischaemic encephalopathy: data from a randomised trial of therapeutic hypothermia. *Arch Dis Child Fetal Neonatal Ed.* 2014;**99**(1):F80–2.

Neonatal Seizures Due to Acute Causes

Elissa Yozawitz and Ronit Pressler

Illustrative Cases

Key Points

- Seizures in the neonatal period are usually acute symptomatic, requiring immediate diagnosis and treatment.
- Common etiologies include hypoxic-ischemic encephalopathy, stroke, and infection in term babies; intraventricular hemorrhage and infection are most common in preterm babies.
- Many neonatal seizures are subclinical, making EEG monitoring a necessity for diagnosis and management.

Introduction

In the neonatal period, the majority of seizures are acute reactive events provoked by insults such as hypoxic-ischemic encephalopathy (HIE), acute metabolic disturbances, infection, inborn error of metabolism, or intracranial hemorrhages. Some etiologies require immediate diagnosis and treatment. Many of these acute, symptomatic seizures resolve once the underlying etiology is corrected or the acute neurological disruption of the causal event subsides. Seizures that persist beyond the neonatal period most often result from long-standing cerebral pathology, such as developmental brain anomalies, inborn errors of metabolism, or as part of a genetic epilepsy syndrome, although these are less common than acute symptomatic causes. The electroencephalogram (EEG), amplitude-integrated EEG (aEEG), or quantitative electroencephalography (QEEG) may aid in rapid diagnosis and treatment of clinical and subclinical seizures [1, 2]. The new International League Against Epilepsy (ILAE) classification for neonatal seizures [3] emphasizes the need for EEG to clarify clinically suspicious movements, as the motor manifestations of seizures in neonates can be discrete [4, 5] or some normal movements and non-ictal abnormal movements may be mistaken for seizures [6]. In the absence of EEG or aEEG, only focal clonic or focal tonic seizures can be diagnosed clinically with at least probable diagnostic certainty [3, 7]. More than half of all seizures are electrographic-only, and consequently the seizure burden may be greatly underestimated without EEG or aEEG. If a clinical correlate is seen, the seizure semiology can have diagnostic value with respect to etiology; for example, clonic seizures are typical for arterial ischemic stroke, while tonic and sequential seizures suggest a genetic etiology [3].

Most EEG patterns in the neonate are nonspecific to the etiology of encephalopathy of seizures. However, even while nonspecific, certain patterns can help direct the diagnostic evaluation. For example, a burst suppression pattern narrows the differential diagnosis for a neonate with seizures considerably. EEG and etiologic correlations are not always straightforward: disorders that cause diffuse pathology can result in focal discharges [8], and focal seizures do not always reflect corresponding anatomical lesions, for example. However, in many cases, neuromonitoring may have specific characteristics that are helpful to direct further workup.

Vascular Causes

Acute Ischemic Stroke

Cerebral vascular disease in neonates can cause acute reactive seizures. Perinatal arterial ischemic stroke (PAIS) occurs in 1 in 2500 live births and is recognized as a common cause of early onset neonatal seizures [9]. Stroke should be suspected when seizures occur in neonates without encephalopathy within the first 48 hours of birth. Clinically, seizures due to ischemic stroke are most often focal clonic movements. EEG may be available for these patients before imaging is possible; there are specific features in the EEG that can aid in the diagnosis when evaluating neonatal seizures.

Acute ischemic neonatal strokes typically involve the middle cerebral artery. Decreased cerebral blood flow in the affected regions leads to focal electrographic changes in the background EEG (Figure 8.1). Focal amplitude suppression is a strong indicator of an infarction [10]. Depending on the size of the infarct, suppression can be quite marked (>50% amplitude reduction). The interictal EEG is typically normal from the contralateral hemisphere. Discrete abnormalities include unilateral absence of sleep–wake cycling or increase of theta (usually most obvious in quite sleep). However, a normal

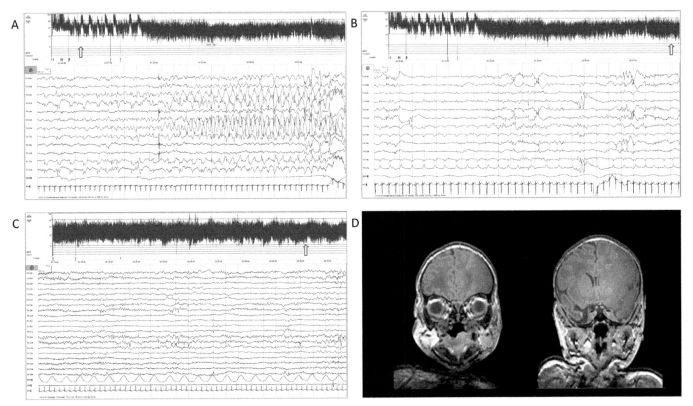

Figure 8.1 cEEG monitoring together with a single cross-cerebral (C3-C4) aEEG channel in a term baby (GA 40+2 weeks) with good Apgar scores, who presented on day of life 2 with clonic seizures. Note that left hemisphere channels are colored in red and right hemisphere channels in blue. Red arrows on the aEEG tracing correspond to the epoch of raw EEG displayed below. A. EEG on day 2 after treatment with phenobarbital captured electrographic-only seizures clearly visible on the aEEG tracing and on the raw EEG over the left central region. B. Seizures responded to second-line anti-seizure medication, but lateralized periodic discharges (LPDs) became apparent on EEG over the right hemisphere, which did not evolve in frequency, amplitude or morphology, therefore these were not considered to represent seizures. C. EEG on day of life 6: Seizures and LPDs have resolved, but background asymmetry is visible with amplitude attenuation and a paucity of faster frequencies over the left hemisphere. D. MRI (coronal T1) confirmed the diagnosis of a large left MCA infarct.

EEG in stroke has also been reported [11]. Depending on the location of the infarct, abnormalities may not be seen in an aEEG. In large central or parietal infarcts, amplitude asymmetry may be apparent when comparing hemispheric aEEG channels. It is not possible to evaluate for this asymmetry using only a cross-hemispheric (single) channel aEEG. Likewise, infarctions in brain regions distal to aEEG electrodes, such as occipital strokes or smaller inferior temporal strokes, may not result in changes in the central and parietal channels used in aEEG.

Periodic discharges may be present on EEG following stroke (Figure 8.1). Persistent, non-evolving, focal sharp waves or focal spike-polyspike waves may be seen at a frequency of 1–2 Hz over the area of infarction [12]. When repetitive focal discharges persist for at least six cycles, they are considered lateralized periodic discharges (LPD, previously called periodic lateralized epileptiform discharges or PLEDs) [13, 14]. These can be of variable amplitude and can be intermixed with seizures. LPDs often fluctuate and may not be present throughout the recording. In contrast to seizures, they do not evolve. The periodic discharges may subsequently evolve to focal electrographic seizures. LPDs are uncommon in neonates and are not diagnostic of stroke when present. At the same time, they

may increase suspicion for focal injury, including stroke, when present.

Quantitative EEG (QEEG) can highlight unilateral ischemia with loss of faster frequencies and increased slowing over the affected area on the spectrograms (Figure 8.2). The asymmetry index can reveal total absolute asymmetry by comparing the asymmetry at each pair of homologous electrodes and summing their absolute valuates to give a total asymmetry score. The alpha/delta ratio is affected and further enhances the abnormality since alpha frequencies decrease and delta increases with ischemia.

With MCA stroke, seizures are typically seen over the central region, often with sharp waves or spike and polyspike discharges in that region. The seizures usually consist of brief discharges of rhythmic spikes at variable frequency. They typically begin as focal 1–2 Hz discharges [15] over the area of infarction. As seizures evolve, the discharges often become biphasic or triphasic [15] but typically remain over the affected hemisphere. Rarely, the seizure may spread to the contralateral hemisphere. In between seizures, the neonate typically remains alert and not encephalopathic, though in severe cases they may be lethargic or comatose.

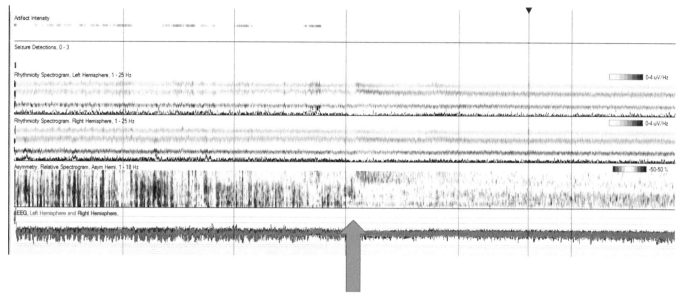

Figure 8.2 QEEG trending panel from a neonate born at 39 weeks gestation with stroke, demonstrating asymmetry. This is most evident in the Asymmetry Spectrogram [middle row], which is predominantly red for the first half of the trend. This reflects that during the first half of the recording period, the neonate was having seizures from the right hemisphere. After treatment [arrow], the seizures resolved. There is a brief period of faster frequencies in the left hemisphere relative to slowing on the right reflected by a denser blue color in the Asymmetry Spectrogram, followed by gradual return to an overall symmetric pattern.

Venous Sinus Thrombosis

More than 40% of childhood cerebral sinovenous thrombosis (CSVT) occurs within the neonatal period, with an incidence of 2–3 per 100,000 children per year [16]. CSVT can cause venous infarction and is often associated with hemorrhage. Seizures are a common manifestation of CSVT. No specific EEG or aEEG changes are typically found in CSVT. In a study by Berfelo et al., 46% of neonates with CSVT exhibited a normal EEG and aEEG with 19% and 13% showing moderately and severely depressed backgrounds, respectively [17]. However, when a focal infarct occurs secondary to CSVT, EEG changes occur that are similar to acute ischemic stroke, due to decreased cerebral perfusion. In animal studies, following CSVT rats have acute and transient EEG depression that is followed by a long-lasting slowing of the electrical activity [18].

Vein of Galen and Other Vascular Malformations

The vein of galen is a rare congenital vascular malformation but is the most common type of arteriovenous malformation in the fetus and neonate. Neonates with vein of Galen malformations can present with seizures or with high output cardiac failure. This and other vascular malformations, including aneurysms, can cause chronic seizures by leaking blood into the surrounding cortex and by causing cortical irritation through mass effect or pulsations. Large arteriovenous malformations create a steal phenomenon and render nearby regions of the brain ischemic. Vascular lesions in utero can result in formation of porencephalic cysts, which in turn can cause neonatal seizures. An EEG or aEEG is not specific to these malformations and shows abnormalities in less than 50% [19]. At the same time, the baseline EEG is abnormal in at least half of cases, typically with focal delta

activity, focal slowing, or a paroxysmal activity [20] over the area of interest.

Intracranial Hemorrhage

Seizures due to subarachnoid, intraparenchymal, or subdural hemorrhage may occur in term neonates. (Hemorrhage in preterm neonates is discussed separately below.) The most common type of intracranial hemorrhage in term neonates is primary subarachnoid hemorrhage, and can be diffuse or focal [21]. In term neonates, intraventricular hemorrhage most often occurs in the setting of cerebral sinovenous thrombosis, and can also be seen with subdural, subependymal, and intraparenchymal hemorrhages. In focal hemorrhages, focal or lateralized abnormalities may appear on EEG or aEEG. There is typically a pronounced unilateral EEG suppression with a marked loss of faster frequencies on the affected side. These EEG changes may be more marked than in patients with ischemic stroke. Ipsilateral to the hemorrhage, delta activity may appear widely, but maximally over the frontotemporal region. EEG may not reveal any epileptiform activity [21]. Clinical seizures can vary from apneic events [22] to clonic seizures. Intraventricular hemorrhage, or any hemorrhage that affects the periventricular white matter, can be associated with central positive sharp waves.

CNS Infection

The signs of meningitis or encephalitis are clinically nonspecific, even as early diagnosis and treatment are crucial. Prenatal and perinatal infections can produce diffuse static neocortical and hippocampal damage. Depending on infection severity, EEG background activity may vary from normal to having varying degrees of abnormality. In the case of CNS infection,

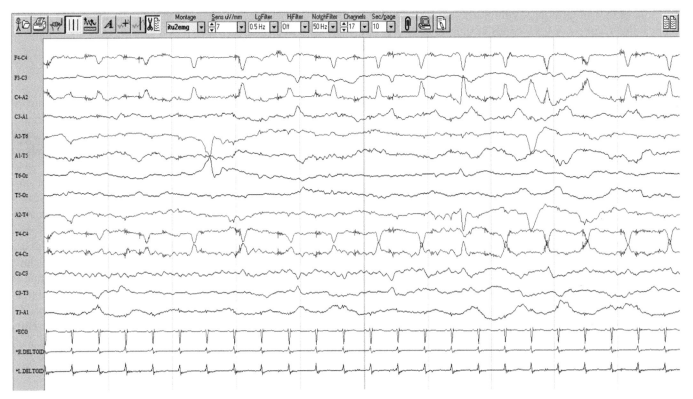

Figure 8.3 EEG from a neonate born at term after uneventful pregnancy via emergent caesarean section for failure to progress. Mother had low-grade fever. While initially in good condition and discharged to home, neonate presented day 5 in shock, with pH 6.9, and hypothermic. The EEG is abnormal with amplitude suppression, paucity of normal maturational pattern, and lateralized periodic discharges over the right central region. PCR for herpes simplex virus was positive.

seizures usually begin by day 3 after birth, except for HSV which more often presents with seizures in the second week. Group B *Streptococcus*, *Listeria*, *Escherichia coli*, and *Streptococcus pneumoniae* CNS infections present from the end of the first week to 3 months of age. The seizures may be subclinical or fragmentary.

Bacterial Meningoencephalitis

Cerebromeningeal infections are responsive for 5–10% of neonatal seizures [23]. The infection can lead to brain edema, vascular thrombosis, or abscess formation. Multiple nonspecific EEG patterns are described in meningoencephalitis. However, complications may reveal more specific abnormalities. Positive Rolandic sharp waves can be seen in deep white matter necrosis. Persistent hemispheric or focal voltage attenuation may be seen in large-vessel infarction or in abscess formation.

Encephalitis typically produces diffuse delta activity. Bursts of intermittent rhythmic delta activity (IRDA) imply involvement of the subcortical gray matter. In acute encephalitis, the degree of slowing usually parallels the severity of the clinical symptoms. The combination of EEG features, including background activity, presence of positive Rolandic sharp waves, presence of seizures, and presence of focal abnormalities, inform the prediction of outcome [24]. Focal neurological deficits may develop as a result of secondary arterial cerebrovascular disease, intracranial hemorrhage, subdural effusion, or developing brain abscess. Amplitude EEG can also aid in

prognostication for these babies. A flat or low-voltage background pattern and electrographic seizures on aEEG have been associated with poor neurological outcome in infants with neonatal sepsis or meningitis, whereas sleep–wake cycling was more likely to be seen in babies with subsequent good outcome [25].

Herpes Simplex Virus

Neonatal herpes simplex encephalitis is a rare but severe neurological condition that requires clinical identification and rapid treatment. Rapid treatment reduces the morbidity and mortality, so clinical suspicion must always be high for this disease. In contrast with adults, most neonatal CNS infection is not localized to the temporal lobes, but rather is diffuse disease secondary to disseminated infection. As such, EEG abnormalities are most often multifocal, rather than the classical temporal periodic discharges described in herpes simplex (HSV) cerebritis in adults. In the less common case of neonatal focal cerebritis, the EEG may show specific changes. The ictal and interictal EEG may be nonspecific at the onset of the disease. Later in the course, the EEG reveals the more classical periodic discharges which begin in the temporal head regions and then may become more diffuse. There is typically focal or multifocal slowing with quasi-periodic discharges that may shift from side to side [26]. When present, lateralized periodic discharges typically appear 2–15 days after the onset of illness (Figure 8.3). They are typically maximal in the temporal/parieto-temporal regions and often consist of waveforms with no more than three phases that are prolonged complexes (approximately 0.5 seconds) that recur every 1–4 seconds for at least six cycles. The amplitudes vary from 500 µV to very subtle changes from the background. The discharge may be spike-like or a sharply contoured delta wave.

Acute Metabolic Disturbances

Electrolyte Disturbances

Electrolyte disturbances can present with neurological manifestations [27]. Acute and severe electrolyte imbalances frequently cause seizures, and seizures may be the sole presenting symptom. Seizures and encephalopathy are especially common in patients with hyponatremia, hypocalcemia, and hypomagnesemia. These changes in blood electrolytes may cause an encephalopathy and consequently diffuse EEG abnormalities. In 1937, Berger first observed slow brain activity induced by hypoglycemia. Typically in acute metabolic encephalopathies, the EEG may demonstrate no change or may demonstrate slowing of background frequencies [28]. Disorganization of the background may develop gradually, and reactivity to external stimulation may be altered [29]. The EEG changes typically correlate with the severity of encephalopathy. While EEG findings are not specific to different etiologies of encephalopathy, some more common patterns have been described. In general, hyponatremia usually produces nonspecific slowing. Hypocalcemia may be associated with a background at first with mainly alpha frequencies that progresses to a theta and delta predominance. In neonates, reversible 3- to 4-Hz spike–wave discharges have been reported [30]. In hypercalcemia, EEG changes include fast activity and bursts of delta and theta slowing that appear when calcium levels reach ~13 mg/dL. When calcium levels normalize, the EEG gradually improves.

Hypoglycemia

Hypoglycemia alters cerebral blood flow and metabolism, which is reflected in the EEG. When compared with controls, hypoglycemic newborns have increased frontal sharp transients in all sleep stages and have less bilateral synchrony [31, 32]. Hypoglycemia may also result in bilateral or unilateral posterior spike and sharp waves in a generalized slow background. The discharges are accentuated with sleep but not with photic stimulation [33]. Several studies have demonstrated that hypoglycemia can cause cortical and subcortical white matter damage, with the posterior parietal and occipital lobes affected most severely [34–36] (Figure 8.4). The level of blood glucose that causes the injury is variable. The epilepsy that develops months or years after symptomatic neonatal hypoglycemia is most often focal epilepsy of occipital origin [37, 38]. A proportion of children also have visual impairment and neurodevelopmental disability, and seizures may become drug resistant.

Brain Injury in Premature Neonates

Intraventricular Hemorrhage

Intraventricular hemorrhage (IVH) is the most frequent form of intracranial hemorrhage in newborns at less than 32 weeks gestation. During this time, bleeding occurs from capillaries in the germinal matrix. There are four grades of IVH that are used to determine the severity of symptoms. In grade I, the bleeding is confined to the germinal matrix. In grade II, there is

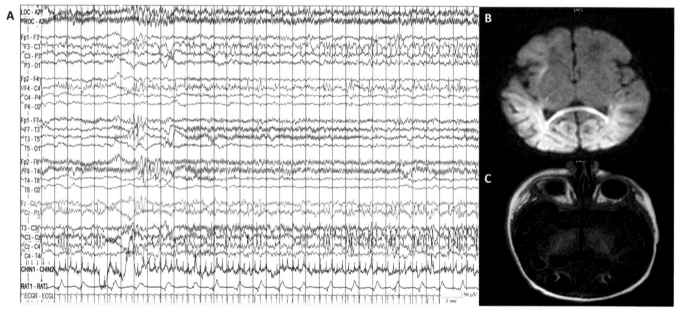

Figure 8.4 Neonate with severe hypoglycemia in the first day of life. Three-day-old baby girl born at 39 weeks following normal pregnancy and delivery. She returned to the hospital 24 hours after discharge because of lethargy and poor feeding. Workup revealed significant hypoglycemia (glucose <20 g/dL). Genetic testing confirmed a pathogenic mutation on the *ABCC8* gene consistent with congenital hyperinsulinism. (A) EEG at the age of 3 days showing a seizure with onset over the left central region (C3) in a bipolar longitudinal montage. (B) MRI at 10 days of life. Diffusion-weighted imaging (DWI) sequence showing restricted diffusion of bilateral occipital lobes as well as splenium of corpus callosum. (C) T1 flair sequence done 1 month after initial MRI showing atrophy of bilateral occipital lobes.

intraventricular bleeding without ventricular enlargement. Grade III consists of larger intraventricular bleeding (>50% of ventricular area or distends ventricle), and grade IV represents intraventricular hemorrhage and blood in the brain tissue around the ventricles [39]. Seizures, mostly electrographic, are more commonly seen in neonates with grade III and IV IVH, both acutely and chronically [40]. Although seizures are thought to be prevalent in premature neonates, they are unlikely to be detected clinically and are most likely underestimated. Lloyd et al. prospectively performed cEEG from as soon as possible after birth for a duration of up to 72 hours in a cohort of 120 newborns <32 weeks gestational age [41]. They found that only 6 infants (5%) had electrographic seizures; five of these had IVH. There do not appear to be any specific EEG features associated with IVH in preterm neonates. The background activity in EEG and aEEG is depressed during the first days of life, and the extent of the depression correlates with the degree of IVH [42]. Watanabe et al. described that the EEG background showed an increasing discontinuity with increasing severity of IVH. The EEG typically is of little diagnostic value but can aid in prognosis [43]. There are acute and chronic EEG changes that correlate with later neurological and cognitive function. Acute stage abnormalities mainly consist of decreased continuity, attenuated faster frequencies, or voltage suppression (Figure 8.5). Chronic state abnormalities consist of dysmature or disorganized patterns [44]. A disorganized background refers to an abnormal morphology of background activities without definite findings of acute stage EEG changes [45]. In order to determine prognosis, serial EEGs are more helpful, as persistent abnormalities are more predictive of prognosis than a single abnormal EEG [46].

There have been conflicting studies regarding the occurrence of positive sharp waves with IVH. Clancy and Tharp found that neonates with grades III and IV hemorrhage had a higher prevalence (69.2%) of central positive sharp waves that were greatest between the 5th and 8th postnatal days [47].

Novotny et al. concluded that central positive sharp waves are not specific for IVH but rather white-matter necrosis which may result from a variety of insults, including IVH [48]. Aso et al. found that the sensitivity of positive sharp waves for white matter lesions was 38% [49].

Post-hemorrhagic hydrocephalus is a major complication after IVH and can be defined as progressive dilation of the ventricular system. With increasing ventricular diameter, aEEG reveals an increased discontinuity without distinguishable sleep–wake cycling in neonates [50]. Therefore, loss of sleep–wake cycling on the aEEG has a high predictive value for the development of post-hemorrhagic hydrocephalus in preterm neonates with IVH [51]. For this reason, in addition to serial head ultrasounds and close clinical monitoring, some centers use serial aEEG once or twice weekly to monitor for early evidence of post-hemorrhagic hydrocephalus, before head circumference increases.

Periventricular Leukomalacia (PVL)

Periventricular leukomalacia (PVL) occurs in 5% of premature neonates. EEG is sensitive in detecting PVL in the neonatal period, though the abnormalities seen are not specific to this etiology; the acute and chronic EEG stage abnormalities present with IVH are also seen with PVL. Positive Rolandic sharp (PRS) waves are commonly seen and may be an early and marker of PVL [52] (Figure 8.5). PRS are sharp transients of positive polarity that appear in the Rolandic region in the centrotemporal area of the brain. Okumura and colleagues found that PRS were always associated with disorganized patterns on the EEG [53]. In another study, he found that among 52 preterm neonates with a disorganized pattern on their EEG, PVL was present in 31 [54]. In contrast, among the 28 neonates with just dysmature EEG patterns, PVL was present in only one neonate. Kidokoro et al. looked at the evolution of EEG changes seen with PVL. In general, the EEG was depressed

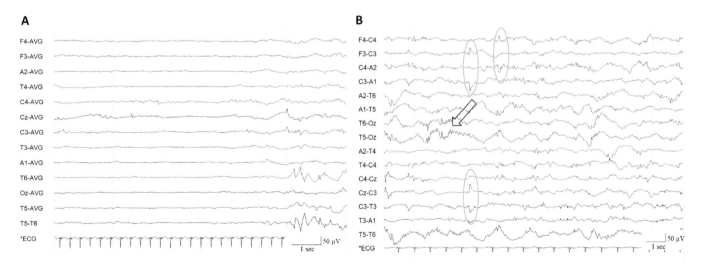

Figure 8.5 EEG from preterm infant born at 29 weeks gestational age. At post-menstrual age (PMA) 32 weeks he had an acute deterioration; cranial ultrasound revealed a grade IV intraventricular hemorrhage. (A) EEG on the day of the deterioration shows diffuse suppression and prolonged inter-burst intervals (equivalent to acute stage abnormality). (B) At PMA of 37 weeks the background activity is continuous but dysmature with too many delta brushes for age [arrow] and positive Rolandic sharp waves independently over both sides [yellow circles], both of which are chronic stage abnormalities.

immediately after birth and improved after a few days. The EEG then developed chronic changes that included a disorganized background with or without frontal and/or occipital sharp waves, positive Rolandic sharp waves, and abnormal delta brushes [55]. The combination of acute and chronic stage abnormalities on the EEG is important to detect neonates with PVL since acute changes are highly sensitive and chronic changes are highly specific – it is the combination of both that is most diagnostically useful [56]. aEEG can be useful in displaying the early changes of amplitude suppression, but is not able to display the more chronic changes of disorganization or sharp waves. Spectral analysis of the EEG may reveal an association between white matter injury and decreased spectral edge frequency [57].

Very Low Birth Weight Neonates

"Very low birth weight" is a term used to describe neonates who are born weighing less than 1,500 grams. Neonates with very low birth weights are most often premature with intrauterine growth restriction (IUGR) and have discontinuous EEG tracings. These neonates are at risk for seizures. Independent risk factors for seizures in these babies include early gestational age, intraventricular hemorrhage, post-hemorrhagic hydrocephalus, sepsis, and necrotizing enterocolitis. Neonates with both sepsis and necrotizing enterocolitis had a 4.6-fold increased risk of seizure [58]. Germinal matrix intraventricular hemorrhage in these babies had an overall incidence of seizures in 46% in an early series, though this was based on clinical observation of suspected seizures and did not include EEG confirmation [59]. In a study of 39 low birth weight neonates, preterm neonates, and small for gestational age neonates had EEG demonstrating similar background abnormalities. Spindle-like fast rhythms were more frequent over the occipital and/or central areas and were more frequent at 31–32 weeks post–conceptional age. A greater number of fast rhythms occurred in REM sleep than in slow wave sleep at 26–32 weeks and was reversed from 33–34 weeks with more fast rhythms in slow wave sleep [60]. The long-term significance of these findings has not been demonstrated.

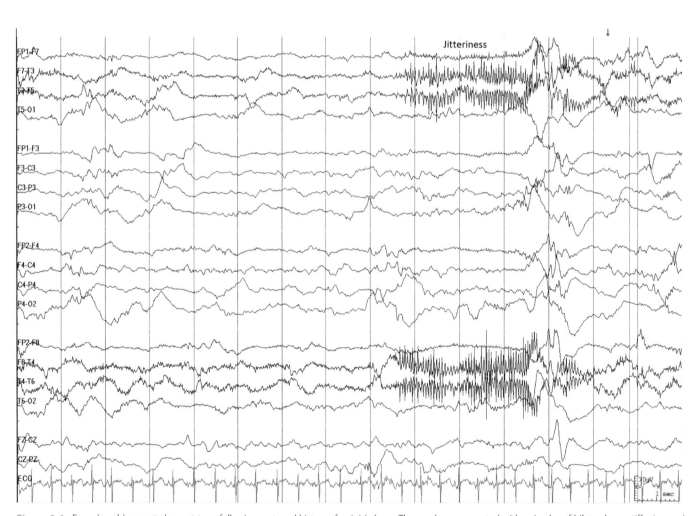

Figure 8.6 Four-day-old neonate born at term following maternal history of opioid abuse. The newborn presented with episodes of bilateral arm stiffening and shaking; these were suppressible. A typical event was marked as "jitteriness" by the bedside nurse. The EEG shows continuous background activity and scattered multifocal sharp waves. The event is shown not to be seizure, but characterized by muscle and movement artifact. cEEG confirmed that the clinical events of concern were not seizure for this child.

Neonatal Abstinence Syndrome

Neonatal abstinence syndrome refers to the constellation of withdrawal symptoms exhibited by the neonate who was exposed to drugs in utero. The onset and nature of symptoms usually varies depending on the specific drug and timing of exposure. Symptoms of withdrawal from heroin typically begin within 24 hours after birth, and from methadone, around 24 to 72 hours of age. Babies exposed to drugs in utero have an increased risk of seizure. At the same time, diagnosis may be challenging as these babies commonly have other abnormal movements that are not seizures, such as jittery movements (Figure 8.6). Seizures have been reported in 2% to 11% of cases during neonatal opioid withdrawal [61]. Withdrawal-associated seizures are often myoclonic, respond to opiates, and have not been shown to increase the risk of adverse long-term outcome [62]. Abnormal EEG without seizures has been reported in greater than 30% of cases of neonatal opioid withdrawal. In a study by Doberczak et al., 17 of 38 babies (45%) with neonatal exposure to cocaine had abnormal EEGs. All the abnormal EEGs showed bursts of sharp waves and spikes, with the majority revealing multifocal abnormalities [63] (Tables 8.1 and 8.2).

Table 8.1 Acute causes of neonatal seizures and accompanying EEG changes in term and preterm neonates

EEG changes	Etiology: Common causes
Abnormal asymmetry	Stroke, venous sinus thrombosis, venous malformation, cerebral contusion, hemorrhage, abscess
Abnormal asynchrony	Meningitis, PVL
Depressed and undifferentiated background	HIE, CNS infection, cerebral hemorrhage, acute metabolic disturbances
Positive Rolandic sharp waves	PVL, intraventricular hemorrhage, meningitis, hydrocephalus, aminoaciduria
Lateralized periodic discharges	Stroke, focal cerebritis
Sharp waves, spikes, polyspikes	Stroke, infection, neonatal abstinence syndrome
Burst suppression	Ohtahara syndrome, early myoclonic epilepsy, inborn error of metabolism, severe HIE

CNS, central nervous system; HIE, hypoxic-ischemic encephalopathy; PVL, periventricular leukomalacia

Table 8.2 Typical EEG features of neonatal seizures due to specific causes

Etiology	Typical time of onset	Type of seizure	EEG pattern
Acute ischemic stroke	12–76 hours after birth	Clonic, contralateral	Focal slowing Focal suppression Lateralized periodic discharges Focal sharp or spike waves Focal seizures
Intracranial infections	Days to weeks after birth	All types	Rolandic sharp waves Rhythmic delta activity Diffuse slowing Focal slowing Lateralized periodic discharges Focal spikes
Intracranial hemorrhage	Subdural: first 1–2 days Subarachnoid: first 5 days	Multifocal, clonic	Focal slowing Focal suppression
Metabolic or electrolyte abnormalities	Hypoglycemia: first 2 days Hyperbilirubinemia: after 3rd day Other electrolytes: any time	All types	Generalized slowing Disorganization

References

1. McCoy B, Hahn CD. Continuous EEG monitoring in the neonatal intensive care unit. *J Clin Neurophysiol.* 2013;**30** (2):106–14.

2. Abend NS, Dlugos DJ, Clancy RR. A review of long-term EEG monitoring in critically ill children with hypoxic-ischemic encephalopathy, congenital heart disease, ECMO, and stroke. *J Clin Neurophysiol.* 2013;**30**(2):134–42.

3. Pressler RM, Cilio MR, Mizrahi EM, et al. The ILAE classification of seizures and the epilepsies: Modification for seizures in the neonate. Position paper by the ILAE Task Force on Neonatal Seizures. *Epilepsia.* 2021;**62**(3):615–28.

4. Boylan GB, Pressler RM, Rennie JM, et al. Outcome of electroclinical, electrographic, and clinical seizures in the newborn infant. *Dev Med Child Neurol.* 1999;**41**(12):819–25.

5. Glass HC. Neonatal seizures: advances in mechanisms and management. *Clin Perinatol.* 2014;**41**(1):177–90.

6. Murray DM, Boylan GB, Ali I, et al. Defining the gap between electrographic seizure burden, clinical expression and staff recognition of neonatal seizures. *Arch Dis Child Fetal Neonatal Ed.* 2008;**93**(3):F187–91.

7. Pellegrin S, Munoz FM, Padula M, et al. Neonatal seizures: case definition & guidelines for data collection, analysis, and presentation of immunization safety data. *Vaccine.* 2019;**37**(52):7596–609.

8. Lombroso CT. Seizures in the newborn period. In Vinken PJ, Bruyn GW, editors. *Handbook of Clinical Neurology.* Volume 15: *The Epilepsies.* Amsterdam: North-Holland; 1974, pp. 189–218.

9. Lynch JK, Nelson KB. Epidemiology of perinatal stroke. *Curr Opin Pediatr.* 2001;**13**(6):499–505.

10. Clancy R, Malin S, Laraque D, Baumgart S, Younkin D. Focal motor seizures heralding stroke in full-term neonates. *Am J Dis Child.* 1985;**139** (6):601–6.

11. Mercuri E, Rutherford M, Cowan F, et al. Early prognostic indicators of outcome in infants with neonatal cerebral infarction: a clinical, electroencephalogram, and magnetic resonance imaging study. *Pediatrics.* 1999;**103**(1):39–46.

12. Scher MS, Beggarly M. Clinical significance of focal periodic discharges in neonates. *J Child Neurol.* 1989;**4** (3):175–85.

13. Tsuchida TN, Wusthoff CJ, Shellhaas RA, et al. American clinical neurophysiology society standardized EEG terminology and categorization for the description of continuous EEG monitoring in neonates: report of the American Clinical Neurophysiology Society critical care monitoring committee. *J Clin Neurophysiol.* 2013;**30**(2):161–73.

14. Herman ST, Abend NS, Bleck TP, et al. Consensus statement on continuous EEG in critically ill adults and children, part II: personnel, technical specifications, and clinical practice. *J Clin Neurophysiol.* 2015;**32**(2):96–108.

15. Walsh BH, Low E, Bogue CO, Murray DM, Boylan GB. Early continuous video electroencephalography in neonatal stroke. *Dev Med Child Neurol.* 2011;**53**(1):89–92.

16. Bonduel M, Sciuccati G, Hepner M et al. Arterial ischemic stroke and cerebral venous thrombosis in children: a 12-year Argentinean registry. *Acta Haematol.* 2006;**115**(3–4):180–5.

17. Berfelo FJ, Kersbergen KJ, van Ommen CH, et al. Neonatal cerebral sinovenous thrombosis from symptom to outcome. *Stroke.* 2010;**41**(7):1382–8.

18. Frerichs KU, Deckert M, Kempski O, et al. Cerebral sinus and venous thrombosis in rats induces long-term deficits in brain function and morphology–evidence for a cytotoxic genesis. *J Cereb Blood Flow Metab.* 1994;**14**(2):289–300.

19. Kelly JJ, Jr., Mellinger JF, Sundt TM, Jr. Intracranial arteriovenous malformations in childhood. *Ann Neurol.* 1978;**3**(4):338–43.

20. Paiva T, Campos J, Baeta E, et al. EEG monitoring during endovascular embolization of cerebral arteriovenous malformations. *Electroencephalogr Clin Neurophysiol.* 1995;**95**(1):3–13.

21. Fenichel GM, Webster DL, Wong WK. Intracranial hemorrhage in the term newborn. *Arch Neurol.* 1984;**41**(1):30–4.

22. Tramonte JJ, Goodkin HP. Temporal lobe hemorrhage in the full-term neonate presenting as apneic seizures. *J Perinatol.* 2004;**24**(11):726–9.

23. Holt DE, Halket S, de Louvois J, Harvey D. Neonatal meningitis in England and Wales: 10 years on. *Arch Dis Child Fetal Neonatal Ed.* 2001;**84**(2):F85–9.

24. Chequer RS, Tharp BR, Dreimane D, et al. Prognostic value of EEG in neonatal meningitis: retrospective study of 29 infants. *PediatrNeurol.* 1992;**8** (6):417–22.

25. ter Horst HJ, van Olffen M, Remmelts HJ, de Vries H, Bos AF. The prognostic value of amplitude integrated EEG in neonatal sepsis and/or meningitis. *Acta Paediatrica.* 2010;**99**(2):194–200.

26. Mizrahi EM, Tharp BR. A characteristic EEG pattern in neonatal herpes simplex encephalitis. *Neurology.* 1982;**32** (11):1215–20.

27. Riggs JE. Neurologic manifestations of electrolyte disturbances. *Neurol Clin.* 2002;**20**(1):227–39, vii.

28. Lin CC. [EEG manifestations in metabolic encephalopathy]. *Acta Neurol Taiwan.* 2005;**14**(3):151–61.

29. Kaplan PW. The EEG in metabolic encephalopathy and coma. *J Clin Neurophysiol.* 2004;**21**(5):307–18.

30. Kossoff EH, Silvia MT, Maret A, Carakushansky M, Vining EP. Neonatal hypocalcemic seizures: case report and literature review. *J Child Neurol.* 2002;**17**(3):236–9.

31. Nunes ML, Penela MM, da Costa JC. Differences in the dynamics of frontal sharp transients in normal and hypoglycemic newborns. *Clin Neurophysiol.* 2000;**111**(2):305–10.

32. Moore AM, Perlman M. Symptomatic hypoglycemia in otherwise healthy, breastfed term newborns. *Pediatrics.* 1999;**103** (4 Pt 1):837–9.

33. Yalnizoglu D, Haliloglu G, Turanli G, Cila A, Topcu M. Neurologic outcome in patients with MRI pattern of damage typical for neonatal hypoglycemia. *Brain Dev.* 2007;**29**(5):285–92.

34. Tam EW, Widjaja E, Blaser SI et al. Occipital lobe injury and cortical visual outcomes after neonatal hypoglycemia. *Pediatrics.* 2008;**122**(3):507–12.

35. Barkovich AJ, Ali FA, Rowley HA, Bass N. Imaging patterns of neonatal hypoglycemia. *AJNR Am J Neuroradiol.* 1998;**19**(3):523–8.

36. Vannucci RC, Vannucci SJ. Hypoglycemic brain injury. *Semin Neonatol.* 2001;**6**(2):147–55.

37. Caraballo RH, Sakr D, Mozzi M, et al. Symptomatic occipital lobe epilepsy following neonatal hypoglycemia. *Pediatr Neurol.* 2004;**31**(1):24–9.

38. Fong CY, Harvey AS. Variable outcome for epilepsy after neonatal

hypoglycaemia. *Dev Med Child Neurol.* 2014;**56**(11):1093–9.

39. Volpe JJ. *Neurology of the Newborn.* 5th ed. Elsevier Health Sciences; 2008.

40. Strober JB, Bienkowski RS, Maytal J. The incidence of acute and remote seizures in children with intraventricular hemorrhage. *Clin Pediatr (Phila).* 1997;**36**(11):643–7.

41. Lloyd RO, O'Toole JM, Pavlidis E, Filan PM, Boylan GB. Electrographic Seizures during the Early Postnatal Period in Preterm Infants. *J Pediatr.* 2017;**187**:18–25 e2.

42. Hellstrom-Westas L, Klette H, Thorngren-Jerneck K, Rosen I. Early prediction of outcome with aEEG in preterm infants with large intraventricular hemorrhages. *Neuropediatrics.* 2001;**32**(6):319–24.

43. Watanabe K, Hakamada S, Kuroyanagi M, Yamazaki T, Takeuchi T. Electroencephalographic study of intraventricular hemorrhage in the preterm newborn. *Neuropediatrics.* 1983;**14**(4):225–30.

44. Watanabe K, Hayakawa F, Okumura A. Neonatal EEG: a powerful tool in the assessment of brain damage in preterm infants. *Brain Dev.* 1999;**21**(6):361–72.

45. Watanabe H. The neonatal electroencephalogram and sleep-cycle patterns. In Eyre J, editor. *The Neurophysiological Examination of the Newborn Infant Clinics in Developmental Medicine.* London: Mac Keith Press; 1992, pp. 11–47.

46. Tharp BR, Scher MS, Clancy RR. Serial EEGs in normal and abnormal infants with birth weights less than 1200 grams–a prospective study with long term follow-up. *Neuropediatrics.* 1989;**20**(2):64–72.

47. Clancy RR, Tharp BR. Positive Rolandic sharp waves in the electroencephalograms of premature neonates with intraventricular hemorrhage. *Electroencephalogr Clin Neurophysiol.* 1984;**57**(5):395–404.

48. Novotny EJ, Jr., Tharp BR, Coen RW, et al. Positive Rolandic sharp waves in the EEG of the premature infant. *Neurology.* 1987;**37**(9):1481–6.

49. Aso K, Abdab-Barmada M, Scher MS. EEG and the neuropathology in premature neonates with intraventricular hemorrhage. *J Clin Neurophysiol.* 1993;**10**(3):304–13.

50. Olischar M, Klebermass K, Kuhle S, et al. Progressive posthemorrhagic hydrocephalus leads to changes of amplitude-integrated EEG activity in preterm infants. *Childs Nerv Syst.* 2004;**20**(1):41–5.

51. Scoppa A, Casani A, Cocca F, et al. aEEG in preterm infants. *J Matern Fetal Neonatal Med.* 2012;**25** Suppl 4:139–40.

52. Baud O, d'Allest AM, Lacaze-Masmonteil T, et al. The early diagnosis of periventricular leukomalacia in premature infants with positive Rolandic sharp waves on serial electroencephalography. *J Pediatr.* 1998;**132**(5):813–7.

53. Okumura A, Hayakawa F, Kato T, Kuno K, Watanabe K. Positive Rolandic sharp waves in preterm infants with periventricular leukomalacia: their relation to background electroencephalographic abnormalities. *Neuropediatrics.* 1999;**30**(6):278–82.

54. Okumura A, Hayakawa F, Kato T, Kuno K, Watanabe K. Developmental outcome and types of chronic-stage EEG abnormalities in preterm infants. *Dev Med Child Neurol.* 2002;**44**(11):729–34.

55. Kidokoro H, Okumura A, Hayakawa F, et al. Chronologic changes in neonatal EEG findings in periventricular leukomalacia. *Pediatrics.* 2009;**124**(3):e468–75.

56. Kubota T, Okumura A, Hayakawa F, et al. Combination of neonatal electroencephalography and ultrasonography: sensitive means of early diagnosis of periventricular leukomalacia. *Brain Dev.* 2002;**24**(7):698–702.

57. Inder TE, Buckland L, Williams CE, et al. Lowered electroencephalographic spectral edge frequency predicts the presence of cerebral white matter injury in premature infants. *Pediatrics.* 2003;**111**(1):27–33.

58. Kohelet D, Shochat R, Lusky A, Reichman B, Israel Neonatal N. Risk factors for seizures in very low birthweight infants with periventricular leukomalacia. *J Child Neurol.* 2006;**21**(11):965–70.

59. Hawgood S, Spong J, Yu VY. Intraventricular hemorrhage. Incidence and outcome in a population of very-low-birth-weight infants. *Am J Dis Child.* 1984;**138**(2):136–9.

60. Watanabe K, Iwase K. Spindle-like fast rhythms in the EEGs of low-birth weight infants. *Dev Med Child Neurol.* 1972;**14**(3):373–81.

61. Hudak ML, Tan RC. Committee on Drugs; Committee on Fetus and Newborn; American Academy of Pediatrics. Neonatal drug withdrawal. *Pediatrics.* 2012;**129**(2):e540–60.

62. Doberczak TM SS, Cutler R, Senie RT, Loucopoulos JA, Kandall SR. One-year follow-up of infants with abstinence-associated seizures. *Arch Neurol.* 1988;**45**(6):649–53.

63. Doberczak TM, Shanzer S, Senie RT, Kandall SR. Neonatal neurologic and electroencephalographic effects of intrauterine cocaine exposure. *J Pediatr.* 1988;**113**(2):354–8.

Neonatal Onset Epilepsy

Akihisa Okumura

Illustrative Cases

Case 9 KCNQ2-Related Seizures

Case 10 Tuberous Sclerosis

Case 11 Hemimegalencephaly

Case 12 Ohtahara Syndrome

Case 13 Zellweger Syndrome

Case 14 Pyridoxine-Dependent Epilepsy

Case 15 Metabolic Encephalopathy

Case 16 Glycine Encephalopathy

Key Points

• Neonatal onset epilepsy is less common than seizures due to acute illness but constitutes an important minority of cases.

• EEG and aEEG are helpful for the diagnosis and management of seizures, and for characterizing the epilepsy syndrome. EEG and aEEG are rarely specific for an underlying genetic, metabolic, or structural cause.

• Neonatal clinical epilepsy syndromes may result from any of multiple distinct etiologies. Conversely, mutations in individual genes have been described to cause variable phenotypes.

Introduction

Neonatal seizures have diverse causes. Most are the result of acute problems, such as hypoxic-ischemic encephalopathy, stroke, central nervous system infection, or electrolyte derangement. Neonatal seizures with acute symptomatic etiologies are excluded from the definition of neonatal onset epilepsy, as acute symptomatic neonatal seizures typically resolve as the acute brain insult stabilizes. As compared to acute symptomatic seizures, neonatal seizures of remote etiologies, including structural, genetic, and metabolic causes, are less common. Approximately 10–15% of neonates with seizures have an underlying neonatal onset epilepsy [1]. Because they are not expected resolve quickly, and reflect a more chronic condition, these seizures are considered neonatal onset epilepsies. The recognition of neonatal epilepsies is important for improving the outcomes of infants, especially those with epileptic encephalopathies, as it allows early detection, precise diagnosis, and appropriate treatment.

Conventional EEG remains the gold standard for the diagnosis of neonatal seizures. In addition, interictal EEG can assist in assessing the severity and type of brain dysfunction in each infant. Amplitude-integrated EEG (aEEG) has been used increasingly in neonatal intensive care units (NICUs) for the diagnosis and monitoring of neonatal seizures. The EEG findings of neonates with seizures are usually dependent upon the abnormalities caused by acute brain insults. However, the EEG findings of neonatal epilepsies can differ substantially, even among patients with the same disorder. As each individual disorder is rare with variable manifestations, it is currently difficult to definitively detail the EEG/aEEG findings in each of the neonatal epilepsies. Rather, some features more commonly seen can be described, with recognition that there is variability between patients. Ongoing research is necessary for the development of a more comprehensive description of the EEG findings in neonatal epilepsies.

Etiology

Many underlying disorders can act as a remote etiology of neonatal seizures. These are classified into structural, genetic, and metabolic types. There is often overlap in phenotypes across multiple etiologies; conversely, mutations in individual genes have been demonstrated to manifest as a variety of phenotypes. Systematic approaches to diagnosis have been suggested for the diagnostic evaluation in neonatal epilepsy [2].

Among the structural causes, various malformations in cortical development are the most common, accounting for 5–9% of neonatal epilepsies [3, 4]. Hemimegalencephaly (also known as unilateral megalencephaly), holoprosencephaly, lissencephaly, focal cortical dysplasia, tuberous sclerosis, schizencephaly, and polymicrogyria are among causes of neonatal epilepsies. Less common causes of neonatal epilepsies are intrauterine acquired lesions, such as porencephaly secondary to in utero periventricular hemorrhage, ulegyria secondary to intrauterine ischemia, and congenital infection. As neuroimaging techniques improve, structural causes of neonatal epilepsy are increasingly recognized.

The list of genetic disorders causing neonatal epilepsies is growing rapidly. As a result of the outstanding methodological progress in genetic analyses, many genes are now known to be associated with neonatal epilepsies. However, the genotype–phenotype correlation in these genes is not always straightforward. *KCNQ2* was first recognized as the causative gene of benign familial neonatal seizures (BFNS) [5], whereas later studies revealed that *KCNQ2* mutations are also found in infants with epileptic encephalopathy of neonatal onset [6]. *SCN2A* mutations were first found in patients with benign familial neonatal–infantile seizures [7].

However, *SCN2A* mutations are also present in some patients with other severe phenotypes, including early infantile epileptic encephalopathy (EIEE), Dravet syndrome, and epilepsy of infancy with migrating focal seizures. Further research is needed to clarify how individual mutations and modifying factors might be associated with specific phenotypes.

Metabolic causes, that is, inborn errors of metabolism, are rare but important causes of neonatal epilepsies. Prompt diagnosis is necessary to start appropriate treatment and potentially prevent irreversible neurodevelopmental sequelae. Metabolic causes of neonatal epilepsies are classified into three different categories: disturbances in neurotransmitter metabolism, disorders of energy production, and biosynthetic defects. In a majority of these disorders, there are biomarkers that can serve as clues to diagnosis: an elevation of glycine level is characteristic of non-ketotic hyperglycinemia, increased sulfite levels are crucial in isolated sulfite oxidase deficiency and molybdenum cofactor deficiency, and an elevation in very long-chain fatty acids is seen in peroxisomal disorders. A detailed discussion of each of these individual disorders is beyond the scope of this chapter (see the review by Dulac et al. [8]); rather, unifying characteristics and EEG findings are discussed below.

The classification of the causes of neonatal epilepsies is not always simple. Inborn errors of metabolism and most of the malformations in cortical development are likely genetic disorders, even if the causative gene is difficult to determine. Similarly, lissencephaly due to *ARX* mutations can be categorized as both a genetic disorder and a structural disorder. Zellweger syndrome is one of the peroxisomal biogenesis disorders caused by mutations in *PEX* genes, which are associated with malformations in cortical development and metabolic disorders, including elevations in very long-chain fatty acids levels. Classifications of the causes of neonatal epilepsy may be revised as knowledge increases about the basic mechanisms of epileptogenicity.

Clinical Manifestations

Studies have attempted to distinguish etiology of neonatal seizures by seizure semiology. Focal clonic seizures are most commonly seen when the etiology is acute provoked illness [9], though importantly, this is not diagnostic. Similarly, myoclonic seizures are particularly common in inborn errors of metabolism or vitamin-dependent epilepsies [10]. Clinical features rarely are specific to a particular gene mutation among the genetic epilepsies [11]. One must always be aware of electroclinical uncoupling in neonates suspected to have seizures. Ictal EEGs show that the majority of seizures are subclinical and not associated with any clinical symptoms. Conversely, many suspicious clinical phenomena such as bicycling/pedaling and crawling are not of cortical origin and do not represent seizures. The diagnosis of seizures based on visual observation of clinical behaviors is unreliable, and misdiagnosis can occur frequently [12]. Thus, the diagnosis of seizures in neonates must be confirmed by some form of EEG.

Electroencephalography

Conventional EEG

Conventional EEG plays an essential role in the diagnosis of neonatal epilepsies. Ictal EEG recordings are necessary to unequivocally determine the presence or absence of seizures. The American Clinical Neurophysiology Society has proposed a standard for neurophysiological monitoring in neonates [13]. Continuous video-EEG with electrodes placed according to the International 10–20 system modified for neonates, is the gold standard for monitoring [14]. Even in infants with neonatal epilepsies, some non-epileptic motor symptoms mimicking epileptic seizures may be observed. When two or more different seizure-like phenomena are seen in one infant, an ictal EEG recording should be performed to determine whether each clinical phenomenon is epileptic or non-epileptic. When non-epileptic seizure-like phenomena are misdiagnosed as epileptic seizures, unnecessary anti-seizure medications may be administered in high doses for a long period, leading to potential adverse effects on the developing brain.

Most seizures in infants with neonatal epilepsies are of focal onset. Focal-onset seizures in neonatal epilepsies are usually characterized by a sudden, repetitive, evolving, and stereotyped ictal EEG pattern with a clear beginning, middle and end, and a minimum duration of 10 seconds [15]. These EEG findings are similar to acute symptomatic seizures in neonates. The minimum seizure duration of 10 seconds is applied by convention for electrographic-only seizures. Brief rhythmic discharges (BRDs) consist of electrographic activity meeting the criteria for a seizure except that they last less than 10 seconds; BRDs occur more often in neonates with pathological findings and often co-exist with subclinical seizures [16]. The site of seizure onset is most commonly in the central and temporal areas, although other locations are not rare. Bilaterally synchronous generalized spike-and-wave complexes are exceedingly rare in neonates. This may be explained by the physiological and anatomical characteristics of the immature brain, including the lack of well-developed dendritic systems, the paucity of synapses, and the poor myelination of axons, which can limit synaptic transmission and reduce widespread recruitment of epileptic networks in the neonate.

Generalized seizures in neonates are limited to epileptic spasms, myoclonic seizures, and tonic seizures. These are typically of brief duration. In these types of seizures when there is a clear clinical correlate to the ictal EEG pattern, the minimum duration of 10 seconds is not required. Interestingly, a Neonatal Seizures Task Force in ILAE stated that newborns have been shown to have seizures with exclusively focal onset [17].

Epileptic spasms: The clinical manifestations and ictal EEG findings of epileptic spasms in neonates are similar to those in older infants. The motor phenomena of epileptic spasms are characterized by brief contractions, typically involving the axial muscles and proximal limb segments, mostly occurring in clusters [18]. They are usually symmetric, but a variety of asymmetric or focal signs can be observed during events [18, 19]. Features of the ictal EEG of epileptic spasms in older infants include (1) fast waves preceding spasms, (2) high-voltage slow

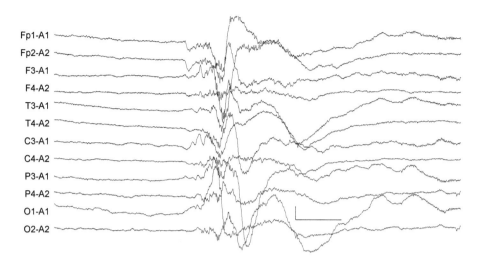

Fp1-A1
Fp2-A2
F3-A1
F4-A2
T3-A1
T4-A2
C3-A1
C4-A2
P3-A1
P4-A2
O1-A1
O2-A2

Figure 9.1 Ictal EEG findings of epileptic spasms in an infant with non-ketotic hyperglycinemia. Fast waves preceded spasms, high-voltage slow waves with positive deflection corresponding to flexor spasms were observed, and desynchronization of electrical activity appeared after spasms. Courtesy of Dr. Tetsuo Kubota, Anjo Kosei Hospital. Calibration, 100 μV, 1 sec.

waves with positive deflection, and (3) desynchronization of electrical activity [18, 19, 20]. This is similar to the epileptic spasms in neonates (Figure 9.1), though there have been no detailed reports on the ictal EEG findings of epileptic spasms specifically in neonates. One recent neurophysiological study in older infants and children suggested that epileptic spasms may be of focal onset: ictal augmentation of high-frequency oscillations was most prominent in a focal seizure onset zone of epileptic spasms [21]. It is unknown whether this also may be the case in neonatal spasms.

Desynchronization of the EEG, characterized by a sudden widespread attenuation of EEG voltage, can be observed in both epileptic and non-epileptic conditions. Thus, desynchronization is inappropriate for the confirmation of epileptic seizures. Desynchronization is seen even in normal neonates in association with arousal during quiet sleep.

Myoclonic seizures: Without an ictal EEG recording, myoclonic seizures are difficult to differentiate from non-epileptic myoclonus. Mizrahi and Kellaway [22] considered myoclonic seizures to be either epileptic or non-epileptic. Ictal video-EEG recordings should be performed when an infant has motor phenomena suspected to be myoclonic seizures, to distinguish them from non-epileptic myoclonus lacking ictal EEG correlate.

Tonic seizures: Generalized tonic seizures are extremely rare in neonates. Mizrahi and Kellaway [22] characterized generalized tonic seizures as mainly non-epileptic in neonates. However, Watanabe et al. [23] reported three neonates with holoprosencephaly having epileptic generalized tonic seizures associated with a typical epileptic recruiting rhythm on EEG. More commonly, focal-onset seizures with tonic posturing or increased muscle tone are misdiagnosed as generalized tonic seizures [24].

Interictal EEG findings are also useful in diagnosing neonatal epilepsies. Unusual patterns of interictal background activity may be observed in infants with seizures due to remote symptomatic etiologies, especially in those with brain malformations. Although there is no evidence associating specific background patterns to outcomes for each of the individual neonatal onset epilepsies, in general, seizures and developmental outcomes

worsen as a function of the severity of the abnormalities in background patterns.

The most prominent abnormality in EEG background activity is a "suppression-burst" pattern (Figure 9.2), the hallmark of EIEE and early myoclonic encephalopathy (EME). It is characterized by higher-voltage bursts of slow waves mixed with multifocal spikes, alternating with an isoelectric suppression phase [25]. A more precise definition of suppression-bust has not been universally established, and the term "suppression-burst" has been used arbitrarily. For this reason, the definition of suppression-burst may differ among researchers. Some consider that the EEG must be isoelectric during the suppression phase to constitute suppression-burst, whereas others may include EEGs with low-voltage but continuous/intermittent activity during the suppression phase. The EEG findings may differ according to neonates' sleep stage; in some infants, a suppression-burst pattern is clearly present during quiet sleep and is less clear during active sleep or wakefulness. While some researchers include such EEG patterns in suppression-burst, in EIEE a true suppression-burst pattern appears consistently and unchangingly during both the awake and asleep states, according to the original report [25]. Complicating matters further, the term "suppression-burst" is sometimes used interchangeably with "burst suppression" to refer to severely suppressed background EEG due to an acute brain insult. The EEGs of infants with severe hypoxic-ischemic encephalopathy may show burst suppression, indicating the presence of severe brain lesions and poor developmental outcomes. The EEG patterns of the suppression-bursts of infants with neonatal epilepsies differ substantially from those of burst suppression seen with severe brain insults. With the suppression-burst pattern of infants with neonatal epilepsies, the amplitude of the EEG activity during the burst phase is usually very high, spikes or sharp waves are abundant, and the duration of suppression phase is around 5–10 seconds [25]. With the burst suppression pattern of infants with severe brain insults, the amplitude of the EEG activity during the burst phase is relatively lower, and the duration of suppression phase is much longer (e.g., 40–60 seconds) [26].

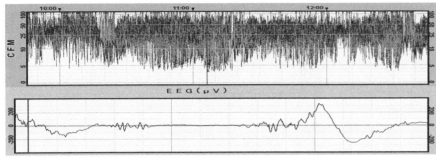

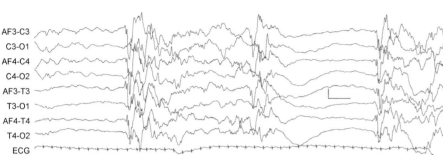

Figure 9.2 EEG and aEEG of suppression-burst pattern of infants with EIEE.
On aEEG, the upper margin was 50–100 μV and the lower margin was 5–10 μV. This differs from the definition of a burst suppression pattern caused by an acute brain insult, which is characterized by a lower margin below 2–3 μV. The corresponding EEG shows high-amplitude bursts with spikes and sharp waves alternating with comparatively suppressed, but not isoelectric, inter-burst intervals. Courtesy of Dr. Toru Okanishi, Seirei Hamamatsu Hospital. Calibration, 100 μV, 1 sec.

Amplitude-Integrated EEG

Multichannel conventional EEG has been the gold standard for the diagnosis of neonatal seizures. However, conventional EEG recording requires the expertise of a trained technologist and experienced neurologists or neurophysiologists which may limit access to EEG in many centers, particularly during nights and weekends. aEEG represents a bedside solution to fill this gap. aEEG is a processed EEG that is filtered and time compressed. aEEG can be applied by personnel with minimal training, including nursing staff and residents, and may be interpreted by persons without neurophysiology training [27].

aEEG findings are classified primarily according to three components: the lower margin, the upper margin, and presence of cycling [28]. The lower margin of an aEEG trace is determined by the minimum amplitude and spacing of peaks in the EEG activities within an EEG segment. The lower margin is lowered when an inter-burst interval becomes longer. The upper margin is defined by the peak-to-peak amplitude of EEG activities within an EEG segment. Cycling represents periodic fluctuation in the width of the aEEG tracing across different sleep and wake states, due to alternation between continuous and discontinuous EEG activity within a sleep cycle [29]. The tracé alternant stage during quiet sleep represents a more discontinuous background corresponding to a wider aEEG tracing, whereas other sleep stages and wakefulness represent a more continuous background, with a narrower aEEG tracing.

On aEEG, seizures may appear as an abrupt rise in the lower margin, often associated with a rise in the upper margin [28]. This is usually true for infants with neonatal epilepsies. However, some exceptional findings may be found. Ito et al. [30] reported downward seizure patterns on an aEEG in an infant with holoprosencephaly. In that infant, interictal EEG showed periodic high-voltage activities, and ictal EEG changes were associated with low-voltage fast rhythms, followed by slow waves of increasing amplitude and decreasing frequency (Figure 9.3). Vilan and colleagues [31] reported a distinctive aEEG pattern among a series of neonates with seizures due to *KCNQ2* mutations. These newborns had a normal aEEG background, with seizures characterized by an abrupt rise of the upper and lower margin, followed by overall amplitude suppression. While not unique to KCNQ2-related epilepsies, this does reflect the typical EEG finding of normal background interrupted by isolated, brief, high-amplitude seizures that are followed by a variable period of post-ictal suppression. EEG/aEEG may show very unusual patterns in infants with severe neonatal epilepsies. Information from the aEEG is complemented by continuous full-array conventional EEG monitoring in infants with neonatal epilepsies.

Burst suppression patterns are also important aEEG findings. Burst suppression in aEEG is defined as discontinuous activity with a lower margin at 0–2 μV without variability and an upper margin with an amplitude > 25 μV [28]; it is observed in infants with severe acute brain insults. Burst suppression in aEEG reflects prolonged inter-burst intervals and short bursts of higher amplitude activity. Notably, these findings can differ from the suppression-burst pattern on aEEG in neonatal epilepsy. Figures 9.2 and 9.4 show aEEG findings of suppression-burst in infants with EIEE and EME. With regard to aEEG in suppression-burst, the upper margin is very high (>100 μV), the lower margin is not markedly lowered (>5–10 μV), and the density of the aEEG trace is thick. These findings are not consistent with the aEEG definition of burst suppression. However, inter-burst intervals are very

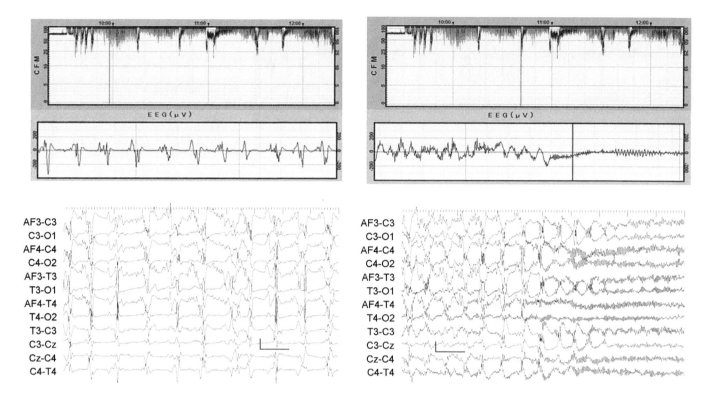

Figure 9.3 Downward seizure pattern on aEEG in infants with holoprosencephaly.
Left. Interictal aEEG and EEG. High-voltage periodic discharges were observed consistently on EEG. On aEEG, both upper and lower margins were markedly elevated.
Right. aEEG and EEG at the beginning of a seizure. Low-voltage fast rhythms were observed from the right centrotemporal area on EEG. aEEG showed downward deflection, due to reduced amplitude of EEG activities associated with a seizure. Courtesy of Dr. Hiroyuki Kidokoro, Nagoya University Graduate School of Medicine. This infant was discussed in Ito et al. 2014. Calibration, 100 μV, 1 sec.

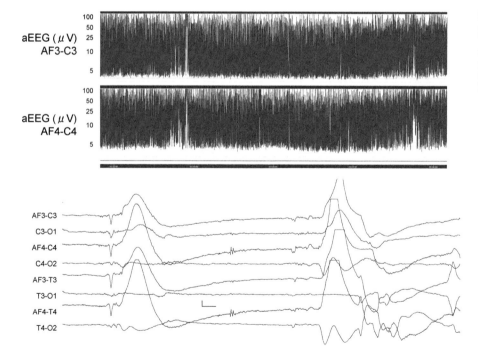

Figure 9.4 EEG and aEEG of suppression-burst pattern of an infant with EME
The infant is the same as that in Figure 9.1. aEEG trace showed an unusual pattern with an upper margin of 50–100 μV and a lower margin of around 5 μV. Courtesy of Dr. Tetsuo Kubota, Anjo Kosei Hospital. Calibration, 100 μV, 1 sec.

long in some infants with EIEE. In such situations, an aEEG trace may resemble a burst suppression due to an acute brain insult, whereas the upper margin will remain higher. The EEG/aEEG findings of infants with neonatal epilepsy

are highly variable; thus, their interpretation should be made with careful consideration for the individual case.

The small number of electrodes, which ranges from three to five in typical aEEG recordings, may limit seizure detection by aEEG. Seizures arising from brain areas distant from the electrodes can be missed. Although placement of electrodes in the frontal head region is easier due to the lack of hair, the frontal location has a lower sensitivity for seizure detection [32]. If only a single-channel aEEG is possible, then a bicentral derivation should be used; however, two-or-more-channel aEEG recordings are recommended for increased sensitivity [33]. Ictal EEG changes can be limited to a narrow, specific area in some infants with neonatal epilepsies, especially those with small focal lesions. Seizures can be missed when an appropriate montage is not applied during aEEG recording. Another limitation of aEEG is that seizures of short duration may not be detected. On aEEG, the EEG signal is plotted as a single vertical line representing a 15-second sample of data. Thus, seizures lasting for a few seconds or less, such as epileptic spasms and myoclonic seizures, may not be visible on aEEG. When aEEG does not show ictal changes during clinical phenomena suspected to be seizures, multichannel conventional EEG should be performed to definitively assess the potential epileptic basis of these phenomena.

Continuous EEG/aEEG Monitoring

Continuous EEG/aEEG monitoring is necessary to determine the efficacy of treatment for neonatal seizures, because electrographic only seizures are very frequent in neonates, especially after administration of anti-seizure medication. Some evidence suggests that seizure burden can be reduced by continuous EEG/aEEG monitoring combined with vigorous treatment of both electroclinical and subclinical seizures in term infants with hypoxic-ischemic encephalopathy [34]. It is uncertain whether a similar therapeutic strategy should be adopted for seizures in infants with neonatal epilepsies. Since subclinical seizures can be observed in infants with neonatal epilepsies, continuous EEG/aEEG monitoring is necessary to objectively determine the efficacy of treatment. However, it is uncertain whether intensive treatment can reduce the seizure burden in infants with neonatal epilepsies, because the seizures in these infants are sometimes highly resistant to the usual anti-seizure medications.

Epilepsy Syndromes

Self-Limited Familial and Non-Familial Neonatal Epilepsy

Benign familial neonatal seizures (BFNS) were first reported in 1964 by Rett and Teubel [35], and have been listed in the International Classification of Epilepsies, Epileptic Syndromes, and Related Disorders since 1989. Now, BFNS has been renamed as self-limited familial neonatal epilepsy (SFNE). In 1998, Singh et al. [5] identified mutations in the KCNQ2 gene in patients with SFNE. In the same year, molecular studies supported the pathogenic role of these mutations [36]. KCNQ2 gene mutations are now known to be the underlying cause of SFNE in a substantial proportion of cases [37]. Subsequently, the KCNQ3 gene was identified as another causative gene of SFNE [38] 1998). Benign non-familial neonatal seizures (BnFNS), renamed as self-limited non-familial neonatal epilepsy (SnFNE), were first described as "fifth day fits" [39]. In some infants with SnFNE, KCNQ2 mutations have been reported. This indicates that the molecular mechanisms of the seizures associated with SFNE and SnFNE may be shared.

The clinical manifestations of SFNE and SnFNE do not differ substantially. The general condition of the infants is good, and physical and neurological examinations are unremarkable. Seizures appear on the second to fifth day of life in most infants, although some infants may have later seizure onset during the first through the third months of life. Seizure manifestations are variable among infants, though focal tonic and clonic seizures are commonly reported. Convulsive movements, automatisms, oculo-facial features, and autonomic signs including desaturation and apnea may be observed. Seizures may differ from seizure to seizure in a single infant. Other types of seizures, such as epileptic spasms and myoclonic seizures, are not characteristic of the clinical syndrome of SFNE. However, they may be seen in more severe phenotypes also associated with KCNQ2 mutations, as described below.

Ictal EEG shows focal seizure onset in infants with SFNE and SnFNE (Figure 9.5). Seizure onset is usually characterized by low-voltage rhythmic activity with or without prior

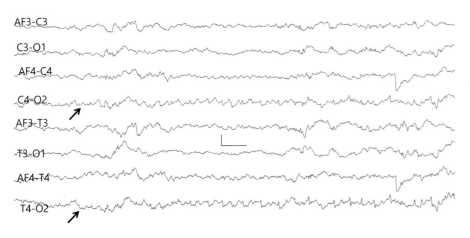

Figure 9.5 Ictal EEG findings from an infant with self-limited non-familial neonatal epilepsy Rhythmic low-voltage spikes were seen in the right occipital area [arrows]. Calibration, 100 μV, 1 sec.

desynchronization. This may evolve to higher amplitude sharp waves or spike-wave discharges. The site of seizure onset may vary in a single infant. Interictal EEG is usually normal. In early publications, a "théta pointu alternant" was reported in infants with SnFNE, characterized by a dominant theta activity, alternating or discontinuous, and unreactive with sharp waves and frequent inter-hemispheric asynchrony [39]. However, this pattern is not specific to SnFNE, and its diagnostic value is unclear. As above, aEEG may demonstrate normal aEEG background with seizures appearing as an abrupt rise of the upper and lower margin, followed by overall amplitude suppression [31].

Seizures in SFNE or SnFNE are presumed to cease in the first year of life without treatment in most cases, although sodium channel blocking drugs, particularly oxcarbazepine, may be effective in controlling seizures until epilepsy remission. Although many infants with SFNE and SnFNE have no long-term sequelae, approximately 15–20% have a recurrence of epilepsy later in life [37, 40]. While for neonates whose clinical syndrome remains consistent with SFNE or SnFNE long-term outcomes are typically good, those with more severe *KCNQ2* disease have variable outcomes. Most infants with SFNE/SnFNE achieve normal psychomotor development and seizure freedom. Recent studies demonstrated that infants with the 20q13.33 microdeletion involving both *KCNQ2* and *CHRNA4* showed a favorable epilepsy phenotype, similar to that of SFNE [41].

Early Infantile Epileptic Encephalopathy (EIEE) and Early Myoclonic Encephalopathy (EME)

Early infantile epileptic encephalopathy (EIEE), also known as Ohtahara syndrome, was first described by Ohtahara et al. [42], and early myoclonic encephalopathy (EME) was first identified by Aicardi and Goutiéres [43]. These two syndromes have been well known as age-dependent epileptic encephalopathies; they are characterized by the EEG feature "suppression-burst." The onset of seizures is mostly within the first month of life. Seizures are highly resistant to antiseizure medication, and neurodevelopmental outcomes are poor.

EIEE

In most patients, EIEE onset is within the first month of life. Encephalopathy is usually present at the onset, and neurological examination reveals abnormal muscle tone: hypotonia or hypertonia.

Originally, epileptic spasms were considered to be the representative seizure type of EIEE [42]. However, recent studies have shown that focal-onset seizures are far more common than epileptic spasms in infants with EIEE, some of whom did not have any epileptic spasms. Focal tonic and myoclonic seizures have been described in several studies.

Ohtahara et al. [44] described a suppression-burst pattern in detail, although no formal definition of suppression-burst has been established. By most definitions, burst phases last for 2–6 seconds and are characterized by very high-voltage slow waves mixed with multifocal spiky discharges. Suppression phases are low amplitude and last for 5–10 seconds. Originally, Ohtahara and Yamatogi [25] emphasized that the suppression-burst pattern in EIEE appeared consistently and was unchanging during both awake and sleep states. However, other investigators found that a suppression-burst pattern may be observed only during sleep in some infants with EIEE. Moreover, some authors seem to categorize as suppression-burst highly discontinuous EEG patterns that are characterized by the alternating appearance of a burst phase and a suppression phase and that have low voltage but continuous/intermittent discharges, although they clearly differ from the original description provided by Ohtahara and colleagues. The presence of the suppression-burst pattern or its analogs indicates severe brain dysfunction as commonly caused by severe epilepsies; it does not reflect a specific underlying pathology.

The etiology of EIEE is often genetic. Mutations in *ARX*, a key gene for the development of interneurons in the fetal brain, were the first genetic cause of EIEE to be identified [45]. A long expansion of the polyalanine residues and a frameshift mutation were identified in infants with EIEE. Mutations in *ARX* can result in many different phenotypes, including X-linked lissencephaly with ambiguous genitalia, EIEE, infantile spasms, and X-linked intellectual disability. *STXBP1* is another gene reported as pathogenic in infants with EIEE [46]. *STXBP1* regulates a late step of neuronal/exocytic fusion, playing an important role in the release of neurotransmitters [47]. Mutations in *STXBP1* have been reported in other types of epileptic encephalopathy, including infantile spasms and Dravet syndrome. *KCNQ2* was found to be a causative gene in SFNE, but screening for *KCNQ2* in a cohort of early-onset epileptic encephalopathy patients revealed *KCNQ2* mutations in 10% [6]. More than 20 additional genes have been reported to be causative for EIEE, and novel genes will likely continue to be identified. The genes related to EIEE are genetically heterogeneous, and their functions vary widely; however, mutations in these many of these genes are also found in patients with clinical phenotypes other than EIEE. Gene panels are increasingly utilized to improve diagnostic yield for patients with EIEE [48].

EME

The onset of EME is within the first month of life. Affected infants may show neurological abnormalities at birth. Altered consciousness, reduced reactivity, and abnormalities of muscle tones are frequent at the onset of seizures. The predominant motor symptom is fragmentary, segmental, or erratic myoclonus. Myoclonus is typically observed in the face or extremities; involves small areas, such as an eyelid or a finger; and often shifts from one area of the body to another randomly. One must be cautious about erratic myoclonus in infants with EME, as it usually lacks ictal EEG correlate, indicating that it is most often not of cortical origin. Axial myoclonus may be preceded by a burst of polyspikes on EEG, but may not be associated with any concurrent ictal EEG change. Focal-onset seizures are common in infants with EME, and epileptic spasms can also occur.

Suppression-burst is the EEG hallmark of EME. Suppression-burst patterns in infants with EME are characterized by burst phases lasting for 1–5 seconds that alternate with a suppression phase lasting for 3–10 seconds [49]. The duration of the burst phase is relatively shorter in EME than in EIEE. Some differences in the suppression-burst pattern between EIEE and EME have been described. Ohtahara et al. [49] noted that the suppression-burst pattern in EME was dependent on sleep–wake state, since the suppression-burst pattern may be seen only or predominantly during sleep. However, Schlumberger et al. [50] stated that this pattern is consistently seen during both wakefulness and sleep, with no differentiation. Furthermore, as with EIEE, suppression-burst is not strictly defined in EME. Thus, the inclusion criteria for EME can differ among investigators.

Inborn errors of metabolism are a common etiology of EME. Increasingly, a genetic etiology has been identified as the basis for the metabolic disorder. Non-ketotic hyperglycinemia is most frequently reported in infants with EME. Other causes of EME include D-glyceric academia, carbamyl phosphate synthetase deficiency, propionic aciduria, molybdenum cofactor deficiency, pyridoxine deficiency, methylmalonic academia, sulfite oxidase deficiency, Menkes disease, and Zellweger syndrome. Unrelated to inborn errors of metabolism, a mutation of the *ERBB4* gene, which is involved in the migration of interneurons to the cortex, has been identified as another potential cause of EME [51]. Mutations in the *SIK1* gene were found in patients with severe developmental epilepsies, including EME [52]. Mutations of *STXBP1*, *PIGA*, and *SLC25A22* have been also reported in infants with EME, as well as in those with EIEE.

Controversy over EIEE and EME

There is a continuing controversy about whether EIEE and EME are two distinct syndromes or whether they fall on a continuum for a single syndrome. Both syndromes are characterized by suppression-burst patterns on EEG. Differences in the suppression-burst patterns of EIEE and EME are not well defined, although some reports emphasize such differences [42, 43, 49]. The difference between the seizure type in EIEE and EME is ambiguous. Focal-onset seizures are very common in both EIEE and EME, and epileptic spasms have also been described in both. Historically, the etiology of EIEE and EME has been considered to differ, whereas recent genetic studies show an overlap of causative genes. Based on these facts, it seems reasonable to consider the possibility that EIEE and EME may fall on a continuum for a single syndrome rather than constitute two distinct syndromes.

Severe Neonatal Epilepsies Other Than EIEE and EME

Severe neonatal epilepsies with genetic etiologies do not always show burst suppression on EEG/aEEG. These are sometimes described simply as severe or malignant neonatal onset epilepsies, encompassing multiple syndromes and etiologies. Some infants with neonatal epilepsies due to *KCNQ2* mutations have encephalopathy and seizures accompanied by an EEG demonstrating focal or multifocal epileptiform discharges without a suppression-burst pattern [53]. Neonatal-onset epilepsies may be observed in infants with 2q24.3 duplication involving both *SCN2A* and *SCN3A*. The EEGs of these patients have been reported to show focal or generalized epileptiform discharges [54]. *KCNT1* mutations can cause neonatal-onset epilepsies as well as epilepsy of infancy with migrating focal seizures without a suppression-burst pattern [55]. Thus, severe neonatal epilepsies other than EIEE and EME are not uncommon and should be recognized as a major clinical entity.

Metabolic Epilepsy

Epilepsy due to inborn errors of metabolism is rare in neonates. Nevertheless, it is important to perform an immediate diagnostic workup if suspected, because some types of metabolic epilepsy can be treated with specific drugs that will be more effective if started earlier. Specific therapeutic interventions can be initiated before the diagnosis of an inborn error of metabolism has been established while awaiting confirmatory results. Neither EEG nor aEEG is diagnostic for inborn errors of metabolism, but they can be useful to assess the severity of brain dysfunction and to detect seizures [56]. EEG/aEEG abnormalities can be a clue that the clinician should consider the possibility of inborn errors of metabolism. In addition, continuous EEG/aEEG monitoring will help to evaluate the efficacy of specific treatments.

Pyridoxine-dependent epilepsy is a severe but eminently treatable autosomal recessive disorder due to mutations in the antiquitin (*ALDH7A1*) gene. Pyridoxine-dependent epilepsy is characterized by multiple seizure types that are refractory to anti-seizure medications. Diagnosis can be made based on elevated CSF, blood, and/or urine levels of a-aminoadipic semialdehyde (AASA). Increasingly, diagnosis is made by direct genetic testing of the *ALDH7A1* gene. Nabbout et al. [57] reported an EEG pattern suggestive of pyridoxine-dependent epilepsy with continuous diffuse high-voltage rhythmic delta slow waves. Periodic jerks may be observed with inconsistent ictal EEG correlation. Attenuation of the epileptiform activities and improvement of the background EEG findings may be observed after intravenous administration of pyridoxine (100–500 mg). However, an ambiguous response to pyridoxine was reported in some genetically confirmed cases [58], thus the diagnosis should not be based solely on this EEG finding. Folinic acid can be added for patients with an incomplete response to pyridoxine.

Pyridoxal 5'-phosphate (PLP) dependency is a distinct condition due to mutations in the *PNPO* gene [59]. The biologically active form of pyridoxine is pyridoxal-5-phosphate (PLP), which is a co-factor for ~100 enzymatic reactions vital for the synthesis, function, and catabolism of neurotransmitters. Diagnosis is made by abnormal CSF metabolite profile, or by direct *PNPO* genetic testing. Clinical manifestations and EEG findings of PLP dependency are indistinguishable from those of pyridoxine-dependent epilepsy. Both have refractory seizures, accompanied by nonseizure abnormal movements

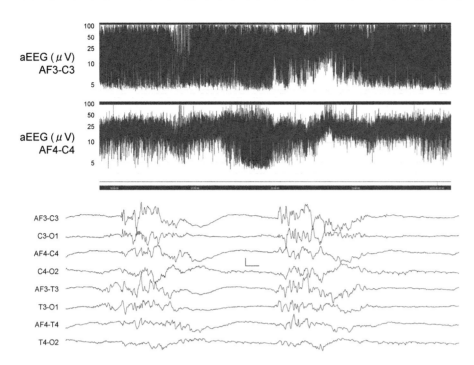

aEEG (μV)
AF3-C3

aEEG (μV)
AF4-C4

AF3-C3
C3-O1
AF4-C4
C4-O2
AF3-T3
T3-O1
AF4-T4
T4-O2

Figure 9.6 EEG and aEEG of unilateral megalencephaly.
The aEEG trace was asymmetrical. In the left hemisphere (the affected hemisphere), an unusual pattern with an upper margin of around 100 μV and a lower margin of around 5 μV was observed. The aEEG trace was less pathological in the right hemisphere. EEG showed an asymmetric suppression-burst pattern with bursts of higher voltage in the left hemisphere. Courtesy of Dr. Tatsuya Fukasawa, Anjo Kosei Hospital. Calibration, 100 μV, 1 sec.

including abnormal eye movements and grimacing [60]. Infants with PLP dependency do not respond to pyridoxine administration and respond only to PLP, at a dose of 30–50 mg/kg per day. For this reason, when pyridoxine-dependent epilepsy is suspected, it may be clinically prudent to initiate treatment with PLP rather than pyridoxine alone.

As mentioned above, early myoclonic encephalopathy is caused by several inborn errors of metabolism, including non-ketotic hyperglycinemia, molybdenum cofactor deficiency, and sulfite oxidase deficiency. Some peroxisomal diseases may present as neonatal epilepsy. Zellweger syndrome, neonatal adrenoleukodystrophy, and D-bifunctional protein deficiency have been reported in infants with neonatal epilepsy. MRI shows characteristic abnormalities in these diseases, such as polymicrogyria or diffusely abnormal gyral patterns, intraventricular/caudothalamic groove cysts, and impaired myelination, which can be diagnostic clues. No specific findings due to peroxisomal disorders have been reported in the conventional EEG or aEEG of patients with neonatal epilepsies.

Neonatal Epilepsies Due to Structural Causes

Various structural abnormalities of the brain can cause neonatal epilepsy. MRI plays a key role in the diagnosis of such abnormalities. EEG findings differ widely according to the type, causative gene, and severity of brain malformation. Specific EEG abnormalities are not diagnostic for specific types of brain malformation, but unusual background EEG patterns have been observed in infants with severe brain malformations.

Unilateral megalencephaly is a representative structural cause of neonatal epilepsy, especially EIEE. Unilateral megalencephaly can be associated with various skin conditions such as epidermal nevus syndrome, hypomelanosis of Ito,

Proteus syndrome, and linear nevus sebaceous syndrome. Conventional EEG in infants with unilateral megalencephaly accompanied by neonatal epilepsies often shows a suppression-burst pattern with high-voltage slow waves mixed with spiky/sharp discharges predominant in the affected hemisphere. aEEG may show marked asymmetry in infants with this condition: in the affected hemisphere, the lower margin is around 5 μV due to the discontinuity of EEG activities, and the upper margin is higher than 50–100 μV, corresponding to high-voltage burst activities (Figure 9.6). The aEEG trace in the other hemisphere varies according to the patient, but it usually shows fewer pathological findings. Early surgical treatment is recommended to improve seizures and developmental outcomes.

Holoprosencephaly is sometimes associated with neonatal epilepsies, although the rate of neonatal epilepsy is unknown. Interictal EEG findings differ substantially among infants. Some infants with holoprosencephaly may have a severely abnormal EEG with high-voltage rhythmic alpha–theta and delta activities, with or without spiky components, whereas others may show mild abnormalities of the EEG background. An unusual downward seizure pattern can be observed on aEEG in infants with holoprosencephaly [30]. At present, the relationship between EEG abnormalities and neuroimaging findings is not understood.

Tuberous sclerosis is another cause of neonatal epilepsy: Kotulska et al. [61] reported that 21 of 421 patients with tuberous sclerosis developed epilepsy during the neonatal period. EEG may reveal epileptiform discharges in the neonatal period, even before the onset of epilepsy. Ikeno et al. [62] reported on an infant with tuberous sclerosis in whom focal-onset seizures without perceivable clinical symptoms were unexpectedly identified on a routine EEG. The MRI findings are diagnostic in these cases.

Acknowledgments

I am deeply grateful to Dr. Toru Kato (Okazaki City Hospital), Dr. Tetsuo Kubota and Dr. Tatsuya Fukasawa (Anjo Kosei Hospital), Dr. Hiroyuki Kidokoro (Nagoya University Graduate School of Medicine), and Dr. Toru Okanishi (Seirei Hamamatsu Hospital) for providing EEG/aEEG samples and important comments about the content.

References

1. Shellhaas RA, Wusthoff CJ, Tsuchida TN, et al; Neonatal Seizure Registry. Profile of neonatal epilepsies: characteristics of a prospective US cohort. *Neurology*. 2017 Aug 29;**89**(9):893–9.

2. Axeen EJT, Olson HE. Neonatal epilepsy genetics. *Semin Fetal Neonatal Med*. 2018 Jun;**23**(3):197–203.

3. Sheth RD, Hobbs GR, Mullett M. Neonatal seizures: incidence, onset and aetiology by gestational age. *J Perinatol*. 1999;**19**:40e3.

4. Tekgul H, Gauvreau K, Soul J, et al. The current etiologic profile and neurodevelopmental outcome of seizures in term newborn infants. *Pediatrics*. 2006;**117**:1270–80.

5. Singh NA, Charlier C, Stauffer D, et al. A novel potassium channel gene, KCNQ2, is mutated in an inherited epilepsy of newborns. *Nat Genet*. 1998;**18**:25–9.

6. Weckhuysen S, Mandelstam S, Suls A, et al. KCNQ2 encephalopathy: emerging phenotype of a neonatal epileptic encephalopathy. *Ann Neurol*. 2012;**71**:15–25.

7. Heron SE, Crossland KM, Andermann E, et al. Sodium-channel defects in benign familial neonatal-infantile seizures. *Lancet*. 2002;**360**:851–2.

8. Dulac O, Plecko B, Gataullina S, et al. Occasional seizures, epilepsy, and inborn errors of metabolism. *Lancet Neurol*. 2014;**13**:727–39.

9. Santarone ME, Pietrafusa N, Fusco L. Neonatal seizures: When semiology points to etiology. *Seizure*. 2020 Aug;**80**:161–5.

10. Nunes ML, Yozawitz EG, Zuberi S, et al; Task Force on Neonatal Seizures, ILAE Commission on Classification & Terminology. Neonatal seizures: Is there a relationship between ictal electroclinical features and etiology? A critical appraisal based on a systematic literature review. *Epilepsia Open*. 2019 Jan 25;**4**(1):10–29; 20.

11. Olson HE, Kelly M, LaCoursiere CM, et al. Genetics and genotype-phenotype correlations in early onset epileptic encephalopathy with burst suppression. *Ann Neurol*. 2017 Mar;**81**(3):419–29.

12. Murray DM, Boylan GB, Ali I, et al. Defining the gap between electrographic seizure burden, clinical expression and staff recognition of neonatal seizures. *Arch Dis Child Fetal Neonatal Ed*. 2008;**93**:F187–91.

13. Shellhaas RA, Chang T, Tsuchida T, et al. The American Clinical Neurophysiology Society's Guideline on Continuous Electroencephalography Monitoring in Neonates. *J Clin Neurophysiol*. 2011;**28**:611–17.

14. Wusthoff CJ. Diagnosing neonatal seizures and status epilepticus. *J Clin Neurophysiol*. 2013;**30**:115–21.

15. Clancy RR, Legido A. The exact ictal and interictal duration of electroencephalographic neonatal seizures. *Epilepsia*. 1987;**28**:537–41.

16. Abend NS, Wusthoff CJ. Neonatal seizures and status epilepticus. *J Clin Neurophysiol*. 2012;**29**:441–8.

17. Pressler RM, Cilio MR, Mizrahi E, et al; The ILAE classification of seizures and the epilepsies. Modification for seizures in the neonate. Position paper by the ILAE Task Force on Neonatal Seizures. Epilepsia. 22021;62(3):615–628.

18. Fusco L, Vigevano F. Ictal clinical electroencephalographic findings of spasms in West syndrome. *Epilepsia*. 1993;**34**:671–8.

19. Watanabe K, Negoro T, Okumura A. Symptomatology of infantile spasms. *Brain Dev*. 2001;**23**:453–66.

20. Vigevano F, Fusco L, Pachatz C. Neurophysiology of spasms. *Brain Dev*. 2001;**23**:467–72.

21. Nariai H, Nagasawa T, Juhász C, et al. Statistical mapping of ictal high-frequency oscillations in epileptic spasms. *Epilepsia*. 2011;**52**:63–74.

22. Mizrahi EM, Kellaway P. *Diagnosis and Management of Neonatal Seizures*. New York: Lippincott-Raven; 1998.

23. Watanabe K, Hara K, Iwase K. The evolution of neurophysiological features in holoprosencephaly. *Neuropaediatrie*. 1976;**7**:19–41.

24. Yamamoto N, Watanabe K, Negoro T, et al. Complex partial seizures in children: ictal manifestations and their relation to clinical course. *Neurology*. 1987;**37**:1379–82.

25. Ohtahara S, Yamatogi Y. Epileptic encephalopathies in early infancy with suppression-burst. *J Clin Neurophysiol*. 2003;**20**:398–407.

26. Watanabe K, Miyazaki S, Hara K, et al. Behavioral state cycles, background EEGs and prognosis of newborns with perinatal hypoxia. *Electroencephalogr Clin Neurophysiol*. 1980;**49**:618–25.

27. Shah NA, Wusthoff CJ. How to use: amplitude-integrated EEG (aEEG). *Arch Dis Child Educ Pract Ed*. 2015;**100**:75–81.

28. Hellström-Westas L, de Vries LS, Rosén I. *An Atlas of Amplitude-Integrated EEGs in the Newborn*, 2nd ed. London: Informa Healthcare; 2003.

29. Kidokoro H, Inder T, Okumura A, et al. What does cyclicity on amplitude-integrated EEG mean? *J Perinatol*. 2012;**32**:565–9.

30. Ito M, Kidokoro H, Sugiyama Y, et al. Paradoxical downward seizure pattern on amplitude-integrated electroencephalogram. *J Perinatol*. 2014;**34**:642–4.

31. Vilan A, Mendes Ribeiro J, Striano P, et al. A distinctive ictal amplitude-integrated electroencephalography pattern in newborns with neonatal epilepsy associated with KCNQ2 mutations. *Neonatology*. 2017;**112**(4):387–93.

32. Wusthoff CJ, Shellhaas RA, Clancy RR. Limitations of single-channel EEG on the forehead for neonatal seizure detection. *J Perinatol*. 2009;**29**:237–42.

33. Kidokoro H, Kubota T, Hayakawa M, et al. Neonatal seizure identification on reduced channel EEG. *Arch Dis Child Fetal Neonatal Ed*. 2013;**98**:F359–61.

34. van Rooij LG, Toet MC, van Huffelen AC, et al. Effect of treatment of subclinical neonatal seizures detected with aEEG: randomized, controlled trial. *Pediatrics*. 2010;**125**: e358–66.

35. Rett A, Teubel R. Neugeborenenkrämpfe im Rahmen einer epileptisch belasten Familie. *Wiener Klinische Wochenschrif*. 1964;**76**:609–13.

36. Biervert C, Schroeder BC, Kubisch C, et al. A potassium channel mutation in neonatal human epilepsy. *Science*. 1998 Jan 16;**279**(5349):403–6.

37. Grinton BE, Heron SE, Pelekanos JT, et al. Familial neonatal seizures in 36 families: clinical and genetic features correlate with outcome. *Epilepsia*. 2015 Jul;**56**(7):1071–80.

38. Charlier C, Singh NA, Ryan SG, et al. A pore mutation in a novel KQT-like potassium channel gene in an idiopathic epilepsy family. *Nat Genet*. 1998;**18**:53–5.

39. Dehan M, Quillerou D, Navelet Y, et al. Convulsions in the fifth day of life: a new syndrome? *Arch Fr Pediatr*. 1977;**34**:730–42. [in French]

40. Ronen GM, Rosales TO, Connolly M, Anderson VE, Leppert M. Seizure characteristics in chromosome 20 benign familial neonatal convulsions. *Neurology*. 1993 Jul;**43**(7):1355–60.

41. Okumura A, Ishii A, Shimojima K, et al. Phenotypes of children with 20q13.3 microdeletion affecting KCNQ2 and CHRNA4. *Epileptic Disord*. 2015;**17**:165–71.

42. Ohtahara S, Ishida T, Oka E, et al. On the specific age-dependent epileptic syndromes: the early-infantile epileptic encephalopathy with suppression-burst. *No To Hattatsu*. 1976;**8**:270–80. [in Japanese]

43. Aicardi J, Goutiéres F. Encéphalopathie myoclonique néonatale. *Rev Electroencephalogr Neurophysiol Clin*. 1978;899–101. [in French]

44. Ohtahara S, Ohtsuka Y, Erba G. Early epileptic encephalopathy with suppression-burst. In Engel J, Jr.,

Pedley T, editors. *Epilepsy: A Comprehensive Textbook*. Volume 3. Philadelphia: Lippincott-Raven; 1998, pp. 2257–61.

45. Kato M, Saitoh S, Kamei A, et al. A longer polyalanine expansion mutation in the ARX gene causes early infantile epileptic encephalopathy with suppression-burst pattern (Ohtahara syndrome). *Am J Hum Genet*. 2007;**81**:361–6.

46. Deprez L, Weckhuysen S, Holmgren P, et al. Clinical spectrum of early-onset epileptic encephalopathies associated with STXBP1 mutations. *Neurology*. 2010 Sep 28;**75**(13):1159–65.

47. Saitsu H, Kato M, Mizuguchi T, et al. De novo mutations in the gene encoding STXBP1 (MUNC18-1) cause early infantile epileptic encephalopathy. *Nat Genet*. 2008;**40**:782–8.

48. Trump N, McTague A, Brittain H, et al. Improving diagnosis and broadening the phenotypes in early-onset seizure and severe developmental delay disorders through gene panel analysis. *J Med Genet*. 2016 May;**53**(5):310–17.

49. Ohtahara S, Ohtsuka Y, Yamatogi Y, Oka E. The early-infantile epileptic encephalopathy with suppression-burst: developmental aspects. *Brain Dev*. 1987;**9**(4):371–6.

50. Schlumberger E, Dulac O, Pluoin P. Early infantile syndrome(s) with suppression-burst: nosological consideration. In Roger J, Bureau M, Drave C, et al., editors. *Epileptic Syndromes of Infancy, Childhood and Adolescence*, 2nd ed. London: John Libbey; 1992, pp. 35–42.

51. Backx L, Ceulemans B, Vermeesch JR, et al. Early myoclonic encephalopathy caused by a disruption of the neuregulin-1 receptor ErbB4. *Eur J Hum Genet*. 2009;**17**: 378–82.

52. Hansen J, Snow C, Tuttle E, et al. De novo mutations in SIK1 cause a spectrum of developmental epilepsies. *Am J Hum Genet*. 2015;**96**:682–90.

53. Weckhuysen S, Ivanovic V, Hendrickx R, et al. Extending the KCNQ2 encephalopathy spectrum: clinical and neuroimaging findings in 17 patients. *Neurology*. 2013;**81**:1697–703.

54. Okumura A, Yamamoto T, Kurahashi H, et al. Epilepsies in children with 2q24.3 deletion/duplication. *J Pediatr Epilepsy*. 2015;**4**:8–16.

55. Ohba C, Kato M, Takahashi N, et al. De novo KCNT1 mutations in early-onset epileptic encephalopathy. *Epilepsia*. 2015;**56**: e121–8.

56. Olischar M, Shany E, Aygün C, et al. Amplitude-integrated electroencephalography in newborns with inborn errors of metabolism. *Neonatology*. 2012;**102**:203–11.

57. Nabbout R, Soufflet C, Plouin P, et al. Pyridoxine dependent epilepsy: a suggestive electroclinical pattern. *Arch Dis Child Fetal Neonatal Ed*. 1999;**81**:F125–9.

58. Bok LA, Maurits NM, Willemsen MA, et al. The EEG response to pyridoxine-IV neither identifies nor excludes pyridoxine-dependent epilepsy. *Epilepsia*. 2010 Dec;**51** (12):2406–11.

59. Mills PB, Camuzeaux SS, Footitt EJ, et al. Epilepsy due to PNPO mutations: genotype, environment and treatment affect presentation and outcome. *Brain*. 2014;**137**:1350–60.

60. Schmitt B, Baumgartner M, Mills PB, et al. Seizures and paroxysmal events: symptoms pointing to the diagnosis of pyridoxine-dependent epilepsy and pyridoxine phosphate oxidase deficiency. *Dev Med Child Neurol*. 2010 Jul;**52**(7):e133–42.

61. Kotulska K, Jurkiewicz E, Domańska-Pakieła D, et al. Epilepsy in newborns with tuberous sclerosis complex. *Eur J Paediatr Neurol*. 2014;**18**:714–21.

62. Ikeno M, Okumura A, Abe S, et al. Clinically silent seizures in a neonate with tuberous sclerosis. *Pediatr Int*. 2016;**58**:58–61.

Management of Status Epilepticus and Recurrent Seizures

Marina Gaínza-Lein, Iván Sánchez Fernández, and Tobias Loddenkemper

Illustrative Cases

Case 20 Cerebral Sinovenous Thrombosis

Case 21 Mitochondrial Encephalomyopathy, Lactic Acidosis, and Stroke-Like Episodes (MELAS)

Case 25 Traumatic Brain Injury

Case 27 Autoimmune Encephalitis

Case 28 Febrile Infection–Related Epilepsy Syndrome (FIRES)

Key Points

- Status epilepticus is a life-threatening and time sensitive emergency.
- Continuous EEG monitoring allows the detection of electrographic seizures and electrographic status epilepticus.
- The treatment of SE consists of benzodiazepines, non-benzodiazepines antiepileptic drugs, and continuous infusions.
- Convulsive and electrographic status epilepticus have been associated with short-term mortality.
- Rapid detection and treatment of status epilepticus could improve outcomes.

Electrographic Seizures and Status Epilepticus

Continuum between Convulsive Status Epilepticus and Electrographic-Only Status Epilepticus

Electrographic status epilepticus is defined as "uninterrupted electrographic seizures lasting 30 minutes or longer, or repeated electrographic seizures totaling more than 30 minutes in any one-hour period" [1]. Electrographic status epilepticus can be classified into convulsive and nonconvulsive status epilepticus. In some patients, these may represent a continuum with two main phases. The first phase is characterized by generalized tonic-clonic seizures that increase sympathetic response, with increased arterial blood pressure and increased cerebral blood flow and cerebral metabolic demand [2, 3]. After approximately 30 minutes of convulsive seizures, the second phase starts, characterized by failure of cerebral autoregulation, decreased cerebral blood flow, metabolic decompensation, and electroclinical uncoupling, defined as the continuation of the electrical seizure activity with fewer correlating clinical manifestations [2, 3]. In clinical practice, a prolonged seizure is often considered status

epilepticus operationally, and treated as such after 5 minutes of continuous seizure [4].

Electrographic seizures can also be divided into convulsive seizures (electroclinical or clinically evident seizures) and nonconvulsive seizures (occult, or EEG-only seizures). Nonconvulsive seizures by definition have no clinical correlate [1, 5] and thus cannot be detected without continuous EEG monitoring (cEEG). Thus, cEEG is required for the accurate diagnosis and optimal management of electrographic seizures and electrographic status epilepticus. Accordingly, its use has increased in the intensive care unit (ICU) [1, 6].

Epidemiology of Electrographic Seizures and Status Epilepticus in the ICU

Convulsive status epilepticus is one of the most common neurological emergencies in childhood [7]. Status epilepticus has an incidence of 6.8–41/100,000 per year in adults and children [8], and the incidence is higher in infants under 1 year of age: 135–156/100,000 per year [8–10].

Considering electrographic seizures, different studies have reported an incidence of 10%–42% among critically ill children who underwent clinically indicated cEEG [11–23]. There is high variability between these studies, which may be explained by small sample sizes and differences in the indications for cEEG between centers [24]. A study by Abend and colleagues of 550 children from 11 tertiary care institutions who underwent clinically indicated cEEG found that electrographic seizures occurred in 30%, of which 38% had electrographic status epilepticus [25]. Another study, led by Claassen, of 570 critically ill adults and children who underwent cEEG monitoring found electrographic seizures in 19% [26]. These relatively high seizure detection rates reflect the highly selected patient populations in these studies, and the incidence of seizures among general ICU populations is likely considerably lower.

Need for cEEG to Recognize Electrographic-Only Seizures

Electrographic seizures with no clinical correlate require cEEG for their detection. The multicenter study by Abend et al. found that among those critically children having seizures, 35% of the electrographic seizures had no accompanying clinical signs [25]. In the Claassen study of critically ill adults and children, 92% of the electrographic seizures were nonconvulsive [26]. Similarly, a study of cEEG monitoring among 236 comatose children and adults who had no clinical signs of status epilepticus found that 8% had nonconvulsive status epilepticus [27]. Even if seizures initially have clinical signs, cEEG is required to determine whether they have resolved: a multicenter study of 98 children with convulsive status epilepticus who underwent cEEG found that 11% continued to have electrographic-only seizures after termination of convulsive seizures [28].

Effect of Seizures and Status Epilepticus on Outcome

The mortality of pediatric status epilepticus ranges from 0%–5% [9, 29–31], lower than the 8%–9% mortality reported in adults [32, 33]. Patients who survive status epilepticus often subsequently have developmental impairments, epilepsy, and recurrent status epilepticus [34, 35]. Younger patients are affected most frequently, with a higher mortality and morbidity. A follow-up study of 193 children with status epilepticus found neurological sequelae in 9.1% of the 186 survivors: 29% of infants younger than 1 year of age, 11% of children 1 to 3 years of age, and 6% of children older than 3 years of age. However, this paralleled the greater incidence of acute neurological disease in the younger age groups. Within each cause of status epilepticus, age did not affect outcome [30, 36].

Electrographic seizures and particularly electrographic status epilepticus have been associated with poor outcomes. A study of 204 comatose children demonstrated that the presence of electrographic seizures independently predicted an unfavorable outcome (severe handicap or vegetative state) after 1 month, while normal EEG background activity predicted survival [18]. In the Abend multicenter study of 550 children who underwent EEG monitoring in the ICU, 13% died. Among that cohort, death was associated with electrographic status epilepticus (OR 2.42), but not with electrographic seizures (OR 1.78) [25]. Death was more common in patients who had electrographic status epilepticus and an acute neurological disorder, but not more common in epilepsy-related disorders. Patients with electrographic status epilepticus also had a longer pediatric ICU stay. Among 200 children who underwent cEEG monitoring in a single pediatric ICU, electrographic status epilepticus (but not electrographic seizures) was associated with higher mortality (OR 5.1) and worsening of their neurological status at ICU discharge (OR 17.3) [23]. Moreover, electrographic seizure burden during critical illness has also been associated with decline in neurological status [37].

Monitoring for Electrographic Seizures and Status Epilepticus

Duration of Monitoring

Several studies have demonstrated that only a small minority of seizures are detected during the first hour of cEEG [11, 26, 38]. A study of 101 critically ill children found that 52% of children experienced their first seizure within the first hour of cEEG, and 87% experienced their first seizure within the first 24 hours

[11]. In a cohort of 570 adults and children undergoing prolonged cEEG monitoring, the first seizure occurred within 24 hours in 88% of patients, during the second day in 5%, and after 48 hours in 7% [26], with comatose patients being more likely to experience seizure onset after 24 hours (OR 4.5). Therefore, although a routine EEG would fail to detect most seizures, 24 hours of monitoring is sufficient to detect seizures among the vast majority of critically ill children at risk.

Financial Aspects and Suggestions for Clinical Care

Longer cEEG detects more seizures, but also consumes limited resources. A study from the United States evaluated the cost-effectiveness of four electrographic seizure identification strategies: no monitoring, monitoring for 1 hour, for 24 hours, or for 48 hours [39]. The authors estimated that the cost of a 1-hour EEG costs $466, 24 hours $1,666, and 48 hours $22,648. At the same time, a 1-hour EEG would identify only 55% of the seizures; this percentage would increase to 85% in 24 hours, but only to 89% in 48 hours. Their results supported monitoring critically ill children for 24 hours [39]. However, some studies showed that comatose patients may need monitoring longer than 24 hours [26], particularly patients with periodic discharges on EEG [26]. There remains a high variability in cEEG practices among institutions [6, 40]. The optimal duration of cEEG monitoring could depend on several factors, such as clinical parameters, initial EEG characteristics, and the available resources, but these are yet not fully understood [41]. From the cost-effectiveness perspective, small variations in the cEEG monitoring strategies can have a major impact on the seizure identification and resource utilization [42]. A recent consensus statement recommended cEEG monitoring for children at risk of seizures for 24–48 hours [43, 44], continuing cEEG monitoring for 24 hours after cessation of electrographic seizures and weaning off anesthetic infusions, and for 48 hours following an acute brain insult in comatose patients.

Quantitative EEG Analysis to Identify Recurrent Seizures

In addition to standard cEEG analysis, QEEG offers a complementary method to facilitate rapid identification of recurrent electrographic seizures at the bedside [1]. QEEG techniques separate the EEG signals into amplitude and frequency, and compress time so that several hours can be displayed in one image, more easily allowing recurrent, paroxysmal changes to be identified (Figure 10.1) [1]. Color density spectral array (CDSA) EEG displays time on the x-axis and frequency on the y-axis, and represents the power (amplitude and frequency) with color; seizures appear in warmer colors [1]. However, if a seizure does not increase substantially in frequency or amplitude, it may not be apparent on CDSA. Conversely, artifacts that increase frequency or power could be mistaken for seizures on CDSA [45]. Thus, while CDSA may facilitate early recognition of seizures, confirmation with review of cEEG is required for definitive diagnosis. Another type of QEEG, amplitude-integrated EEG, represents time on the x-axis and amplitude on the y-axis, with seizures displayed as upward

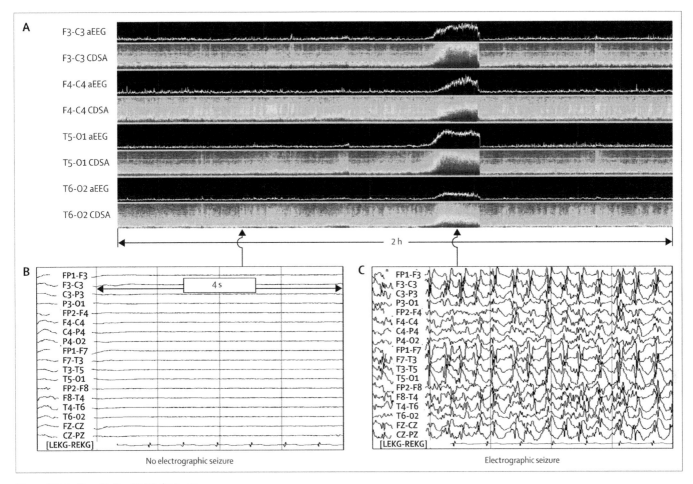

Figure 10.1 Quantitative EEG techniques.
EEG from a 13-year-old boy resuscitated from cardiac arrest with hypoxic-ischemic brain injury.
(A) A 2-hour color density spectral array (CDSA) and amplitude-integrated EEG (aEEG). Time progresses along the x-axis and amplitude is shown on the y-axis. For CDSA, power is shown in color. (B) The EEG background is low amplitude and slow, and thus both the aEEG and CDSA trends show low-amplitude activity. (C) During an electrographic seizure, amplitude and frequency are increased.
Reproduced from Electrographic seizures and status epilepticus in critically ill children and neonates with encephalopathy, Abend, N. S., et al., *Lancet Neurol.* 2013;**12** (12): pp. 1170–9, Copyright 2016, with permission from Elsevier. [109]

arches on the y-axis [1] (Figure 10.1). These QEEG trends may be displayed in conjunction to allow easier seizure recognition.

The advantage of quantitative EEG techniques is that they save time as compared to visual analysis of cEEG, and seizures may be identified at the bedside by non-electroencephalographers [1]. However, when using QEEG alone, seizures may be missed and some non-ictal events are misdiagnosed as seizure [45–47]. A study including 84 CDSA images reviewed by 8 encephalographers showed a sensitivity of 65% and specificity of 92% for seizure identification, with a 10% rate of false positives [45]. In a different study, 2 electrographers evaluated 27 CDSA and amplitude-integrated EEG displays. The median sensitivity for seizure identification was 83% using CDSA and 82% with amplitude-integrated EEG. However, when analyzing individual recordings the sensitivity ranged from 0% to 100%. Use of either technique led to a false positive about every 17–20 hours [46].

Quantitative EEG techniques are a great improvement toward a more rapid identification of many, but not all seizures [45, 46]. Similarly, with reliance on QEEG in isolation, false positives could be unnecessarily treated. Thus, while QEEG

may be used to identify suspected seizures, confirmation with raw cEEG is still needed [1, 45, 48].

Distinguishing Seizures from Periodic/Rhythmic Patterns

Seizures can be difficult to differentiate from other rhythmic and periodic EEG patterns prevalent among critically ill patients. The American Clinical Neurophysiology Society (ACNS) has defined periodic as "a periodic repetition of a waveform with relatively uniform morphology and duration with a quantifiable interdischarge interval between consecutive waveforms and recurrence of the waveform at nearly regular intervals." Discharges are defined as "waveforms with no more than 3 phases (i.e. crosses the baseline no more than twice) or any waveform lasting 0.5 seconds or less, regardless of number of phases" [49]. Periodic discharges frequently occur in critically ill neurological patients, and they have been classified into different types, such as lateralized periodic discharges (LPDs), bilateral independent periodic discharges (BIPDs), or generalized periodic discharges (GPDs)

The Ictal-Interictal-Injury Continuum

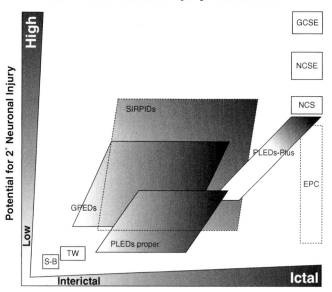

Figure 10.2 The ictal-interictal-injury continuum.
This figure represents different clinical electrographic diagnoses on the ictal-interictal continuum (x-axis). The y-axis represents the potential for secondary neuronal injury, and based on this, the likely importance of aggressive treatment. It is important to consider that if any of these patterns were to have clinical correlate, they would be considered ictal. However, presence of a clinical correlate would not necessarily confer higher chances of neuronal injury. Also, the terminology proposed by the 2012 ACNS guideline recommends the use of generalized periodic discharges (GPDs) instead of GPEDs, lateralized periodic discharges (LPDs) instead of PLEDs, continuous 2 per second GPDs with triphasic morphology instead of TW [49].
EPC, epilepsia partialis continua; GCSE, generalized convulsive status epilepticus; GPEDs, generalized periodic epileptiform discharges; NCS, nonconvulsive seizures; NCSE, nonconvulsive status epilepticus; PLEDs, periodic lateralized epileptiform discharges; S-B, suppression-burst; SIRPIDs, stimulus-induced rhythmic, periodic, or ictal discharges; TW, triphasic waves.
Reproduced from Which EEG patterns warrant treatment in the critically ill? reviewing the evidence for treatment of periodic epileptiform discharges and related patterns, Chong, D. J. and L. J. Hirsch, *J Clin Neurophysiol.* 2005;**22**(2): pp. 79–91, Copyright 2016, with permission from Wolters Kluwer Health, Inc. [50].

[49, 50]. Most of these have uncertain clinical significance on their own, but they are associated with an increased risk for seizures [49, 50].

The Ictal-Interictal Continuum

Periodic discharges have been interpreted as ictal, interictal, and postictal [51–58], or as predictors of electrographic seizures [26]. The lack of a clear distinction between seizures and other rhythmic and periodic EEG patterns has led to the concept of "ictal-interictal continuum," representing the uncertainty in distinguishing the potential ictal nature of these patterns and their associated clinical consequences [59] (Figure 10.2). There is currently no consensus for how these patterns should be treated due to our lack of understanding of their potential to cause neuronal injury [60].

Treatment of Status Epilepticus

As in any other emergency, the first step in the treatment of status epilepticus is stabilization: secure the airway and ensure

breathing and circulation. Current protocols recommend a rapid stepwise progression of treatment [43, 61–63]. As illustrated in Figure 10.3, the first-line treatments are benzodiazepines (BZDs), which should be administered within the first 5 to 10 minutes [43, 61, 63] of seizure onset, and by 20 minutes as suggested by the American Epilepsy Society (AES) guideline [62]. If the seizure persists, the first dose can be repeated. The second-line treatment is a non-BZD anti-seizure medicine (ASM) that should be started after 10 minutes [43, 61] and by 20 minutes [62]. If two non-BZD ASM doses do not control the status epilepticus, or if the duration is longer than 40 minutes [62] or 30–70 minutes [43, 61], the initiation of anesthetic drugs via continuous infusions is recommended [43, 61, 62]. These protocols are based on limited available data, and there is no clear evidence to guide third-line therapy [62].

Benzodiazepines

Benzodiazepines (BZDs) are relatively safe, rapid-acting, widely available, and effective drugs that have multiple routes of administration. The most commonly used initial therapy is intravenous lorazepam [7], which in a study of 182 children with status epilepticus had 3.7 (95% CI: 1.7–7.9) times greater likelihood of seizure cessation than rectal diazepam [64]. BZDs should be administered in the pre-hospital setting by caregivers or emergency medical services providers. A double-blind trial with 205 adults showed that patients who received pre-hospital treatment with lorazepam or diazepam had fewer respiratory or circulatory complications than patients treated with placebo [65]. Also, a meta-analysis demonstrated that intravenous lorazepam was at least as effective as intravenous diazepam, with fewer adverse effects [66].

Current guidelines recommend the use of intramuscular midazolam, intravenous lorazepam, or intravenous diazepam as first-line treatment of status epilepticus (level A, four class I randomized controlled trials [RCTs]) [62]. In the pre-hospital setting, alternative initial therapies are rectal diazepam, intranasal midazolam, and buccal midazolam (level B) [62]. In neonates, the most commonly used first-line medication is phenobarbital. Appropriate dosing of the BZD is important, as under-dosing in the emergency room is common among patients who fail to respond to BZD [67] and has been associated with ICU admission [68]. BZD should be administered as a single full dose, and intravenous lorazepam and diazepam can be repeated at full doses once (level A, two class I, one class II RCTs) [62] (Table 10.1). The most common adverse effect of BZDs is respiratory depression (level A) [62]; there is no substantial difference in this between BZD types (level B) [62]. Other adverse effects are sedation, cardiac dysrhythmia, and ataxia [7] (Table 10.1).

Non-benzodiazepine ASMs

If status epilepticus continues, the second-line treatment should be started 20 minutes from seizure onset [43, 61–63]. There are several non-benzodiazepine ASMs available, such as fosphenytoin (level U), valproic acid (level B, one class II study), levetiracetam (level U), or phenobarbital (level B, one class II study) [62]. Recent evidence suggests children with

Immediate management
Non-Invasive airway protection and gas exchange with head positioning.
Intubation if needed.
Monitoring O_2 saturation, blood pressure heart rate, temperature.
Finger stick blood glucose.
Peripheral IV access.
Medical and neurological examination.
Labs: BMP, magnesium, phosphate, CBC, LFT, coagulation tests, ABG, anticonvulsant levels.

Emergent Initial Therapy (given immediately)
IV: Lorazepam 0.1 mg/Kg IV (max 4 mg)–may repeat if seizures persist.
No IV:
Diazepam 2–5 years 0.5 mg/kg, 6–11 years 0.3 mg/kg, ≥12 years 0.2 g/kg (max 20 mg)
Midazolam IM if 13–40 kg then 5 mg. If >40 kg then 10 mg.
Intranasal 0.2 mg/kg.
Buccal 0.5 mg/kg.
Consider whether out-of-hospital benzodiazepines have been administered when considering how many doses to administer.

Urgent management
Additional diagnostic testing as Indicated: LP, CT, MRI, toxicology labs, Inborn errors of metabolism.
Consider EEG monitoring (evaluate for psychogenic status epilepticus or persisting EEG-only seizures).
Neurological consultation.

Urgent control therapy
Phenytoin 20 mg/kg IV (may give another 10 mg/kg if needed)–may cause arrhythmia, hypotension, purple glove syndrome.
OR Fosphenytoin 20 PE/kg IV (may be given another 10 PE/kg if needed).
OR consider phenobarbital, valproate sodium, or levetiracetam.

If <2 years, consider pyridoxine 100mg IV.

Refractory status epilepticus

If seizure continue after benzodiazepines and a second anti-seizure medication, the patient is in refractory status epilepticus regardless of elapsed time.

Continue management as make plans for ICU admission/transfer. Expect need for continuous EEG monitoring once clinically evident seizures terminate to evaluate for persisting EEG-only seizures.

Administer another urgent control anticonvulsant or proceed to pharmacological coma.
Levetiracetam 20–60 mg/kg IV
Valproate Sodium 20–40 mg/kg IV–contraindicated if liver disease, thrombocytopenia, or possible metabolic disease.
Phenobarbital 20–40 mg/kg IV–may cause respiratory depression and hypotension.

Pharmacological coma medications
Midazolam 0.2 mg/kg bolus (max 10 mg) and then initiate infusion at 0.1 mg/kg/hr. Titrate up as needed.
Pentobarbital 5 mg/kg bolus and then initiate infusion at 0.5 mg/kg/hour. Titrate up as needed.
Other options: Isoflurane

Pharmacological coma management
Titrate to either seizure suppression or burst suppression based on EEG monitoring.
Continue pharmacological coma for 24–48 hours.
Modify anti-seizure medications so additional seizure coverage is in place for influsion wean.
Continue diagnostic testing and Implementation of etiology-directed therapy.

Add-on options
Medications: phenytoin, phenobarbital, levetiracetam, valproate sodium, topiramate, lacosamide, ketamine, pyridoxine,
Other: epilepsy surgery, ketogenic diet, vagus nerve stimulator, Immunomodulation, hypothermia, electroconvulsive therapy.

Figure 10.3 Example of a pediatric status epilepticus evaluation and management pathway. ABG, arterial blood gas; BMP, basic metabolic panel; CBC, complete blood count; CT, computerized tomography; EEG, electroencephalography; IM, intramuscular; IV, intravenous; LFT, liver function tests; LP, lumbar puncture; PE, phenytoin equivalents.
Reproduced from Abend, N. S. and T. Loddenkemper, Pediatric status epilepticus management, *Curr Opin Pediatr.* 2014;**26**(6): pp. 668–74, Copyright 2016, with permission from Wolters Kluwer Health, Inc. [63]

status epilepticus refractory to benzodiazepines respond similarly to these medications; there are no data to support one as superior to the others [69–71].

An RCT (class II) of 100 children and adults with seizures that were refractory to BZD therapy compared IV valproic acid with IV phenytoin and found no difference between both in their efficacy (88% vs 84%) or adverse events [72]. Another RCT with 60 children compared valproate and phenobarbital, and found no difference in efficacy (valproate 90% vs phenobarbital 77%, p=0.19), but the patients in the valproate group had fewer adverse effects than those who received phenobarbital (24% vs 74%, p<0.001) [73]. A retrospective study included 167 adults with status epilepticus who were treated with phenytoin, valproate, and levetiracetam after BZD [74]. Valproate failed to control the status epilepticus in 25.4%, phenytoin in 41%, and levetiracetam in 48% of cases [74]. After adjusting for status epilepticus severity, levetiracetam failed more often than valproate (OR 2.69), but there was no difference in the efficacy of phenytoin compared to valproate and levetiracetam [74]. A different RCT randomized 68 patients with status epilepticus to receive valproate or phenytoin. Valproate aborted 66% of the seizures vs 42% in the phenytoin group (one-sided p=0.046) [75]. When the drug was used as a second choice in the refractory patients, valproate aborted 79% of the seizures while phenytoin 25% [75]. Also, there were difference on the adverse effect rate (one-sided p=0.004) [75].

Currently, the most common drug used as second-line treatment is fosphenytoin (or phenytoin), and the second option is usually phenobarbital [7, 43, 61]. However, these choices are mostly based on tradition, and current data show these drugs are not superior to newer ASMs, such as valproate and levetiracetam. The current AES guideline recommends the use of fosphenytoin, valproic acid, or levetiracetam as a second-line treatment [62]. Doses and common adverse effects are summarized in Table 10.1.

Table 10.1 Recommended initial doses and adverse effects
Recommended initial doses, maximum doses, routes, and main adverse effects for the first-, second-, and third-line medication of status epilepticus [7, 43]

Drug	Dose	Maximum dose	Route and rate	Main adverse effects
Benzodiazepines				
Lorazepam	0.1 mg/kg	4 mg	IV	Hypotension Respiratory depression
Diazepam	0.2–0.5 mg/kg 2–5 years, 0.5 mg/kg; 6–11 years, 0.3 mg/kg; >12 years, 0.2 mg/kg	20 mg	Rectal	Hypotension Respiratory depression
Diazepam	0.15–0.2 mg/kg	10 mg	IV	Hypotension Respiratory depression
Midazolam	0.2–0.3 mg/kg	10 mg	Nasal	Respiratory depression Hypotension
Midazolam	If 13–40 kg, 5mg; If >40 kg, 10 mg	10 mg	IM	Respiratory depression Hypotension
Phenobarbital	15 mg/kg	Single dose	IV	CNS and respiratory depression as well as hypotension
Non-BZD ASM				
Phenytoin	20 mg/kg at 1 mg/kg/min	50 mg/min	IV	Local tissue necrosis. Hypotension Arrhythmias
Fosphenytoin	20 PE/kg	150 mg PE/min	IV	Local tissue necrosis. Hypotension Arrhythmias
Valproate	40 mg/kg	3 000 mg/dose	IV 1.5–3 mg/kg/min	Hepatic failure and pancreatitis. Dose related increase in serum transaminases, Stevens–Johnson syndrome, and thrombocytopenia
Levetiracetam	60 mg/kg	4 500 mg/dose	IV 2–5 mg/kg/min	Agitation. Occasional phenytoin equivalents with overdosing
Phenobarbital	15 mg/kg	Maximum dose	Iv 50–100 mg/min	CNS and respiratory depression, hypotension

Continuous infusion

Midazolam	0.1–0.3 mg/kg, 2 mg/min (max. 10 mg bolus)	Breakthrough SE: 0.1–0.2 mg/kg bolus, increase CI rate by 0.05–0.1 mg/kg/h every 3–4 h.	0.05–2 mg/kg/h CI	Respiratory depression, hypotension
Pentobarbital	3 to 15 mg/kg, <50 mg/min	Breakthrough SE: 5 mg/kg bolus, increase CI rate by 0.5–1 mg/kg/h every 12 h	0.5–5 mg/kg/h CI	CNS and respiratory depression, hypotension, cardiac depression
Propofol	1–2 mg/kg (<65 mcg/kg/min)	Breakthrough SE: Increase CI rate by 5–10 mcg/kg/min every 5 min or 1 mg/kg bolus plus CI Titration	30–200 mcg/kg/min CI	Sedation, respiratory depression, hypotension. Propofol infusion syndrome may lead to cardiovascular compromise. Rhabdomyolysis, metabolic acidosis, renal failure (PRIS)
Thiopental	2–7 mg/kg, <50 mg/min	Breakthrough SE: 1–2 mg/kg bolus, increase CI rate by 0.5–1 mg/kg/h every 12 h	0.5–5 mg/kg/h CI	Hypotension Respiratory depression Cardiac depression

mg, milligrams; kg, kilograms; h, hour; min, minutes; IM, intramuscular; IV, intravenous; PE, phenytoin equivalents; ASM, anti-seizure medicine; BZDs, benzodiazepines; CI, continuous infusion; CNS, central nervous system; PRIS, propofol-related infusion syndrome; SE, status epilepticus.

Time to Treatment

Current status epilepticus treatment protocols recommend a timely and stepwise progression of the treatment of SE [43, 61, 62]. The rationale for this is that the longer the seizure, the worse the response to the treatment. BZDs act through binding and activation of the gamma-aminobutyric acid A receptor (GABA$_A$R), and this receptor internalizes during prolonged seizures, which leads to a loss of GABA-mediated inhibition [76, 77]. There is also an increase in the number of postsynaptic N-methyl-D-aspartate (NMDA) receptors, leading to an increase in excitation [78]. Animal models and clinical studies have demonstrated progressive refractoriness to BZD with treatment delay [79–81]. Delayed treatment is associated with prolonged seizures [31, 64, 81], and longer seizures have been associated with worse outcome [82, 83].

A prospective study of 81 patients demonstrated that longer time to the first three doses of BZD was correlated with longer status epilepticus duration [31]. Treatment delays were associated with intermittent refractory status epilepticus and out-of-hospital refractory status epilepticus [84]. A study of 240 episodes of convulsive status epilepticus in children showed that for every minute of delay in arrival to hospital patients had a 5% increased risk of prolonged status epilepticus (>60 minutes) [64]. In a series of 154 adult patients, a treatment before 30 minutes from seizure onset was associated with 80% of response to the first-line medication, while the response was less than 40% when they were treated after 2 hours [85]. A different study with 157 children with status epilepticus also showed a delayed response when patients were treated after 30 minutes [81].

The main outcome predictors for status epilepticus are age, etiology, and status epilepticus duration [30, 35, 83, 86]. The only factor that can be modified is the status epilepticus duration by using a faster treatment [31]. However, the treatment of status epilepticus is commonly delayed both in the pre-hospital and in-hospital setting [31]. In contrast with the time line recommended by guidelines and summarized in Figure 10.3, a multicenter study showed that the median (p25-p75) time to the first BZD was 28 (6–67) minutes and 69 (40–120) minutes to the first non-BZD ASM [31]. Treatment for status epilepticus should be initiated as quickly as possible.

Refractory Status Epilepticus

Status epilepticus is defined as refractory when it does not respond to the administration of two antiepileptic drugs with different mechanisms of action, i.e., one benzodiazepine and on non-BZD ASMs, independent of seizure duration [7, 43, 87, 88]. Status epilepticus is often refractory; in a series of 68 children with status epilepticus, 55.9% had refractory status epilepticus [89]; a different study with 154 children showed that 39% had refractory status epilepticus [90].

Continuous Infusions

After administering BZD and non-BZD ASM, the third-line treatment is continuous infusions of ASMs or anesthetic therapies [7, 43, 62]. The most common drugs used for continuous infusions are midazolam and pentobarbital, though largely on

convention rather than a strong evidence base [62]. Similarly, there is little evidence to direct precisely when to start a continuous infusion [43]. Some guidelines recommend to start continuous infusion relatively early [43, 62]; for example, the AES guideline recommends to start continuous infusion if seizure persists 40 minutes from seizure onset [62].

Many patients with status epilepticus may be require treatment with a third-line medication. A multicenter study with 542 children with status epilepticus found that 33% of patients had ongoing seizures after 40 minutes in the emergency department [91]. Status epilepticus terminated after first-line treatment in 42% of the children, after second-line treatment in 35%, and after continuous infusions in 22% [91]. In another study in children with status epilepticus, out of 240 episodes, 44 (18%) required anesthesia to terminate the seizures.

The most commonly used third-line medications are thiopental, midazolam, pentobarbital, or propofol [62]. All require cEEG monitoring. Table 10.1 shows the doses, suggested infusion rates, and main adverse effects of the most commonly used drugs (mostly respiratory depression and hypotension), as well as the treatment for breakthrough status epilepticus or recurrent seizures during infusion. The third-line treatment should always be started with close cardiopulmonary monitoring and with preparations for the possibility of intubation, mechanical ventilation, and blood pressure management. In addition to these potential adverse effects, some drug-specific effects have been described. Midazolam infusion in neonates resulting in myoclonus has been observed at higher doses [92]. Propofol has been used more frequently in the adult population, but the risk for propofol infusion syndrome in children is high and therefore not recommended in the pediatric ICU by some institutions [61].

cEEG Monitoring to Evaluate Burst Suppression and Depth of Anesthesia

Some treatment guidelines recommend titrating continuous infusions not only to seizure suppression but also to burst suppression on the EEG for 12–48 hours [7, 43, 93] (Figure 10.4). The aim for inducing burst suppression is to aid in preventing seizure recurrence once weaning the continuous infusions [7]. An RCT sought to compare drugs, but only recruited 24 out of the 150 patients needed, showing no difference between drugs in achieving burst suppression [88]. A retrospective study included 35 episodes of status epilepticus in adults treated with phenobarbital. Patients with a more intensive suppression of the EEG had fewer relapses (p=0.049), and there was a trend toward lower mortality as compared to a less intensive suppression (p=0.076) [94]. A review of 28 studies with 169 refractory status epilepticus cases treated with pentobarbital, midazolam, or propofol showed that burst suppression was associated with lower frequency of breakthrough seizures (4% vs 56%) but a higher frequency of hypotension (76% vs 29%) [95]. A different study with 22 adults with refractory status epilepticus who received continuous infusions showed that burst suppression was associated with good seizure control (83.3% in burst

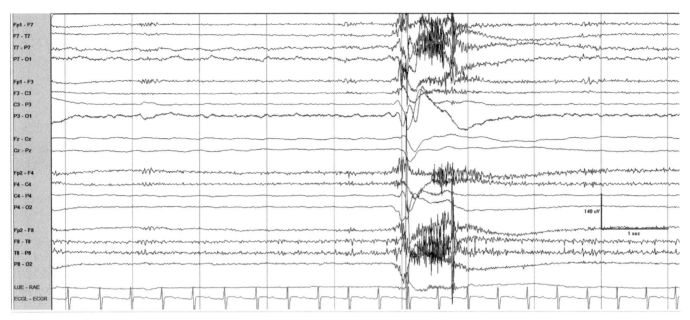

Figure 10.4 EEG example of burst suppression.
Example of burst suppression with bursts of generalized and multifocal spikes separated by periods of voltage attenuation.

suppression versus 62.5%), but not with outcome or prolonged hospital stay [96]. However, a retrospective study with 63 refractory status epilepticus episodes showed that patients had a better functional outcome when the treatment aimed seizure control (16 episodes) and not burst suppression (27 episodes) (p=0.01) [97].

Continuous EEG monitoring assists in medication titration and infusion rate adjustment required to achieve and maintain EEG background suppression while minimizing adverse effects [98]. Continuous EEG should also be used during the withdrawal of continuous infusions. The main adverse effects of continuous infusions, apart from respiratory depression, are hypotension, renal failure, cardiac depression, and hepatic dysfunction [7, 43]; these can be limited by using the lowest dose of continuous infusions needed to achieve burst suppression [98]. Infrequent and relatively short electrographic-only seizures may require a less aggressive approach in some situations where seizure suppression may compromise cardiovascular stability or the overall patient situation.

Other Therapies and Emerging Treatments

If the status epilepticus continues after using continuous infusion, it is considered super refractory status epilepticus. The most commonly used definition is "status epilepticus that continues for 24 hours or more after the onset of anesthesia,

including those cases in which the status epilepticus recurs on the reduction or withdrawal of anesthesia" [99]. In these patients, other therapies can be tried, but their efficacy is mainly supported by case reports of small case series limited by many potential confounders and simultaneous treatments [99]. One option is ketamine, which is an NMDA receptor antagonist. A multicenter study showed that ketamine contributed to the control of seizures in 32% of the cases; mortality was lower when the status epilepticus was controlled within 24 hours of ketamine initiation [100]. The ketogenic diet [101, 102] and hypothermia [103, 104] have also shown some efficacy in small case series. Patients who have an identifiable focus and refractory status epilepticus could be candidates for resective epilepsy surgery [105], or in the absence of focal epileptogenesis, corpus callosotomy may be considered [106]. Patients with suspected or confirmed autoimmune encephalitis may be treated with immunotherapy such as steroids, intravenous immunoglobulins, or plasma exchange [107, 108]. However, even in confirmed cases the response to treatment is variable [107, 108]. These alternative therapies are often used after several other treatments, with concomitant continuous infusions; large multicenter studies are needed to clarify their efficacy, especially in children. In the future, such targeted therapies could improve the treatment of status epilepticus.

References

1. Abend NS, Chapman KE, Gallentine WB, et al. Electroencephalographic monitoring in the pediatric intensive care unit. *Curr Neurol Neurosci Rep.* 2013;**13**(3):330.

2. Lothman E. The biochemical basis and pathophysiology of status epilepticus. *Neurology.* 1990;**40**(5 Suppl 2):13–23.

3. Meldrum BS, Horton RW. Physiology of status epilepticus in primates. *Arch Neurol.* 1973;**28**(1):1–9.

4. Lowenstein DH, Bleck T, Macdonald RL. It's time to revise the definition of status epilepticus. *Epilepsia.* 1999;**40**(1):120–2.

5. Tsuchida TN, Wusthoff CJ, Shellhaas RA, et al. American clinical neurophysiology society standardized EEG terminology and categorization for

the description of continuous EEG monitoring in neonates: report of the American Clinical Neurophysiology Society critical care monitoring committee. *J Clin Neurophysiol.* 2013;**30** (2):161–73.

6. Sanchez SM, Carpenter J, Chapman KE, et al. Pediatric ICU EEG monitoring: current resources and practice in the United States and Canada. *J Clin Neurophysiol.* 2013;**30**(2):156–60.

7. Loddenkemper T, Goodkin HP. Treatment of pediatric status epilepticus. *Curr Treat Options Neurol.* 2011;**13**(6):560–73.

8. Chin RF, Neville BG, Scott RC. A systematic review of the epidemiology of status epilepticus. *Eur J Neurol.* 2004;**11**(12):800–10.

9. DeLorenzo RJ, Hauser WA, Towne AR, et al. A prospective, population-based epidemiologic study of status epilepticus in Richmond, Virginia. *Neurology.* 1996;**46**(4):1029–35.

10. Hesdorffer DC, Logroscino G, Cascino G, Annegers JF, Hauser WA. Incidence of status epilepticus in Rochester, Minnesota, 1965–1984. *Neurology.* 1998;**50**(3):735–41.

11. Abend NS, Gutierrez-Colina AM, Topjian AA, et al. Nonconvulsive seizures are common in critically ill children. *Neurology.* 2011;**76** (12):1071–7.

12. Hosain SA, Solomon GE, Kobylarz EJ. Electroencephalographic patterns in unresponsive pediatric patients. *Pediatr Neurol.* 2005;**32**(3):162–5.

13. Jette N, Claassen J, Emerson RG, Hirsch LJ. Frequency and predictors of nonconvulsive seizures during continuous electroencephalographic monitoring in critically ill children. *Arch Neurol.* 2006;**63**(12):1750–5.

14. Abend NS, Dlugos DJ. Nonconvulsive status epilepticus in a pediatric intensive care unit. *Pediatr Neurol.* 2007;**37**(3):165–70.

15. Alehan FK, Morton LD, Pellock JM. Utility of electroencephalography in the pediatric emergency department. *J Child Neurol.* 2001;**16**(7):484–7.

16. Shahwan A, Bailey C, Shekerdemian L, Harvey AS. The prevalence of seizures in comatose children in the pediatric intensive care unit: a prospective video-EEG study. *Epilepsia.* 2010;**51** (7):1198–204.

17. Williams K, Jarrar R, Buchhalter J. Continuous video-EEG monitoring in pediatric intensive care units. *Epilepsia.* 2011;**52**(6):1130–6.

18. Kirkham FJ, Wade AM, McElduff F, et al. Seizures in 204 comatose children: incidence and outcome. *Intensive Care Med.* 2012;**38**(5):853–62.

19. Abend NS, Topjian A, Ichord R, et al. Electroencephalographic monitoring during hypothermia after pediatric cardiac arrest. *Neurology.* 2009;**72** (22):1931–40.

20. Tay SK, Hirsch LJ, Leary L, et al. Nonconvulsive status epilepticus in children: clinical and EEG characteristics. *Epilepsia.* 2006;**47** (9):1504–9.

21. Greiner HM, Holland K, Leach JL, et al. Nonconvulsive status epilepticus: the encephalopathic pediatric patient. *Pediatrics.* 2012;**129**(3):e748–55.

22. Saengpattrachai M, Sharma R, Hunjan A, et al. Nonconvulsive seizures in the pediatric intensive care unit: etiology, EEG, and brain imaging findings. *Epilepsia.* 2006;**47**(9):1510–18.

23. Topjian AA, Gutierrez-Colina AM, Sanchez SM, et al. Electrographic status epilepticus is associated with mortality and worse short-term outcome in critically ill children. *Crit Care Med.* 2013;**41**(1):215–23.

24. Abend NS. Electrographic status epilepticus in children with critical illness: epidemiology and outcome. *Epilepsy Behav.* 2015;**49**:223–7.

25. Abend NS, Arndt DH, Carpenter JL, et al. Electrographic seizures in pediatric ICU patients: cohort study of risk factors and mortality. *Neurology.* 2013;**81**(4):383–91.

26. Claassen J, Mayer SA, Kowalski RG, Emerson RG, Hirsch LJ. Detection of electrographic seizures with continuous EEG monitoring in critically ill patients. *Neurology.* 2004;**62** (10):1743–8.

27. Towne AR, Waterhouse EJ, Boggs JG, et al. Prevalence of nonconvulsive status epilepticus in comatose patients. *Neurology.* 2000;**54**(2):340–5.

28. Sanchez Fernandez I, Abend NS, Arndt DH, et al. Electrographic seizures after convulsive status epilepticus in children and young adults: a retrospective multicenter study. *J Pediatr.* 2014;**164**(2):339–46 e1-2.

29. Loddenkemper T, Syed TU, Ramgopal S, et al. Risk factors associated with death in in-hospital pediatric convulsive status epilepticus. *PLoS ONE.* 2012;**7**(10):e47474.

30. Maytal J, Shinnar S, Moshe SL, Alvarez LA. Low morbidity and mortality of status epilepticus in children. *Pediatrics.* 1989;**83**(3):323–31.

31. Sanchez Fernandez I, Abend NS, Agadi S, et al. Time from convulsive status epilepticus onset to anticonvulsant administration in children. *Neurology.* 2015;**84**(23):2304–11.

32. Coeytaux A, Jallon P, Galobardes B, Morabia A. Incidence of status epilepticus in French-speaking Switzerland: (EPISTAR). *Neurology.* 2000;**55**(5):693–7.

33. Knake S, Rosenow F, Vescovi M, et al. Incidence of status epilepticus in adults in Germany: a prospective, population-based study. *Epilepsia.* 2001;**42**(6):714–18.

34. Martinos MM, Yoong M, Patil S, et al. Early developmental outcomes in children following convulsive status epilepticus: a longitudinal study. *Epilepsia.* 2013;**54**(6):1012–19.

35. Raspall-Chaure M, Chin RF, Neville BG, Scott RC. Outcome of paediatric convulsive status epilepticus: a systematic review. *Lancet Neurol.* 2006;**5**(9):769–79.

36. Sahin M, Menache CC, Holmes GL, Riviello JJ. Outcome of severe refractory status epilepticus in children. *Epilepsia.* 2001;**42**(11):1461–7.

37. Payne ET, Zhao XY, Frndova H, et al. Seizure burden is independently associated with short term outcome in critically ill children. *Brain.* 2014;**137** (Pt 5):1429–38.

38. Schreiber JM, Zelleke T, Gaillard WD, et al. Continuous video EEG for patients with acute encephalopathy in a pediatric intensive care unit. *Neurocrit Care.* 2012;**17**(1):31–8.

39. Abend NS, Topjian AA, Williams S. How much does it cost to identify a critically ill child experiencing electrographic seizures? *J Clin Neurophysiol.* 2015;**32**(3):257–64.

40. Abend NS, Dlugos DJ, Hahn CD, Hirsch LJ, Herman ST. Use of EEG monitoring and management of non-convulsive seizures in critically ill patients: a survey of neurologists. *Neurocrit Care.* 2010;**12** (3):382–9.

41. Payne ET, Hahn CD. Continuous electroencephalography for seizures

and status epilepticus. *Curr Opin Pediatr.* 2014;**26**(6):675–81.

42. Gutierrez-Colina AM, Topjian AA, Dlugos DJ, Abend NS. Electroencephalogram monitoring in critically ill children: indications and strategies. *Pediatr Neurol.* 2012;**46**(3):158–61.

43. Brophy GM, Bell R, Claassen J, et al. Guidelines for the evaluation and management of status epilepticus. *Neurocrit Care.* 2012;**17**(1):3–23.

44. Herman ST, Abend NS, Bleck TP, et al. Consensus statement on continuous EEG in critically ill adults and children, part II: personnel, technical specifications, and clinical practice. *J Clin Neurophysiol.* 2015;**32**(2):96–108.

45. Pensirikul AD, Beslow LA, Kessler SK, et al. Density spectral array for seizure identification in critically ill children. *J Clin Neurophysiol.* 2013;**30**(4):371–5.

46. Stewart CP, Otsubo H, Ochi A, et al. Seizure identification in the ICU using quantitative EEG displays. *Neurology.* 2010;**75**(17):1501–8.

47. Shah DK, Mackay MT, Lavery S, et al. Accuracy of bedside electroencephalographic monitoring in comparison with simultaneous continuous conventional electroencephalography for seizure detection in term infants. *Pediatrics.* 2008;**121**(6):1146–54.

48. Shellhaas RA, Chang T, Tsuchida T, et al. The American Clinical Neurophysiology Society's Guideline on Continuous Electroencephalography Monitoring in Neonates. *J Clin Neurophysiol.* 2011;**28**(6):611–17.

49. Hirsch LJ, LaRoche SM, Gaspard N, et al. American Clinical Neurophysiology Society's Standardized Critical Care EEG Terminology: 2012 version. *J Clin Neurophysiol.* 2013;**30**(1):1–27.

50. Chong DJ, Hirsch LJ. Which EEG patterns warrant treatment in the critically ill? Reviewing the evidence for treatment of periodic epileptiform discharges and related patterns. *J Clin Neurophysiol.* 2005;**22**(2):79–91.

51. Ronner HE, Ponten SC, Stam CJ, Uitdehaag BM. Inter-observer variability of the EEG diagnosis of seizures in comatose patients. *Seizure.* 2009;**18**(4):257–63.

52. Brenner RP, Schaul N. Periodic EEG patterns: classification, clinical correlation, and pathophysiology. *J Clin Neurophysiol.* 1990;**7**(2):249–67.

53. Garzon E, Fernandes RM, Sakamoto AC. Serial EEG during human status epilepticus: evidence for PLED as an ictal pattern. *Neurology.* 2001;**57**(7):1175–83.

54. Treiman DM, Walton NY, Kendrick C. A progressive sequence of electroencephalographic changes during generalized convulsive status epilepticus. *Epilepsy Res.* 1990;**5**(1):49–60.

55. Yemisci M, Gurer G, Saygi S, Ciger A. Generalised periodic epileptiform discharges: clinical features, neuroradiological evaluation and prognosis in 37 adult patients. *Seizure.* 2003;**12**(7):465–72.

56. Garcia-Morales I, Garcia MT, Galan-Davila L, et al. Periodic lateralized epileptiform discharges: etiology, clinical aspects, seizures, and evolution in 130 patients. *J Clin Neurophysiol.* 2002;**19**(2):172–7.

57. Brenner RP. Is it status? *Epilepsia.* 2002;**43** (Suppl 3):103–13.

58. Fushimi M, Matsubuchi N, Sekine A, Shimizu T. Benign bilateral independent periodic lateralized epileptiform discharges. *Acta Neurol Scand.* 2003;**108**(1):55–9.

59. Koren JP, Herta J, Pirker S, et al. Rhythmic and periodic EEG patterns of "ictal-interictal uncertainty" in critically ill neurological patients. *Clin Neurophysiol.* 2016;**127**(2):1176–81.

60. Claassen J. How I treat patients with EEG patterns on the ictal-interictal continuum in the neuro ICU. *Neurocrit Care.* 2009;**11**(3):437–44.

61. Wilkes R, Tasker RC. Pediatric intensive care treatment of uncontrolled status epilepticus. *Crit Care Clin.* 2013;**29**(2):239–57.

62. Glauser T, Shinnar S, Gloss D, et al. Evidence-based guideline: treatment of convulsive status epilepticus in children and adults: report of the Guideline Committee of the American Epilepsy Society. *Epilepsy Curr.* 2016;**16**(1):48–61.

63. Abend NS, Loddenkemper T. Pediatric status epilepticus management. *Curr Opin Pediatr.* 2014;**26**(6):668–74.

64. Chin RF, Neville BG, Peckham C, et al. Wade A, Bedford H, Scott RC. Treatment of community-onset, childhood convulsive status epilepticus: a prospective, population-based study. *Lancet Neurol.* 2008;**7**(8):696–703.

65. Alldredge BK, Gelb AM, Isaacs SM, et al. A comparison of lorazepam, diazepam, and placebo for the treatment of out-of-hospital status epilepticus. *N Engl J Med.* 2001;**345**(9):631–7.

66. Appleton R, Macleod S, Martland T. Drug management for acute tonic-clonic convulsions including convulsive status epilepticus in children. *Cochrane Database Syst Rev.* 2008(3):CD001905.

67. Sathe AG, Tillman H, Coles LD, et al. Underdosing of benzodiazepines in patients with status epilepticus enrolled in established status epilepticus treatment trial. *Acad Emerg Med.* 2019;**26**(8):940–3.

68. Chin RF, Verhulst L, Neville BG, Peters MJ, Scott RC. Inappropriate emergency management of status epilepticus in children contributes to need for intensive care. *J Neurol Neurosurg Psychiatry.* 2004;**75**(11):1584–8.

69. Chamberlain JM, Kapur J, Shinnar S, et al. Efficacy of levetiracetam, fosphenytoin, and valproate for established status epilepticus by age group (ESETT): a double-blind, responsive-adaptive, randomised controlled trial. *Lancet.* 2020;**395**(10231):1217–24.

70. Dalziel SR, Borland ML, Furyk J, et al. Levetiracetam versus phenytoin for second-line treatment of convulsive status epilepticus in children (ConSEPT): an open-label, multicentre, randomised controlled trial. *Lancet.* 2019;**393**(10186):2125–34.

71. Lyttle MD, Rainford NEA, Gamble C, et al. Levetiracetam versus phenytoin for second-line treatment of paediatric convulsive status epilepticus (EcLiPSE): a multicentre, open-label, randomised trial. *Lancet.* 2019; **393**(10186):2135–45.

72. Agarwal P, Kumar N, Chandra R, et al. Randomized study of intravenous valproate and phenytoin in status epilepticus. *Seizure.* 2007;**16**(6):527–32.

73. Malamiri RA, Ghaempanah M, Khosroshahi N, et al. Efficacy and safety of intravenous sodium valproate versus phenobarbital in controlling convulsive status epilepticus and acute prolonged convulsive seizures in children: a randomised trial. *Eur J Paediatr Neurol.* 2012;**16**(5):536–41.

74. Alvarez V, Januel JM, Burnand B, Rossetti AO. Second-line status epilepticus treatment: comparison of phenytoin, valproate, and

levetiracetam. *Epilepsia*. 2011;**52**(7):1292–6.

75. Misra UK, Kalita J, Patel R. Sodium valproate vs phenytoin in status epilepticus: a pilot study. *Neurology*. 2006;**67**(2):340–2.

76. Goodkin HP, Yeh JL, Kapur J. Status epilepticus increases the intracellular accumulation of GABAA receptors. *J Neurosci*. 2005;**25**(23):5511–20.

77. Naylor DE, Liu H, Wasterlain CG. Trafficking of GABA(A) receptors, loss of inhibition, and a mechanism for pharmacoresistance in status epilepticus. *J Neurosci*. 2005;**25**(34):7724–33.

78. Naylor DE, Liu H, Niquet J, Wasterlain CG. Rapid surface accumulation of NMDA receptors increases glutamatergic excitation during status epilepticus. *Neurobiol Dis*. 2013;**54**:225–38.

79. Mazarati AM, Baldwin RA, Sankar R, Wasterlain CG. Time-dependent decrease in the effectiveness of antiepileptic drugs during the course of self-sustaining status epilepticus. *Brain Res*. 1998;**814**(1–2):179–85.

80. Goodkin HP, Liu X, Holmes GL. Diazepam terminates brief but not prolonged seizures in young, naive rats. *Epilepsia*. 2003;**44**(8):1109–12.

81. Eriksson K, Kalviainen R. Pharmacologic management of convulsive status epilepticus in childhood. *Expert Rev Neurother*. 2005;**5**(6):777–83.

82. DeLorenzo RJ, Garnett LK, Towne AR, et al. Comparison of status epilepticus with prolonged seizure episodes lasting from 10 to 29 minutes. *Epilepsia*. 1999;**40**(2):164–9.

83. Logroscino G, Hesdorffer DC, Cascino GD, et al. Long-term mortality after a first episode of status epilepticus. *Neurology*. 2002;**58**(4):537–41.

84. Sanchez Fernandez I, Gainza-Lein M, Abend NS, et al. Factors associated with treatment delays in pediatric refractory convulsive status epilepticus. *Neurology*. 2018;**90**(19):e1692-e701.

85. Lowenstein DH, Alldredge BK. Status epilepticus at an urban public hospital in the 1980s. *Neurology*. 1993; **43** (3 Pt 1): 483–8.

86. Sutter R, Kaplan PW, Ruegg S. Outcome predictors for status epilepticus–what really counts. *Nat Rev Neurol*. 2013;**9**(9):525–34.

87. Sanchez Fernandez I, Abend NS, Agadi S, et al. Gaps and opportunities in refractory status epilepticus research in children: a multi-center approach by the Pediatric Status Epilepticus Research Group (pSERG). *Seizure*. 2014;**23**(2):87–97.

88. Rossetti AO, Lowenstein DH. Management of refractory status epilepticus in adults: still more questions than answers. *Lancet Neurol*. 2011;**10**(10):922–30.

89. Koul R, Chacko A, Javed H, Al Riyami K. Eight-year study of childhood status epilepticus: midazolam infusion in management and outcome. *J Child Neurol*. 2002;**17**(12):908–10.

90. Lambrechtsen FA, Buchhalter JR. Aborted and refractory status epilepticus in children: a comparative analysis. *Epilepsia*. 2008;**49**(4):615–25.

91. Lewena S, Pennington V, Acworth J, et al. Emergency management of pediatric convulsive status epilepticus: a multicenter study of 542 patients. *Pediatr Emerg Care*. 2009;**25**(2):83–7.

92. Zaw W, Knoppert DC, da Silva O. Flumazenil's reversal of myoclonic-like movements associated with midazolam in term newborns. *Pharmacotherapy*. 2001;**21**(5):642–6.

93. Meierkord H, Boon P, Engelsen B, et al. EFNS guideline on the management of status epilepticus in adults. *Eur J Neurol*. 2010;**17**(3):348–55.

94. Krishnamurthy KB, Drislane FW. Depth of EEG suppression and outcome in barbiturate anesthetic treatment for refractory status epilepticus. *Epilepsia*. 1999;**40**(6):759–62.

95. Claassen J, Hirsch LJ, Emerson RG, Mayer SA. Treatment of refractory status epilepticus with pentobarbital, propofol, or midazolam: a systematic review. *Epilepsia*. 2002;**43**(2):146–53.

96. Kang BS, Jung KH, Shin JW, et al. Induction of burst suppression or coma using intravenous anesthetics in refractory status epilepticus. *J Clin Neurosci*. 2015;**22**(5):854–8.

97. Hocker SE, Britton JW, Mandrekar JN, Wijdicks EF, Rabinstein AA. Predictors of outcome in refractory status epilepticus. *JAMA Neurol*. 2013;**70**(1):72–7.

98. Friedman D, Claassen J, Hirsch LJ. Continuous electroencephalogram monitoring in the intensive care unit. *Anesth Analg*. 2009;**109**(2):506–23.

99. Ferlisi M, Shorvon S. The outcome of therapies in refractory and super-refractory convulsive status epilepticus and recommendations for therapy. *Brain*. 2012;**135**(Pt 8):2314–28.

100. Gaspard N, Foreman B, Judd LM, et al. Intravenous ketamine for the treatment of refractory status epilepticus: a retrospective multicenter study. *Epilepsia*. 2013;**54**(8):1498–503.

101. Nabbout R, Mazzuca M, Hubert P, et al. Efficacy of ketogenic diet in severe refractory status epilepticus initiating fever induced refractory epileptic encephalopathy in school age children (FIRES). *Epilepsia*. 2010;**51**(10):2033–7.

102. Fung EL, Chang SK, Yam KK, Yau PY. Ketogenic diet as a therapeutic option in super-refractory status epilepticus. *Pediatrics and Neonatol*. 2015;**56**(6):429–31.

103. Corry JJ, Dhar R, Murphy T, Diringer MN. Hypothermia for refractory status epilepticus. *Neurocrit Care*. 2008;**9**(2):189–97.

104. Lin JJ, Lin KL, Hsia SH, Wang HS. Therapeutic hypothermia for febrile infection-related epilepsy syndrome in two patients. *Pediatr Neurol*. 2012;**47**(6):448–50.

105. Vendrame M, Loddenkemper T. Surgical treatment of refractory status epilepticus in children: candidate selection and outcome. *Semin Pediatr Neurol*. 2010;**17**(3):182–9.

106. Greiner HM, Tillema JM, Hallinan BE, et al. Corpus callosotomy for treatment of pediatric refractory status epilepticus. *Seizure*. 2012;**21**(4):307–9.

107. Petit-Pedrol M, Armangue T, Peng X, et al. Encephalitis with refractory seizures, status epilepticus, and antibodies to the GABAA receptor: a case series, characterisation of the antigen, and analysis of the effects of antibodies. *Lancet Neurol*. 2014;**13**(3):276–86.

108. Suleiman J, Brilot F, Lang B, Vincent A, Dale RC. Autoimmune epilepsy in children: case series and proposed guidelines for identification. *Epilepsia*. 2013;**54**(6):1036–45.

109. Abend NS, Wusthoff CJ, Goldberg EM, Dlugos DJ. Electrographic seizures and status epilepticus in critically ill children and neonates with encephalopathy. *Lancet Neurol*. 2013;**12**(12):1170–9.

Screening for Seizures in At-Risk Pediatric Patients

Adam Wallace and Eric T. Payne

Illustrative Cases

Key Points

- Seizures are common among encephalopathic critically ill children.
- Continuous EEG monitoring is required to diagnose seizures in this vulnerable population, as most seizures lack any definitive clinical signs.
- The etiology for seizures in this at-risk population is extremely heterogeneous and does not require the presence of an acute brain injury.
- Certain clinical and EEG characteristics can help predict the risk for seizures and the duration of EEG monitoring.

Introduction

Neurological injury is extremely common among children admitted to the pediatric intensive care unit (PICU) [1]. These children have longer lengths of stay and higher mortality rates compared to their non-neurologically affected critically ill peers, with seizures and status epilepticus occupying the most common neurological diagnoses [1]. Observational studies of children undergoing continuous EEG (cEEG) monitoring in the PICU have identified electrographic seizures in 7%–46% [2–10], and status epilepticus in 1%–23% [2–7]. Importantly, the vast majority (>70%) of these EEG-confirmed seizures are subclinical, lacking any clear clinical signs [11], thus necessitating the use of cEEG to detect and

treat them. Further, EEG-confirmed status epilepticus can be *entirely* subclinical; hence, without cEEG monitoring, some children with status epilepticus can be completely missed [11].

The importance of recognizing and treating seizures in this vulnerable pediatric population is supported by a growing body of evidence suggesting that seizures, both clinical and subclinical, negatively impact short- and long-term clinical outcomes [6, 12–16]. Indeed, an increasing seizure burden is independently associated with worsened neurological decline, including patients with MRI-negative brain injury [6]. While aggressive management of seizures in the PICU has not yet been shown to improve outcomes, the available data strongly suggest that seizures, and an increasing seizure burden, are harmful to the developing brain. Hence, titrating anti-seizure medications to achieve control of EEG-confirmed seizures may modulate or attenuate the secondary, independent brain injury associated with an increased electrographic seizure burden.

Continuous EEG monitoring offers the only noninvasive means to detect subclinical seizures and to confirm whether paroxysmal events suspicious for seizures (autonomic, motor, etc.), do in fact represent clinical seizure activity. As clinically based prediction of seizures is difficult and unreliable [17–19], cEEG monitoring is required to ascertain whether clinical paroxysms of concern truly represent seizure activity. This information can help to avoid unnecessary administration of anti-seizure medications and their potentially harmful sequelae [20]. Further, administration of short-acting paralytics during cEEG monitoring can help to confirm true cortical seizures (i.e., cortical myoclonus vs. non-cortical hiccups).

While critically ill children with encephalopathy and acute brain injury are at highest risk for seizures, seizures can occur even in the absence of MRI-confirmed brain injury [5, 6]. This chapter will discuss the evidence to support screening for seizures in specific disease states encountered in the PICU population where clinical and subclinical seizures are common. We will begin by outlining the *key clinical and EEG risk factors* for the development of seizures shared by children admitted to the PICU across all etiologies. We will then discuss the *etiology-specific* risk factors. Finally, considerations related to the *timing and duration* of cEEG monitoring will be discussed.

Risk Factors for Seizures in Critically Ill Children

Across several large observational studies of pediatric patients admitted to the PICU who underwent cEEG monitoring,

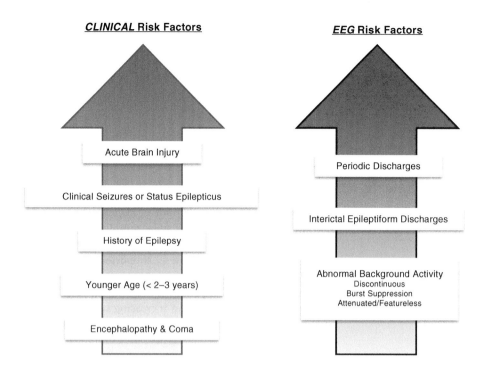

CLINICAL Risk Factors

Acute Brain Injury

Clinical Seizures or Status Epilepticus

History of Epilepsy

Younger Age (< 2–3 years)

Encephalopathy & Coma

EEG Risk Factors

Periodic Discharges

Interictal Epileptiform Discharges

Abnormal Background Activity
Discontinuous
Burst Suppression
Attenuated/Featureless

Figure 11.1 Clinical and EEG risk factors associated with the development of electrographic clinical and subclinical seizures among pediatric patients admitted to the ICU. This figure is based on information from large retrospective and prospective observational studies of critically ill children undergoing cEEG monitoring [2–7, 9, 10, 23].

certain clinical and electrographic risk factors are consistently associated with the development of clinical and subclinical seizures (Figure 11.1).

Encephalopathy and Coma

An extremely important risk factor for seizure occurrence among all PICU patients is the presence of *encephalopathy*, or an altered mental state. This encephalopathy can be secondary to an underlying brain injury, ongoing subclinical or dyscognitive seizure activity, or iatrogenically induced by sedative and paralytic medications. Encephalopathic patients are particularly vulnerable to subclinical seizures or seizures with subtle clinical correlate, as their encephalopathy masks clear clinical expression of their seizures. Indeed, most observational studies assessing the frequency of seizures in PICU patients are performed on patients with some degree of explained or unexplained encephalopathy [2, 3, 5, 6]. When sedative or paralytic medications are used, the accuracy of one's clinical exam becomes limited. In these instances, the presence of additional clinical risk factors can direct the need to initiate cEEG monitoring, while the initial few hours of EEG background activity (discussed below) can help to direct cEEG monitoring duration.

Acute Brain Injury

The presence of an *acute brain injury* is not only the single most important prognostic factor in determining neurological outcomes among critically ill children, but is also *the most important risk factor* for the development of clinical and subclinical seizures [6]. While not all acute brain injuries (i.e., infection, trauma, stroke) carry the same degree of seizure risk, the presence (or suspicion) of an acute brain injury in a critically ill child, particularly one with concomitant

encephalopathy, is highly associated with electrographic seizures. Etiology-specific electrographic seizure risks are described in more detail below.

Clinical Seizures and Status Epilepticus

Not surprisingly, the presence or suspicion of *clinical seizures* and/or convulsive status epilepticus increases the risk for developing subsequent clinical and subclinical seizures. Retrospective studies have observed electrographic seizures in as many as 70%–79% of those who experienced clinical seizures prior to cEEG monitoring [2, 4]. Similarly, nonconvulsive status epilepticus was preceded by an early clinical seizure in 92% of patients [21]. Clinical seizures need not reach the severity of status epilepticus, as single convulsions are an independent risk factor for the development of subclinical seizures [2, 3, 9].

Younger Age

Younger children, especially children less than 2–3 years old, are at increased risk for developing seizures in the ICU [3–6, 10]. This is especially important given evidence that the young brain is particularly vulnerable to injury [22]. While pediatric patients are generally felt to be at a higher risk for subclinical seizures than adults, data suggest that there is an even greater risk of seizures with decreasing age within the pediatric population. Specifically, with each year of increasing age there was a 7% decrease in the odds for seizure occurrence [3]. Indeed, this trend continues into the neonatal period, a demographic highly prone to (subclinical) seizures (detailed in Chapter 8). This association between younger age and increased seizure frequency is particularly true for some of the specific acute brain injury etiologies (i.e., trauma, stroke) as discussed later in this chapter.

Electrographic Risk Factors

Once cEEG monitoring is initiated, several electrographic risk factors, when present, are consistently associated with a higher likelihood of seizure development [11]. These include: (1) the presence of interictal epileptiform discharges; (2) the presence of periodic discharges (both lateralized and generalized); and (3) an abnormal background activity – particularly discontinuous, burst suppressed and attenuated/featureless backgrounds.

Focal interictal discharges and lateralized periodic discharges suggest an increased propensity toward focal seizures arising from the area(s) where these discharges are observed on EEG. Among children, periodic discharges likely carry a higher risk for seizure occurrence compared to non-periodic interictal epileptiform discharges [23]. Among adult patients undergoing cEEG monitoring, a continuous background with generalized slowing and the *absence* of interictal and periodic discharges during the first few hours of cEEG monitoring is quite predictive that the patient will *not* develop seizures [24, 25]. This is likely true of pediatric patients as well, but has not been studied as such. These EEG risk factors are therefore quite helpful in determining the appropriate duration of cEEG monitoring, which can be particularly useful when EEG resources are limited.

Etiology-Specific Risk Factors for Seizures

The following sections describe the risk for electrographic seizures among critically ill children categorized by primary etiology (Figure 11.2). Among the observational studies assessing seizures in children admitted to the ICU who underwent cEEG monitoring, the etiologies were quite heterogeneous, and specific details are often not available [2–7, 9, 10, 23]. Most of these studies were retrospective and classified each patient's etiology after the fact, with the primary etiologies frequently categorized differently among studies. Further, whether or not the cEEG-confirmed seizures had clinical correlate (subclinical vs clinical) for a specific etiology category was largely unreported. Thus, consolidating the available literature for etiology-specific electrographic seizure risk is challenging and subject to limitations. Consider also that one acute neurological diagnosis does not preclude the existence of others (i.e., an encephalopathic child with acute bacterial meningitis, encephalopathy, clinical status epilepticus, who subsequently develops multifocal ischemic strokes) – many studies specified only a single primary etiology.

Acute Convulsive Status Epilepticus and/or Pre-Existing Epilepsy

Convulsive status epilepticus during the acute phase of illness is a common indication for cEEG monitoring in the PICU setting [26]. This is for good reason, given that even when treated appropriately, the clinical correlate to a patient's seizures frequently becomes subtle or entirely absent, a phenomenon termed uncoupling. Cohorts of adults and children with convulsive status epilepticus placed on cEEG monitoring after "resolution" of convulsive status epilepticus have very high rates of subsequent subclinical seizures, including many with continued nonconvulsive status epilepticus [27, 28]. In a series of 98 children with convulsive status epilepticus, 32 children developed electrographic seizures, including 11 patients with subclinical-only seizures [28]. It is worth re-iterating that status epilepticus can be *entirely* subclinical and missed without cEEG monitoring [6, 28].

Patients with a history of epilepsy are also at a higher risk for developing electrographic seizures during their PICU admission, many of whom present with increased seizure frequency [2, 5, 6, 9]. In one series, patients with an "acute presentation of epilepsy" were found to be the highest risk group, with 50% of patients developing subclinical seizures [9]. Similarly, in the largest cohort of PICU patients monitored with cEEG, 48% of patients with a diagnosis of epilepsy had electrographic seizures [5].

As such, serious consideration for cEEG monitoring should be given to any patient who presents to a PICU with convulsive status epilepticus or an exacerbation of their pre-existing epilepsy, even if there is apparent resolution of clinical seizure activity. Cessation of clinical seizures and convulsive status epilepticus should not be considered definitive seizure resolution. A slow return to cognitive baseline or the presence of concomitant risk factors (i.e., presence of an acute brain injury) further supports the need for cEEG monitoring in this population to rule out subclinical seizures including nonconvulsive status epilepticus.

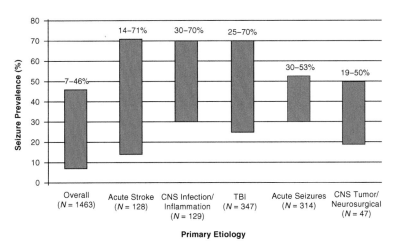

Figure 11.2 Prevalence of electrographic seizures among critically ill children undergoing cEEG monitoring stratified by primary etiology. Data were consolidated from multiple pediatric cohort studies as follows: (1) Overall [2–7, 9, 10, 23]; (2) Acute Stroke [3–6, 41]; (3) CNS Infection/Inflammation [2–6, 10]; (4) TBI [2–6, 10, 29, 30]; (5) Acute Seizures [2–6, 10]; (6) CNS Tumor/Neurosurgical [2, 3, 5, 6, 10]. Acute stroke, acute ischemic stroke, intracerebral hemorrhage, and cerebral sinus venous thrombosis; CNS, central nervous system; TBI, traumatic brain injury; acute seizures, new onset seizures or seizure exacerbation among patients with pre-existing epilepsy.

Traumatic Brain Injury

Traumatic brain injury (TBI) is a very important risk factor for the development of electrographic seizures among critically ill children – many of whom present with persistent encephalopathy [5, 29–33]. Among large observational cohort studies of critically ill children admitted to the ICU who underwent cEEG monitoring, 25%–70% of patients with TBI had electrographic seizures which were frequently subclinical [2–6, 10].

Retrospective and prospective clinical studies focused on critically ill children with TBI have shown that early post-traumatic seizures (seizures within 7 days of injury) are a common acute complication, occurring in up to 44% of children monitored with cEEG [29, 30, 34, 35]. Subclinical seizures were very common among these patients, with 93% of patients with cEEG-confirmed seizures experiencing at least one subclinical seizure [30], and 16%–18% experiencing nonconvulsive status epilepticus [29, 30].

Among children with TBI who underwent cEEG monitoring, the risk of seizures was further increased in those who suffered from *abusive head trauma* [29, 30, 34–36], with subclinical-only seizures and nonconvulsive status epilepticus even more commonly observed. Further, *younger age* (generally <1–2 years) is repeatedly shown to be an independent risk factor for the development of early post-traumatic (subclinical) seizures [29, 30, 32, 34–36]. Perhaps not coincidentally, these younger patients are most likely to have also suffered an abusive head trauma. Other clinical characteristics that further increase the risk of cEEG-confirmed seizures among children following TBI include those with *severe injury* [32, 34, 35], as well as the presence of *ischemia* [36], and subdural or intra-axial *hemorrhages* [29, 35].

Critically ill children suffering from TBI may be particularly vulnerable to seizure-induced brain injury, as adult evidence suggests electrographic seizures are associated with increases in intracranial pressure and may cause increasing cerebral metabolic stress [37].

Given the particularly high incidence of seizures (often subclinical) in these children, many pediatric centers have adopted protocols which include cEEG monitoring and prophylactic treatment with anti-seizure medications [38].

Acute Stroke

Seizures are a common initial presenting sign of stroke in children, particularly among those admitted to a PICU [39–42]. This includes children with acute ischemic stroke, cerebral sinus venous thrombosis, and intracerebral hemorrhage. Clinical studies specifically assessing the frequency of seizures within the acute setting of pediatric stroke have demonstrated that 22%–49% of patients seize in the early post-stroke period (up to 2 weeks following injury), with a large majority of seizures occurring within the first 24 hours [43, 44]. Most commonly, these seizures affect younger children [39, 40, 45].

Among critically ill children with acute stroke (all subtypes) who underwent cEEG monitoring, 14%–71% of patients had electrographic seizures including some with nonconvulsive status epilepticus [3–6, 39–41]. Most of these patients experienced at least some subclinical seizures.

Central Nervous System Infections

Central nervous system infections have the potential to directly cause cortical irritability sufficient to provoke seizures or can indirectly produce seizures through secondary injury (i.e., acute stroke). In one cohort, seizures occurred in 55 of 116 children with bacterial meningitis (47%) [46]. While the data are limited, electrographic seizures were observed in 28%–70% of PICU patients with concomitant CNS infections who underwent cEEG monitoring [2–5]. Among pediatric patients with encephalitis, subclinical seizures and nonconvulsive status epilepticus are common [47–49].

Neurological Autoimmune Disease

Autoimmune encephalitis is being increasingly recognized as an important cause of encephalopathy and seizures in the PICU setting. Among the large observational studies of critically ill children undergoing cEEG monitoring, only one study subcategorized patients as "CNS inflammation or autoimmune disease" and included 24 patients, 8 (33%) of whom had electrographic seizures [5]. Patients with CNS vasculitis are not well described in the literature with respect to electrographic seizure prevalence, but certainly those patients with additional clinical risk factors such as concomitant encephalopathy or acute strokes should undergo cEEG monitoring given their risk described above.

Seizures, including status epilepticus, are very commonly associated with anti- N-methyl-D-aspartate (NMDA) receptor encephalitis in children (50%–77%) [50, 51] and in adults (61%) [52], with the majority experiencing some subclinical seizures [51, 52]. The presence of an "extreme delta-brush" EEG pattern is suggestive of anti-NMDA receptor encephalitis and may warrant extended cEEG monitoring; however, extreme delta brushes appear to be less common in children [52].

Although conditions such as acute disseminated encephalomyelitis (ADEM) and acute hemorrhagic leukoencephalitis (AHLE) are associated with seizures in affected children [53–55], data are lacking on their prevalence during cEEG monitoring. Among children with ADEM, seizures are commonly (35%) the presenting clinical feature [53]. In a series of patients with ADEM, 28% had electrographic seizures, with a trend toward increased seizures among those with more severe degrees of encephalopathy [54].

Brain Tumors and Post-Neurosurgery

Limited data exist to describe the prevalence of electrographic seizures among critically ill children with a brain tumor or post-neurosurgical intervention. Among the 47 patients described across several observational studies, 59% experienced electrographic seizures [2, 3, 5, 6, 10]. The greatest risk for electrographic seizures is likely in the acute post-operative period and among those with persistent unexplained encephalopathy or other concomitant risk factors.

Post-Cardiac Arrest +/− Therapeutic Hypothermia

Children with congenital heart disease are at risk for developing electrographic seizures in the acute post-operative period, often following surgeries that include deep hypothermia with circulatory arrest [56–59]. Certain congenital heart defects may confer a higher risk of electrographic seizures than others (i.e., single-ventricle physiology vs cyanotic lesion) [57]. These patients are of course at risk for secondary ischemic and hemorrhagic brain injuries. Similarly, patients undergoing treatment with ECMO, often treated with concomitant sedative or paralytic medications, are at high risk for electrographic seizures [60].

Among a small cohort of critically ill children with cardiac arrest who underwent therapeutic hypothermia, electrographic seizures, including subclinical seizures and status epilepticus, were common [61]. Interestingly, the EEG risk factors for seizures described above (i.e., burst suppression background pattern) were particularly predictive for this cohort of children. Importantly, some children in this study began experiencing electrographic seizures during the rewarming phase of therapeutic hypothermia, suggesting the need to extend cEEG monitoring until normothermia is attained [62]. This topic is covered in greater detail in Chapter 15.

Posterior Reversible Encephalopathy Syndrome

Posterior reversible encephalopathy syndrome (PRES) is a vascular mediated disease observed in critically ill children which carries an 87%–96% risk of seizures [63, 64]. As encephalopathy is generally a required feature to make the diagnosis of PRES, these patients are at high risk for clinical and subclinical seizures. In the largest single series of pediatric patients with PRES, 21 of 27 patients presented with status epilepticus, 11 of those with nonconvulsive status epilepticus [64].

Sepsis and Other Systemic Illness

Despite their apparent lack of a direct brain injury, critically ill children admitted with a primary systemic illness who undergo cEEG monitoring (i.e., sepsis and other systemic infections) are also at risk for developing electrographic seizures [5, 6]. Many of these patients have no evidence of injury on brain MRI. Sepsis in particular is associated with a higher risk for electrographic seizures in children [5] and adults [65]. In the large observational study of 550 PICU patients monitored with cEEG, electrographic seizures were present in 11 of 19 patients (58%) with sepsis [5]. Among children with acute liver failure and mild to severe hepatic encephalopathy, seizures are common and often subclinical [66]. Therefore, the presence of an overt acute brain injury is not necessary for critically ill children to experience electrographic seizures.

Additional systemic illnesses that may pose an increased risk of electrographic seizures include: significant electrolyte abnormalities or hypoglycemia, inborn errors of metabolism, and intoxication syndromes [5, 6, 23]. Intoxication secondary to antidepressant medication poses a particular risk for developing seizures [67]. No specific literature exists regarding the prevalence of subclinical seizures in these conditions. Of course, most, if not all, of these patients will have acute encephalopathy.

Timing and Duration of Continuous EEG Monitoring

Unfortunately, etiology-specific evidence is lacking to inform the timing and duration of cEEG monitoring among subgroups of critically ill children. None of the large observational studies of critically ill children monitored with cEEG assessed the timing of electrographic seizure occurrence by etiology [2–10]. As such, recommendations with respect to cEEG monitoring timing and duration to confirm electrographic seizures apply to the high-risk, critically ill pediatric population as a whole, with a few etiology-specific considerations already discussed above under their respective etiology (Figure 11.3).

Among critically ill adults, cEEG monitoring consensus guidelines exist and suggest that EEG should be applied within an hour of onset of status epilepticus and should continue for at least 48 hours or until 24 hours after the last seizure, whichever comes later [68]. Large practice variability exists among pediatric centers that perform cEEG monitoring [69]. However, the observational pediatric cEEG monitoring studies indicate that <50% of patients who experience electrographic seizures do so within the first hour of cEEG monitoring [2–4, 6, 7, 9], whereas 80%–87% have them within the first 24 hours of cEEG monitoring [2–4, 6, 7, 9, 10]. As such, *24–48 hours of cEEG monitoring is often sufficient* to detect seizures among high-risk children.

The use of anti-seizure medication, particularly continuous infusions, will of course greatly impact seizure occurrence. Continuous EEG monitoring is certainly necessary throughout the titration of anti-seizure medications to treat refractory status epilepticus. It should likely be continued for 24 hours after the last electrographic seizure is captured *and* the infusion has been weaned off. Clearly clinical context remains important. For example, if a patient's mental status improves such that the clinical assessment of seizures becomes reliable, cEEG monitoring may no longer be necessary. Since the risk for electrographic seizures may change over the duration of a critically ill child's ICU admission, the need for cEEG monitoring should also be re-evaluated according to changes in clinical status. For example, the appearance of new clinical paroxysms suspicious for seizures may necessitate repeat cEEG monitoring until the paroxysms of concern are captured and properly diagnosed.

EEG background activity can also help to guide the length of cEEG monitoring (Figure 11.1). Adult studies have assessed the value of the baseline EEG recording to predict subsequent electrographic seizures. A recent study indicated that if 2 hours of baseline cEEG monitoring demonstrate a continuous background and no epileptiform discharges the probability of developing subsequent seizures is only 5% [24]. Similar predictive modelling in children is currently lacking. However, when EEG risk factors are absent, a critically ill child may not require a full 24–48 hours of cEEG monitoring, especially if resources are limited. Conversely, cEEG monitoring may need

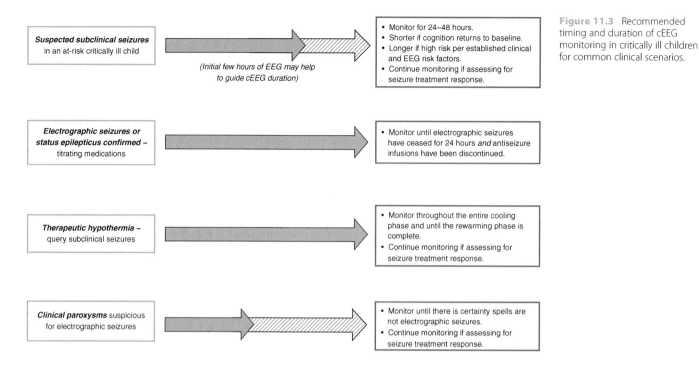

Figure 11.3 Recommended timing and duration of cEEG monitoring in critically ill children for common clinical scenarios.

to be extended in critically ill children when important EEG risk factors (i.e., periodic discharges) are present, particularly if clinical suspicion remains high.

Conclusions

Critically ill pediatric children with a wide variety of diagnoses are at risk for developing electrographic seizures. These clinical and subclinical seizures are difficult to diagnose on clinical grounds alone, and therefore necessitate cEEG monitoring. Status epilepticus can be entirely nonconvulsive. Certain clinical and electrographic risk factors are highly associated with the development of electrographic seizures and may help to guide cEEG monitoring timing and duration. A high index of suspicion is required to detect and treat electrographic seizures and to avoid potentially harmful anti-seizure medications when unnecessary. Ultimately, the hope is that prompt recognition and treatment of electrographic seizures may modulate, or even attenuate, the independent brain injury associated with seizures.

References

1. Bell MJ, Carpenter J, Au AK, et al. Development of a pediatric neurocritical care service. *Neurocriti Care.* 2009;**10**(1):4–10.

2. Jette N, Claassen J, Emerson RG, Hirsch LJ. Frequency and predictors of nonconvulsive seizures during continuous electroencephalographic monitoring in critically ill children. *Arch Neurol.* 2006;**63**(12):1750–5.

3. Abend NS, Gutierrez-Colina AM, Topjian AA, et al. Nonconvulsive seizures are common in critically ill children. *Neurology.* 2011;**76**(12):1071–7.

4. Schreiber JM, Zelleke T, Gaillard WD, et al. Continuous video EEG for patients with acute encephalopathy in a pediatric intensive care unit. *Neurocrit Care,* 2012;**17**(1):31–8.

5. Abend NS, Arndt DH, Carpenter JL, et al. Electrographic seizures in pediatric ICU patients: cohort study of risk factors and mortality. *Neurology.* 2013;**81**(4):383–91.

6. Payne ET, Zhao XY, Frndova H, et al. Seizure burden is independently associated with short term outcome in critically ill children. *Brain.* 2014;**137**(Pt 5):1429–38.

7. Shahwan A, Bailey C, Shekerdemian L, Harvey AS. The prevalence of seizures in comatose children in the pediatric intensive care unit: a prospective video-EEG study. *Epilepsia* 2010;**51** (7):1198–1204.

8. Kirkham FJ, Wade AM, McElduff F, et al. Seizures in 204 comatose children: incidence and outcome. *Intensive Care Med.* 2012;**38**(5):853–62.

9. McCoy B, Sharma R, Ochi A, et al. Predictors of nonconvulsive seizures among critically ill children. *Epilepsia.* 2011;**52**(11):1973–8.

10. Williams K, Jarrar R, Buchhalter J. Continuous video-EEG monitoring in pediatric intensive care units. *Epilepsia.* 2011;**52**(6):1130–6.

11. Payne ET, Hahn CD. Continuous electroencephalography for seizures and status epilepticus. *Current Opin Pediatr.* 2014;**26**(6):675–81.

12. Bellinger DC, Wypij D, Rivkin MJ, et al. Adolescents with d-transposition of the great arteries corrected with the arterial switch procedure: neuropsychological assessment and structural brain imaging. *Circulation.* 2011;**124** (12):1361–9.

13. Gaynor JW, Jarvik GP, Gerdes M, et al. Postoperative electroencephalographic seizures are associated with deficits in executive function and social behaviors at 4 years of age following cardiac surgery in infancy. *J Thorac Cardiovasc Surg.* 2013;**146**(1):132–7.

14. Topjian AA, Gutierrez-Colina AM, Sanchez SM, et al. Electrographic status epilepticus is associated with mortality and worse short-term outcome in critically ill children. *Crit Care Med.* 2013;**41**(1):215–23.

15. Wagenman KL, Blake TP, Sanchez SM, et al. Electrographic status epilepticus and long-term outcome in critically ill children. *Neurology.* 2014;**82** (5):396–404.

16. Srinivasakumar P, Zempel J, Trivedi S, et al. Treating EEG seizures in hypoxic ischemic encephalopathy: a randomized controlled trial. *Pediatrics.* 2015;**136**(5):e1302–9.

17. Malone A, Ryan CA, Fitzgerald A, et al. Interobserver agreement in neonatal seizure identification. *Epilepsia.* 2009;**50**(9):2097–2101.

18. Payne ET, McBain K, Sharma R, et al. Ability of ICU bedside caregivers to predict seizures among children who undergo continuous EEG monitoring. *Ann Neurol.* 2016;**80**(suppl 20):s316.

19. Dang LT, Shellhaas RA. Diagnostic yield of continuous video electroencephalography for paroxysmal vital sign changes in pediatric patients. *Epilepsia.* 2016;**57**(2):272–8.

20. Barberio M, Reiter PD, Kaufman J, Knupp K, Dobyns EL. Continuous infusion pentobarbital for refractory status epilepticus in children. *J Child Neurol.* 2012;**27**(6):721–6.

21. Greiner HM, Holland K, Leach JL, et al. Nonconvulsive status epilepticus: the encephalopathic pediatric patient. *Pediatrics.* 2012;**129** (3):e748–55.

22. Holmes GL. The long-term effects of neonatal seizures. *Clin Perinatol.* 2009;**36**(4):901–14, vii–viii.

23. Payne E, McBain K, Hutchison JS, et al. Detecting seizures among comatose children: interim results. *J Clin Neurophysiol.* 2013;226.

24. Westover MB, Shafi MM, Bianchi MT, et al. The probability of seizures during EEG monitoring in critically ill adults. *Clin Neurophysiol.* 2015;**126**(3):463–71.

25. Shafi MM, Westover MB, Cole AJ, et al. Absence of early epileptiform abnormalities predicts lack of seizures on continuous EEG. *Neurology.* 2012;**79** (17):1796–1801.

26. Sanchez SM, Arndt DH, Carpenter JL, et al. Electroencephalography monitoring in critically ill children: current practice and implications for future study design. *Epilepsia.* 2013;**54** (8):1419–27.

27. DeLorenzo RJ, Waterhouse EJ, Towne AR, et al. Persistent nonconvulsive status epilepticus after the control of convulsive status epilepticus. *Epilepsia.* 1998;**39**(8):833–40.

28. Sanchez Fernandez I, Abend NS, Arndt DH, et al. Electrographic seizures after convulsive status epilepticus in children and young adults: a retrospective multicenter study. *J Pediatr.* 2014;**164**(2):339–46 e331–2.

29. Arndt DH, Lerner JT, Matsumoto JH, et al. Subclinical early posttraumatic seizures detected by continuous EEG monitoring in a consecutive pediatric cohort. *Epilepsia.* 2013;**54**(10):1780–8.

30. O'Neill BR, Handler MH, Tong S, Chapman KE. Incidence of seizures on continuous EEG monitoring following traumatic brain injury in children. *J Neurosurg. Pediatrics.* 2015;**16**(2):167–76.

31. Moreau JF, Fink EL, Hartman ME, et al. Hospitalizations of children with neurologic disorders in the United States. *Pediatr Crit Care Med.* 2013;**14** (8):801–10.

32. Chiaretti A, De Benedictis R, Polidori G, et al. Early post-traumatic seizures in children with head injury. *Childs Nerv Syst.* 2000;**16**(12):862–6.

33. Hahn YS, Fuchs S, Flannery AM, Barthel MJ, McLone DG. Factors influencing posttraumatic seizures in children. *Neurosurgery.* 1988;**22** (5):864–7.

34. Arango JI, Deibert CP, Brown D, et al. Posttraumatic seizures in children with severe traumatic brain injury. *Childs Nerv Syst.* 2012;**28**(11):1925–9.

35. Liesemer K, Bratton SL, Zebrack CM, Brockmeyer D, Statler KD. Early post-traumatic seizures in moderate to severe pediatric traumatic brain injury: rates, risk factors, and clinical features. *J Neurotrauma.* 2011;**28**(5):755–62.

36. Hasbani DM, Topjian AA, Friess SH, et al. Nonconvulsive electrographic seizures are common in children with abusive head trauma. *Pediatr Crit Care Med.* 2013;**14**(7):709–15.

37. Vespa PM, Miller C, McArthur D, et al. Nonconvulsive electrographic seizures after traumatic brain injury result in a delayed, prolonged increase in intracranial pressure and metabolic crisis. *Crit Care Med.* 2007;**35** (12):2830–6.

38. Gallentine WB. Utility of continuous EEG in children with acute traumatic brain injury. *J Clin. Neurophysiol.* 2013 **30**(2):126–33.

39. Abend NS, Beslow LA, Smith SE, et al. Seizures as a presenting symptom of acute arterial ischemic stroke in childhood. *J Pediatr.* 2011;**159**(3):479–83.

40. Singh RK, Zecavati N, Singh J, et al. Seizures in acute childhood stroke. *J Pediatr.* 2012;**160**(2):291–6.

41. Payne E, Yau I, Frndova H, et al. Prevalence of acute seizures and subsequent epilepsy among critically-ill children with acute ischemic stroke. *Ann Neurol.* 2016;S337.

42. Beslow LA, Abend NS, Gindville MC, et al. Pediatric intracerebral hemorrhage: acute symptomatic seizures and epilepsy. *JAMA Neurol.* 2013;**70**(4):448–54.

43. Yang JS, Park YD, Hartlage PL. Seizures associated with stroke in childhood. *Pediatr Neurol.* 1995;**12**(2):136–8.

44. Lee JC, Lin KL, Wang HS, et al. Seizures in childhood ischemic stroke in Taiwan. *Brain Dev.* 2009;**31**(4):294–9.

45. Zimmer JA, Garg BP, Williams LS, Golomb MR. Age-related variation in presenting signs of childhood arterial ischemic stroke. *Pediatr Neurol.* 2007;**37**(3):171–5.

46. Chang CJ, Chang HW, Chang WN, et al. Seizures complicating infantile and childhood bacterial meningitis. *Pediatr Neurol.* 2004;**31**(3):165–71.

47. Gold JJ, Crawford JR, Glaser C, et al. The role of continuous electroencephalography in childhood encephalitis. *Pediatr Neurol.* 2014;**50** (4):318–23.

48. Carrera E, Claassen J, Oddo M, et al. Continuous electroencephalographic monitoring in critically ill patients with central nervous system infections. *Arch Neurol.* 2008;**65**(12):1612–18.

49. Fujita K, Nagase H, Nakagawa T, et al. Non-convulsive seizures in children with infection-related altered mental status. *Pediatr Int.* 2015;**57**(4):659–64.

50. Florance NR, Davis RL, Lam C, et al. Anti-*N*-methyl-D-aspartate receptor (NMDAR) encephalitis in children and adolescents. *Ann Neurol.* 2009;**66** (1):11–18.

51. Sands TT, Nash K, Tong S, Sullivan J. Focal seizures in children with anti-NMDA receptor antibody encephalitis. *Epilepsy Res.* 2015;**112**:31–6.

52. Schmitt SE, Pargeon K, Frechette ES, et al. Extreme delta brush: a unique EEG pattern in adults with anti-NMDA receptor encephalitis. *Neurology.* 2012;**79**(11):1094–1100.

53. Tenembaum S, Chamoles N, Fejerman N. Acute disseminated encephalomyelitis: a long-term follow-up study of 84 pediatric patients. *Neurology.* 2002;**59**(8):1224–31.

54. Fridinger SE, Alper G. Defining encephalopathy in acute disseminated encephalomyelitis. *J Child Neurol.* 2014;**29**(6):751–5.

55. Payne ET, Rutka JT, Ho TK, Halliday WC, Banwell BL. Treatment leading to dramatic recovery in acute hemorrhagic leukoencephalitis. *J Child Neurol.* 2007;**22**(1):109–13.

56. Bellinger DC, Jonas RA, Rappaport LA, et al. Developmental and neurologic status of children after heart surgery with hypothermic circulatory arrest or low-flow cardiopulmonary bypass. *N Eng J Med.* 1995;**332**(9):549–55.

57. Clancy RR, Sharif U, Ichord R, et al. Electrographic neonatal seizures after infant heart surgery. *Epilepsia.* 2005;**46**(1):84–90.

58. Andropoulos DB, Mizrahi EM, Hrachovy RA, et al. Electroencephalographic seizures after neonatal cardiac surgery with high-flow cardiopulmonary bypass. *Anesth Analg.* 2010;**110**(6):1680–5.

59. Latal B, Wohlrab G, Brotschi B, et al. Postoperative amplitude-integrated electroencephalography predicts four-year neurodevelopmental outcome in children with complex congenital heart disease. *J Pediatr.* 2016;**178**:55–60 e51.

60. Piantino JA, Wainwright MS, Grimason M, et al. Nonconvulsive seizures are common in children treated with extracorporeal cardiac life support. *Pediatr Crit Care Med.* 2013;**14**(6):601–9.

61. Abend NS, Topjian A, Ichord R, et al. Electroencephalographic monitoring during hypothermia after pediatric cardiac arrest. *Neurology.* 2009;**72**(22):1931–40.

62. Abend NS, Dlugos DJ, Clancy RR. A review of long-term EEG monitoring in critically ill children with hypoxic-ischemic encephalopathy, congenital heart disease, ECMO, and stroke. *J Clin Neurophysiol.* 2013;**30**(2):134–42.

63. Chen TH, Lin WC, Tseng YH, et al. Posterior reversible encephalopathy syndrome in children: case series and systematic review. *J Child Neurol.* 2013;**28**(11):1378–86.

64. Cordelli DM, Masetti R, Ricci E, et al. Life-threatening complications of posterior reversible encephalopathy syndrome in children. *Eur J Paediatri Neurol.* 2014;**18**(5):632–40.

65. Oddo M, Carrera E, Claassen J, Mayer SA, Hirsch LJ. Continuous electroencephalography in the medical intensive care unit. *Crit Care Med.* 2009;**37**(6):2051–6.

66. Press C, Morgan L, Mills M, et al. Spectral electroencephalogram analysis for the evaluation of encephalopathy grade in children with acute liver failure. *Pediatr Criti Care Med.* 2017;**18**(1):64–72.

67. Finkelstein Y, Hutson JR, Freedman SB, Wax P, Brent J, Toxicology Investigators Consortium Case R. Drug-induced seizures in children and adolescents presenting for emergency care: current and emerging trends. *Clin Toxicol.* 2013;**51**(8):761–6.

68. Brophy GM, Bell R, Claassen J, et al. Guidelines for the evaluation and management of status epilepticus. *Neurocrit Care.* 2012;**17**(1):3–23.

69. Sanchez SM, Carpenter J, Chapman KE, et al. Pediatric ICU EEG monitoring: current resources and practice in the United States and Canada. *J Clin Neurophysiol.* 2013;**30**(2):156–60.

Chapter 12

Monitoring for Impending Ischemia

Ersida Buraniqi and Tobias Loddenkemper

Illustrative Cases

Case 31 Multimodality Monitoring of Acute Stroke

Case 32 Multimodal Neurological Monitoring: Ventilation and Cerebral Perfusion

Key Points

- EEG reflects neuronal metabolism and activity; changes in cerebral perfusion are quickly followed by changes in the EEG.
- While EEG is most often used to identify early ischemia in adults with subarachnoid hemorrhage, it may also be useful in patients with ischemic stroke and moyamoya disease.
- Quantitative EEG is particularly useful to identify changes in the EEG background that may indicate ischemia.

The use of electrophysiological methods to monitor patients for cerebral ischemia is based on the observation that electrical brain activity is exquisitely dependent on adequate cerebral perfusion. The effect of ischemia on the EEG is dependent on the degree, duration, and rate of hypoperfusion, as well as on the cerebral metabolic rate, which itself can be influenced by sedation and body temperature. Under normal physiological conditions, cerebral blood flow is approximately 750 mL per minute, equivalent to 15% to 20% of cardiac output. This equates to 50 to 54 mL of blood per 100 g of brain tissue per minute. In conditions of mild to moderate ischemia (15–35 mL/100 g per minute), synaptic transmission becomes compromised [1, 2]. As an example, inhibitory neurons are likely to be more affected by ischemia, resulting from a decrease in excitation from changes in the glutamatergic synapse [2, 3], or intrinsic dysfunction [4]. This may explain the increased synchronization often observed in patients with severe hypoxic damage with generalized period discharges [3, 5]. EEG potentials are mainly generated by the summation of postsynaptic currents of pyramidal cells in the supragranular and infragranular cortical layers and depends also partially on thalamic input to the granular layer (layer IV) [6]. The cortical neurons involved in the synaptic networks sustaining the EEG signal are exquisitely sensitive to ischemia, such that a decrease in cerebral perfusion below a certain threshold is quickly followed by changes in neuronal metabolism and activity that are reflected at the level of the EEG [7–14] (Table 12.1).

Simplified EEG montages are widely and successfully used for EEG monitoring under ICU conditions, although general recommendations regarding the best montage and number of electrodes for ischemia monitoring are still lacking [15, 16].

Table 12.1 Relationship between cerebral flow and metabolic, neurophysiological, and EEG changes

CBF (mL × 100 g-1 × min-1)	Metabolic changes	Neurophysiological changes	EEG changes
35–50	Decline in protein synthesis	Synaptic transmission failure	Normal
25–35	Anaerobic metabolism, increase in glucose consumption and lactate concentration Energetic failure: decline in glucose consumption and in ATP and phosphocreatine levels	Spontaneous neurotransmitter release (including glutamate)	Attenuation of fast (alpha and beta) activity
10–25	Na+/K + ATPase failure Anoxic depolarization and ionic disturbances: increase in extracellular potassium	Axonal transmission failure	Slowing than progressive attenuation of all activities (isoelectric)
5–10	Cytotoxic edema		Isoelectric
<5	Irreversible infarction		Isoelectric

ATP, adenosine triphosphate; Na+/K+ ATPase, sodium/potassium adenosine triphosphate; CBF, cerebral blood flow.

The key to the discrimination of EEG changes triggered by delayed cerebral ischemia (DCI) from changes due to other causes is the recognition of vasospasm as a predominantly focal event [17]. Although some selective neuronal loss starts very early, EEG changes occur before reversible clinical findings and well before macroscopic infarction [9,12]. EEG changes occur as early as 10 seconds after the onset of a significant decrease in cerebral perfusion [12], in comparison to abnormalities in diffusion-weighted imaging MRI that appear after at least 12 minutes of ischemia [18]. This allows EEG to serve as an early indicator of ischemia, before clinical signs may be apparent, and potentially before permanent injury occurs.

Continuous EEG monitoring (cEEG) is increasingly used in intensive care units (ICU) to detect nonconvulsive seizures and status epilepticus and to monitor their treatment [19]. cEEG provides continuous, real-time information on brain activity and could thus disclose changes suggestive of impeding ischemia before infarction occurs, thus creating a window of opportunity for intervention to prevent irreversible injury. Visual inspection of every single page of a recording remains the gold standard of EEG interpretation. At the same time, it is time-consuming and requires the remote or on-site presence of an expert neurophysiologist, which precludes its use as a continuous real-time solution. Though this method of EEG interpretation may be suited for the detection of subtle transient abnormalities, it may overlook progressive changes that reflect ischemia evolving slowly over more than several hours. Visual interpretation can be assisted by quantitative EEG analysis (QEEG), as illustrated in Figure 12.1. Various methods of QEEG exist and some are currently available in commercial software. Of these methods, spectral frequency analysis has received the most attention in the field of DCI detection. Beyond large vessel ischemia, DCI may also be a consequence of other mechanisms such as cortical spreading depression or microcirculatory dysfunction undetectable by transcranial Doppler (TCD) [20]. Approximately 20% of DCI after SAH are not detected clinically or are identified too late, mostly due to impaired clinical assessment in high Hunt and Hess scale-grade, comatose

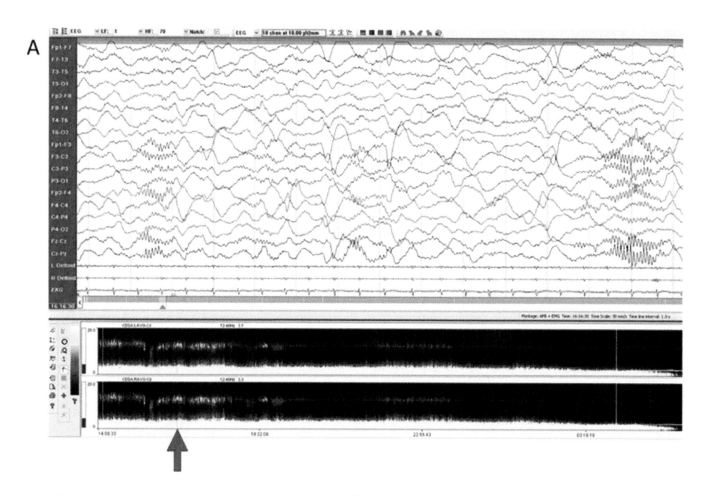

Figure 12.1 Slowly evolving global ischemia is best visualized by quantitative EEG.
Continuous EEG performed in a 7-year-old girl who sustained traumatic brain injury with a depressed skull fracture. While in the ICU, she experienced a sudden progressive decline in her level of consciousness. Conventional EEG recording (top) and quantitative EEG tracings (bottom) depicting 15 hours of left and right hemispheric average data. Arrows indicates the corresponding times on raw EEG. (A) Sleep spindles visible on raw EEG are represented by as horizontal bands of increased power on color density spectral array (CDSA). (B) Over time sleep spindles disappear and background activity becomes increasingly attenuated, represented by gradual decrease in power on CDSA and aEEG until there is no discernable electrocerebral activity. (Figure courtesy Cecil Hahn)

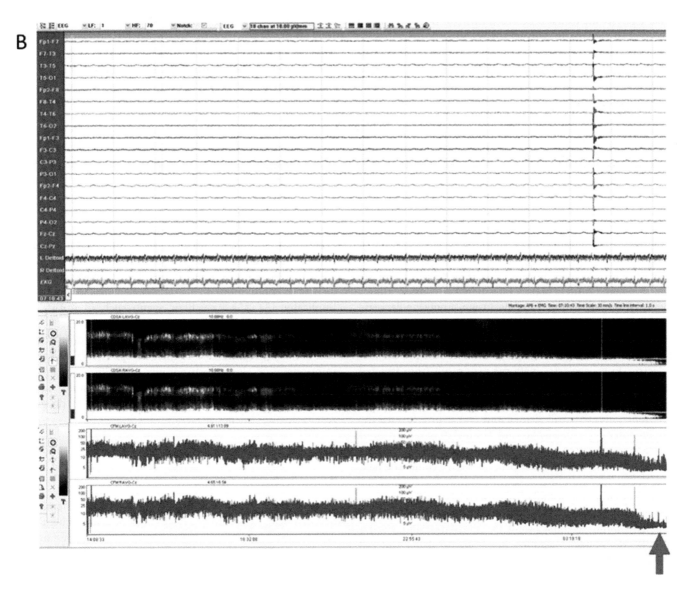

Figure 12.1 (cont.)

subarachnoid hemorrhage (SAH) patients [20]. Therefore, early detection of imminent ischemia to prevent infarction remains challenging.

EEG Features Indicative of Impending Ischemia

The normal awake EEG is characterized by the presence of abundant fast activity in the alpha (8–13 Hz) and, to a lesser extent, beta (14–25 Hz) range, mostly generated by postsynaptic activity of cortical pyramidal cells. In contrast, slow activity, and in particular delta activity, is the hallmark of slow wave sleep and pathological conditions, including focal and diffuse brain dysfunction. The complex EEG signal consists of overlapping sinusoidal waveforms of different frequencies, which can be decomposed into their component parts using Fourier transformation in order to quantify the relative power within each of the canonical frequency bands (delta, theta, alpha, and

beta). The ratio of delta to alpha power has been found to be of particular utility in ischemia monitoring. Several studies report a strong correlation between cerebral blood flow and the frequency content of the EEG: lower blood flow rates were associated with higher delta and theta content and lower alpha and beta content. For example, one group found a high probability for patients to develop DCI when the alpha–delta ratio decreased by >10% in six consecutive recordings or by >50% in a single recording [22]. Furthermore, Stuart et al. reported the alpha–delta ratio to be most predictive for DCI in intracortical EEG [23]. Vespa studied 32 patients with low grade (Hunt–Hess grades I–III) aneurysmal SAH [24]. A six-channel montage (F3-T3, F4-T4, T3-P3, T4-P4, P3-O1, and P4-O2) was used to display the trend of relative alpha power (calculated every 2 minutes) in 8- to 12-hour pages. These trends were subjected to semiquantitative visual scoring of the variability of relative alpha power (relative alpha variability [RAV]) using a four-point scale. Variability was also quantitatively measured.

Visual analysis identified a decrease in RAV in 15 of the 19 patients with vasospasm. Changes in RAV preceded abnormalities of intracranial artery velocities by at least 2 days in 10 patients and occurred the same day in five. A possible explanation for the temporal dissociation of the EEG and TCD findings may be illustrated by the work of Machado et al.: that work applied QEEG to patients with middle cerebral artery (MCA) ischemic strokes and found delta power increases to be related to the ischemic core while the tissue at risk, penumbra, and edema were characterized by alpha and theta alterations [25]. In this context, the alpha/delta ratio could be a valuable parameter to estimate the prognosis and predict the patient's functional outcome [26] while the alpha power may be the superior parameter to prevent infarction by initiating countermeasures.

Although the diminution of alpha power as a marker of DCI has not yet been confirmed by other studies, some evidence supports alpha power as a sensitive and specific predictor of DCI in the context of pathophysiological considerations. A typical response to diminished perfusion supply is a decrease in fast activities (alpha and beta) followed by an increase in slow activities in the delta band, depending on the severity and duration of ischemia [27, 28]. In severe cases, EEG can become isoelectric. Even isoelectric patterns may result from isolated synaptic failure and may be reversible. If ischemia is more severe and perfusion drops below 10 mL/100 g per minute, membrane potentials will change and may evolve toward the Donnan potential, typically around 215 to 220 mV. This non-zero membrane potential in situations in which all adenosine triphosphate (ATP)-dependent processes have come to a halt, in particular the sodium-potassium pumps, results from the presence of large, intracellular, negatively charged macromolecules that cannot pass the membrane. This is accompanied by an increase in intracellular osmolality, and extracellular water will enter the neuron, resulting in cytotoxic edema and cell death [29, 30]. In this situation, EEG rhythms will permanently disappear [31]. Claassen et al. found a strong correlation between a decrease of the alpha–delta power ratio and DCI (a sensitivity of 100% and a specificity of 76%) by analyzing artifact-free clips visually preselected by experienced electroencephalographers [22]. Vespa et al. also chose a continuous approach and identified the relative alpha (RA) variability as the most sensitive (100%) indicator of imminent ischemia [16]. Although highly sensitive, RA variability not only corresponded exclusively to vasospasm or DCI but also dropped significantly as a consequence of a variety of other conditions, for example, increase of intracranial pressure (ICP) or herniation, causing low specificity (50%). In conclusion, this widespread experience gathered in adults, particularly those with SAH, should inform similar work in the pediatric population, where many of these techniques still require validation.

Pitfalls in EEG Interpretation

Maintenance of high-quality EEG monitoring over several days under ICU conditions is difficult and labor intensive [32], since artifacts unavoidably contaminate EEG recordings in the ICU. The EEG is also sensitive to other disturbances of brain activity, such as metabolic disorders, sedation, intoxication, increased intracranial pressure, temperature, or ischemia, and can potentially be used as a tool to monitor cerebral function and perfusion. There have been ways to address these shortcomings by using a reduced but multichannel montage that could be maintained over days with limited effort. This montage was still able to reliably detect focal EEG changes. In addition, an efficient automatic artifact rejection technique can be implemented, which was evaluated extensively in previous studies [21].

In general, the effects of general anesthesia on skull and intracranial electroencephalographic activity are poorly understood. Several studies of electroencephalography during anesthesia have identified distinct "arousal" electroencephalogram patterns of change in response to a noxious stimulus [33]. How anesthetics differ in their ability to modulate noxious stimulation-evoked electroencephalogram activation is unclear, although direct depression of the ascending transmission of noxious input to the thalamocortical pathways was implicated [34, 35]. Anesthetic agents such as nitrous oxide and sevoflurane were reported to decrease interictal spikes during electrocorticography [36, 37]. Several studies indicate that fentanyl may decrease or increase spike frequency during intra-operative electrocorticography [38, 39]. Sedation with propofol induces higher-frequency background activity, which does not appear to interfere with electrocorticography results during epilepsy surgery [40].

Applications of Ischemia Monitoring

Acute Ischemic Stroke

There are two major categories of strokes: ischemic and hemorrhagic. Approximately 80% of strokes are ischemic and 20% hemorrhagic. Within these two major categories are subcategories of possible etiologies that fit under ischemic, including cardioembolism, large vessel thrombosis, and lacunar strokes. EEG has been explored for prognostication in acute stroke for over 40 years [41]. Serial EEG recordings have been studied for their potential utility to predict the course during recovery. Several quantitative EEG features have been proposed, often based on ratios of the power in the alpha, theta, or delta band [27]. Others have used the pairwise-derived brain symmetry index (pdBSI) and the (delta + theta)/ (alpha + beta) ratio (DTABR) as a prognostic index for dependency, disability, or death at 6 months after stroke [26]. The pdBSI is a slight modification of the spatial BSI. It does not estimate the normalized difference between the mean spectral densities of each hemisphere, but the normalized difference between the spectral densities of each bipolar signal from each hemisphere. This makes the pdBSI more sensitive for focal EEG asymmetries. Continuous quantitative EEG monitoring using the BSI was shown to correlate with the clinical neurological condition (measured with the National Institute of Health Stroke Scale) of patients with hemispheric stroke [5], and was successfully used to monitor the effects of intravenous thrombolysis [42]. Reliable measurement of EEG activity in the very low-frequency range, that is, below 0.5 Hz (infraslow activity), including phenomena associated with spreading depressions or depolarizations, could also be of clinical relevance. There exists unequivocal neurophysiological evidence that spreading depressions or depolarizations (SD) occurs in patients with acute stroke, and contributes to lesion progression [43]. However, measurement of SD through the intact skull is challenging and associated with several fundamental difficulties [44]. At present, only electrocorticography with subdural or intraparenchymal electrodes has reliably recorded spreading depolarizations in patients with structural brain damage [45, 46, 47]. It has also been shown in microdialysis studies that changes in brain metabolism such as an increase in lactate–pyruvate ratio and decreased brain tissue oxygenation preceding imaging are proof of ischemia. EEG could be a powerful tool to capture these changes at an early stage [48], and warrants further study.

Secondary Stroke Prevention in Moyamoya Disease

Moyamoya disease is an arteriopathy of uncertain etiology, characterized by progressive stenosis of the intracranial internal carotid arteries and their proximal branches [49, 50]. The decreased blood supply to the brain resulting from this arterial narrowing predisposes patients to ischemic stroke, whereas fragile collateral vessels are prone to hemorrhage, especially in adults [49, 51, 52]. Although the course of moyamoya disease varies in its rate from slow to fulminant, it is invariably progressive in the vast majority of patients, and typically results in severe stroke burden and death. Although no treatment is known to reverse the primary disease process, surgical revascularization can prevent strokes by improving blood flow to the affected brain [53]. The majority of surgical techniques use a branch of the unaffected external carotid artery (usually the parietal branch of the superficial temporal artery of the scalp) as a source of new blood supply to the ischemic hemisphere. Many variations of this general approach have been described. During pial synangiosis, the arachnoid mater is widely opened, and the superficial temporal artery is sutured to the surface of the brain [53]. In total, 220 consecutive patients were included in an EEG monitoring study during intracranial procedures for moyamoya, with a median age of 8 years (range, 0.5–33 years); the vast majority (n=201) were younger than 21 years [54]. Electroencephalogram slowing was evident in 100 cases (45.5%). Slowing was generalized in 64% of cases, but was preceded by unilateral changes in 13%. The detection of slowing, either unilaterally or bilaterally, was independent of the presence of unilateral or bilateral disease. Specifically, in the nine patients with persistent slowing, EEG changes were associated with suturing the superficial temporal artery to the brain surface in seven cases, the opening of the arachnoid mater in one case, and with the initial craniotomy in one case. Systemic arterial hypertension frequently accompanied EEG slowing, especially when EEG slowing was more pronounced. Whether this hypertension developed immediately before or after the EEG slowing is unclear, because these instances were not recorded on the same monitor. No significant correlation was evident between intra-operative EEG changes and outcomes. EEG monitoring, using a modified montage to accommodate the craniotomy incision, was

successfully achieved in all cases, demonstrating the technical feasibility of this approach (even in the setting of bilateral craniotomies). Slowing coincided with specific operative manipulations, most commonly while suturing the donor vessel to the pia, and during closure of the craniotomy. Slowing generally occurred bilaterally and was independent of the side of intervention. The presence, length, and severity of observed EEG slowing was not predictive of perioperative ischemic events. Slowing was more common in children younger than 10 years. The detection of bilateral EEG slowing during unilateral surgery, and its incidence during specific surgical steps, may indicate a pain-related phenomenon. Slowing occurred during certain maneuvers that are likely to trigger pain, such as suturing the meninges and applying pressure on the brain surface when the bone flap is replaced. These data demonstrated that the use of intra-operative EEG can be helpful in identifying episodes of cerebral ischemia, potentially allowing surgeons and anesthesiologists to respond quickly with measures to improve cerebral blood flow to prevent infarction [54]. However, the relationship between these intra-operative EEG findings, the occurrence of perioperative ischemia and outcomes require further study.

Subarachnoid Hemorrhage

Subarachnoid hemorrhage (SAH), usually resulting from the spontaneous hemorrhage of a brain aneurysm, accounts for approximately 5% of all strokes [55]. The annual incidence of SAH is 10/100,000 worldwide. In patients with severe SAH, in-hospital mortality rates range from 34% (in patients with Hunt and Hess grade IV, stupor) to 52% (in patients with Hunt and Hess grade V, coma); however, these rates were approximately twice as high three decades ago [56]. Approximately 4.5%–8% of patients will either present with seizures or develop seizures as a result of SAH. Thirty percent of patients with subarachnoid hemorrhage experience delayed cerebral ischemia or delayed ischemic neurological decline (DIND) [57, 58]. Delayed cerebral ischemia (DCI) is one of the most significant complications in the days after an acute aneurysmal SAH [59]. Therefore, ischemia has a decisive impact on mortality and functional outcome after aneurysmal subarachnoid hemorrhage (SAH) [60]. The EEG sensitively mirrors metabolic deterioration and disturbed neuronal activity following reduced cerebral blood flow [7, 61]. EEG changes such as flattening of the EEG signal and loss of higher frequencies are found to occur rapidly if cerebral blood flow decreases below 0.16–0.17 ml g/1 min [62, 63]. Literature reports continuous EEG monitoring as a promising approach for early detection of imminent DCI in SAH patients [15, 16, 22, 64, 65].

Future Directions: Portable Devices for Monitoring and Automated Signal Processing

Secondary ischemic injury is common after acute brain injury and can be evaluated with the use of neuro-monitoring devices. Transcranial Doppler ultrasonography (TCD) and transcranial color-coded duplex sonography (TCCS) are important devices to monitor cerebral blood flow in critically ill patients. Results may indicate vasospasm and delayed ischemic neurological deficits after aneurysmal subarachnoid hemorrhage. TCD and TCCS may be beneficial in identifying vasospasm after traumatic brain injury; however, they have shortcomings in identifying some secondary ischemic risks. Similarly, noninvasive imaging of ischemia lacks the immediacy that allows for early intervention or real-time feedback. Other devices have been used to monitor for ischemia or ischemia risk. Implantable thermal diffusion flowmetry probes may provide real-time continuous quantitative assessment of ischemic risks. Non-implantable ischemia sensors, such as externally measured electrical (ECG) monitoring and microprocessor control, may be useful. However, such devices monitor multiple external sites using wire leads placed upon the chest wall and are not designed for implantation. Implantable devices require that issues of size, power consumption, biocompatibility, and robustness over time be optimized alongside sensing performance, a non-trivial task. Implantable sensors exist, but those designed to detect ischemia are rare. Currently no implantable sensors detect tissue ischemia directly, but rather predict the presence of ischemia based upon electrical (ECG), blood pressure, local pH, and/or physical (acceleration during contraction) characteristics of the heart. For each of the devices above, ischemia is measured only by indirect and unreliable indicators. Furthermore, such devices are targeted to monitor for cardiac ischemia rather than ischemia in other tissues.

Of promise is an implantable ischemia detection system recently shown to provide real-time information regarding local tissue ischemia in high-risk patients. It uses broadband light for determination of tissue ischemia using spectroscopy, and in particular differential spectroscopy, which allows for compensation of light scattering by tissues [66]. Other near-infrared spectroscopy (NIRS) devices have been applied for rapid screening of intracranial bleeding [67]. These include portable NIRS scanners that may identify hemorrhage prior to CT in the acute setting. NIRS devices identify hemorrhage by detecting hemoglobin in the brain using its light-absorbing properties. While these tools show promise, better and more developed methods of continuous cerebral blood flow monitoring are needed to limit secondary ischemic injury in the neurocritical care unit.

References

1. Bolay H, Reuter U, Dunn AK, et al. Intrinsic brain activity triggers trigeminal meningeal afferents in a migraine model. *Nat Med.* 2002 Feb;**8**(2):136–42.

2. Hofmeijer J, van Putten MJ. Ischemic cerebral damage: an appraisal of synaptic failure. *Stroke.* 2012 Feb;**43**(2):607–15.

3. Tjepkema-Cloostermans MC, Hindriks R, Hofmeijer J, van Putten MJ. Generalized periodic discharges after acute cerebral ischemia: reflection of selective synaptic failure? *Clin Neurophysiol.* 2014 Feb;**125**(2):255–62.

4. Paz JT, Huguenard JR. Microcircuits and their interactions in epilepsy: is the focus out of focus? *Nat Neurosci.* 2015 Mar;**18**(3):351–9.

5. van Putten MJ, Tavy DL. Continuous quantitative EEG monitoring in hemispheric stroke patients using the brain symmetry index. *Stroke.* 2004 Nov;**35**(11):2489–92.

6. Berenyi A, Belluscio M, Mao D, Buzsaki G. Closed-loop control of epilepsy by transcranial electrical stimulation. *Science.* 2012 Aug 10;**337**(6095):735–7.

7. Astrup J, Siesjo BK, Symon L. Thresholds in cerebral ischemia – the ischemic penumbra. *Stroke.* 1981 Nov-Dec;**12**(6):723–5.

8. Boysen G, Ladegaard-Pedersen HJ, Henriksen H, et al. The effects of PaCO2 on regional cerebral blood flow and internal carotid arterial pressure during carotid clamping. *Anesthesiology.* 1971 Sep;**35**(3):286–300.

9. Hossmann KA. Viability thresholds and the penumbra of focal ischemia. *Ann Neurol.* 1994 Oct;**36**(4):557–65.

10. Ingvar DH, Sjolund B, Ardo A. Correlation between dominant EEG frequency, cerebral oxygen uptake and blood flow. *Electroencephalogr Clin Neurophysiol.* 1976 Sep;**41**(3):268–76.

11. Nagata K. Topographic EEG mapping in cerebrovascular disease. *Brain Topogr.* 1989 Fall-Winter;**2**(1-2):119–28.

12. Sharbrough FW, Messick JM, Jr., Sundt TM, Jr. Correlation of continuous electroencephalograms with cerebral blood flow measurements during carotid endarterectomy. *Stroke.* 1973 Jul-Aug;**4**(4):674–83.

13. Sundt TM, Jr., Sharbrough FW, Piepgras DG, et al. Correlation of cerebral blood flow and electroencephalographic changes during carotid endarterectomy: with results of surgery and hemodynamics of cerebral ischemia. *Mayo Clin Proc.* 1981 Sep;**56**(9):533–43.

14. Trojaborg W, Boysen G. Relation between EEG, regional cerebral blood flow and internal carotid artery pressure during carotid endarterectomy. *Electroencephalogr Clin Neurophysiol.* 1973 Jan;**34**(1):61–9.

15. Labar DR, Fisch BJ, Pedley TA, Fink ME, Solomon RA. Quantitative EEG monitoring for patients with subarachnoid hemorrhage. *Electroencephalogr Clin Neurophysiol.* 1991 May;**78**(5):325–32.

16. Vespa PM, Nuwer MR, Juhasz C, et al. Early detection of vasospasm after acute subarachnoid hemorrhage using continuous EEG ICU monitoring. *Electroencephalogr Clin Neurophysiol.* 1997 Dec;**103**(6):607–15.

17. Miller CM, Palestrant D. Distribution of delayed ischemic neurological deficits after aneurysmal subarachnoid hemorrhage and implications for regional neuromonitoring. *Clinical Neurol Neurosurg.* 2012 Jul;**114**(6):545–9.

18. Kohno K, Ohta S, Kohno K, et al. Early detection of cerebral ischemic lesion using diffusion-weighted MRI. *J Comput Assist Tomogr.* 1995 Nov-Dec;**19**(6):982–6.

19. Friedman D, Claassen J, Hirsch LJ. Continuous electroencephalogram monitoring in the intensive care unit. *Anesth Analg.* 2009 Aug;**109**(2):506–23.

20. Schmidt JM, Wartenberg KE, Fernandez A, et al. Frequency and clinical impact of asymptomatic cerebral infarction due to vasospasm after subarachnoid hemorrhage. *J Neurosurg.* 2008 Dec;**109**(6):1052–9.

21. Hopfengartner R, Kerling F, Bauer V, Stefan H. An efficient, robust and fast method for the offline detection of epileptic seizures in long-term scalp EEG recordings. *Clin Neurophysiol.* 2007 Nov;**118**(11):2332–43.

22. Claassen J, Hirsch LJ, Kreiter KT, et al. Quantitative continuous EEG for detecting delayed cerebral ischemia in patients with poor-grade subarachnoid hemorrhage. *Clin Neurophysiol*. 2004 Dec;**115**(12):2699–2710.

23. Stuart RM, Schmidt M, Kurtz P, et al. Intracranial multimodal monitoring for acute brain injury: a single institution review of current practices. *Neurocrit Care*. 2010 Apr;**12**(2):188–98.

24. Vespa PM. Acute presentation and early intensive care of acute aneurysmal subarachnoid hemorrhage. *J Stroke Cerebrovasc Dis*. 1997 Apr-May;**6**(4):230–4.

25. Machado C, Cuspineda E, Valdes P, et al. Assessing acute middle cerebral artery ischemic stroke by quantitative electric tomography. *Clin EEG Neurosci*. 2004 Jul;**35**(3):116–24.

26. Sheorajpanday RV, Nagels G, Weeren AJ, van Putten MJ, De Deyn PP. Quantitative EEG in ischemic stroke: correlation with functional status after 6 months. *Clin Neurophysiol*. 2011 May;**122**(5):874–83.

27. Finnigan SP, Rose SE, Walsh M, et al. Correlation of quantitative EEG in acute ischemic stroke with 30-day NIHSS score: comparison with diffusion and perfusion MRI. *Stroke*. 2004 Apr;**35**(4):899–903.

28. Foreman B, Claassen J. Quantitative EEG for the detection of brain ischemia. *Crit Care*. 2012;**16**(2):216.

29. Rungta RL, Choi HB, Tyson JR, et al. The cellular mechanisms of neuronal swelling underlying cytotoxic edema. *Cell*. 2015 Apr 23;**161**(3):610–21.

30. Stokum JA, Gerzanich V, Simard JM. Molecular pathophysiology of cerebral edema. *J Cereb Blood Flow Metab*. 2016 Mar;**36**(3):513–38.

31. Zandt BJ, ten Haken B, van Dijk JG, van Putten MJ. Neural dynamics during anoxia and the "wave of death." *PLoS ONE*. 2011;**6**(7):e22127.

32. Young GB, Campbell VC. EEG monitoring in the intensive care unit: pitfalls and caveats. *J Clin Neurophysiol*. 1999 Jan;**16**(1):40–5.

33. MacKay EC, Sleigh JW, Voss LJ, Barnard JP. Episodic waveforms in the electroencephalogram during general anaesthesia: a study of patterns of response to noxious stimuli. *Anaesth Intensive Care*. 2010 Jan;**38**(1):102–12.

34. Leduc ML, Atherley R, Jinks SL, Antognini JF. Nitrous oxide depresses electroencephalographic responses to repetitive noxious stimulation in the rat. *Br J Anaesth*. 2006 Feb;**96**(2):216–21.

35. Antognini JF, Carstens E, Sudo M, Sudo S. Isoflurane depresses electroencephalographic and medial thalamic responses to noxious stimulation via an indirect spinal action. *Anesth Analg*. 2000 Nov;**91**(5):1282–8.

36. Sato Y, Sato K, Shamoto H, Kato M, Yoshimoto T. Effect of nitrous oxide on spike activity during epilepsy surgery. *Acta Neurochir (Wien)*. 2001 Dec;**143**(12):1213–15; discussion 1215–16.

37. Endo T, Sato K, Shamoto H, Yoshimoto T. Effects of sevoflurane on electrocorticography in patients with intractable temporal lobe epilepsy. *J Neurosurg Anesth*. 2002 Jan;**14**(1):59–62.

38. Asano E, Benedek K, Shah A, et al. Is intraoperative electrocorticography reliable in children with intractable neocortical epilepsy? *Epilepsia*. 2004 Sep;**45**(9):1091–9.

39. Manninen PH, Burke SJ, Wennberg R, Lozano AM, El Beheiry H. Intraoperative localization of an epileptogenic focus with alfentanil and fentanyl. *Anesth Analg*. 1999 May;**88**(5):1101–6.

40. Herrick IA, Craen RA, Gelb AW, et al. Propofol sedation during awake craniotomy for seizures: electrocorticographic and epileptogenic effects. *Anesth Analg*. 1997 Jun;**84**(6):1280–4.

41. Kaste M, Waltimo O. Prognosis of patients with middle cerebral artery occlusion. *Stroke*. 1976 Sep-Oct;**7**(5):482–5.

42. de Vos CC, van Maarseveen SM, Brouwers PJ, van Putten MJ. Continuous EEG monitoring during thrombolysis in acute hemispheric stroke patients using the brain symmetry index. *J ClinNeurophysiol*. 2008 Apr;**25**(2):77–82.

43. Dreier JP, Major S, Pannek HW, et al. Spreading convulsions, spreading depolarization and epileptogenesis in human cerebral cortex. *Brain*. 2012 Jan;**135**(Pt 1):259–75.

44. Drenckhahn C, Winkler MK, Major S, et al. Correlates of spreading depolarization in human scalp electroencephalography. *Brain*. 2012 Mar;**135**(Pt 3):853–68.

45. Dohmen C, Sakowitz OW, Fabricius M, et al. Spreading depolarizations occur in human ischemic stroke with high incidence. *Ann Neurol*. 2008 Jun;**63**(6):720–8.

46. Dreier JP, Woitzik J, Fabricius M, et al. Delayed ischaemic neurological deficits after subarachnoid haemorrhage are associated with clusters of spreading depolarizations. *Brain*. 2006 Dec;**129**(Pt 12):3224–37.

47. Jeffcote T, Hinzman JM, Jewell SL, et al. Detection of spreading depolarization with intraparenchymal electrodes in the injured human brain. *Neurocrit Care*. 2014 Feb;**20**(1):21–31.

48. Helbok R, Madineni RC, Schmidt MJ, et al. Intracerebral monitoring of silent infarcts after subarachnoid hemorrhage. *Neurocrit Care*. 2011 Apr;**14**(2):162–7.

49. Scott RM, Smith ER. Moyamoya disease and moyamoya syndrome. *N Engl J Med*. 2009 Mar 19;**360**(12):1226–37.

50. Suzuki J, Takaku A. Cerebrovascular "moyamoya" disease. Disease showing abnormal net-like vessels in base of brain. *Arch Neurol*. 1969 Mar;**20**(3):288–99.

51. Hallemeier CL, Rich KM, Grubb RL, Jr., et al. Clinical features and outcome in North American adults with moyamoya phenomenon. *Stroke*. 2006 Jun;**37**(6):1490–6.

52. Yilmaz EY, Pritz MB, Bruno A, Lopez-Yunez A, Biller J. Moyamoya: Indiana University Medical Center experience. *Arch Neurol*. 2001 Aug;**58**(8):1274–8.

53. Smith ER, Scott RM. Surgical management of moyamoya syndrome. *Skull Base*. 2005 Feb;**15**(1):15–26.

54. Vendrame M, Kaleyias J, Loddenkemper T, et al. Electroencephalogram monitoring during intracranial surgery for moyamoya disease. *Pediatr Neurol*. 2011 Jun;**44**(6):427–32.

55. Cahill J, Calvert JW, Zhang JH. Mechanisms of early brain injury after subarachnoid hemorrhage. *J Cereb Blood Flow Metab*. 2006 Nov;**26**(11):1341–53.

56. Komotar RJ, Schmidt JM, Starke RM, et al. Resuscitation and critical care of poor-grade subarachnoid hemorrhage. *Neurosurgery*. 2009 Mar;**64**(3):397–410; discussion 410–391.

57. Al-Tamimi YZ, Orsi NM, Quinn AC, Homer-Vanniasinkam S, Ross SA. A

review of delayed ischemic neurologic deficit following aneurysmal subarachnoid hemorrhage: historical overview, current treatment, and pathophysiology. *World Neurosurg.* 2010 Jun;**73**(6):654–67.

58. Suarez JI. Treatment of ruptured cerebral aneurysms and vasospasm after subarachnoid hemorrhage. *Neurosurg Clin N Am.* 2006 Sep;**17** Suppl 1:57–69.

59. Roos YB, de Haan RJ, Beenen LF, et al. Complications and outcome in patients with aneurysmal subarachnoid haemorrhage: a prospective hospital based cohort study in the Netherlands. *J Neurol Neurosurg Psychiatry.* 2000 Mar;**68**(3):337–41.

60. Vergouwen MD, Fang J, Casaubon LK, et al. Higher incidence of in-hospital complications in patients with clipped versus coiled ruptured intracranial aneurysms. *Stroke.* 2011 Nov;**42** (11):3093–8.

61. O'Gorman RL, Poil SS, Brandeis D, et al. Coupling between resting cerebral perfusion and EEG. *Brain Topogr.* 2013 Jul;**26**(3):442–57.

62. Sundt TM, Jr., Sharbrough FW, Anderson RE, Michenfelder JD. Cerebral blood flow measurements and electroencephalograms during carotid endarterectomy. *J Neurosurg.* 1974 Sep;**41**(3): 310–20.

63. Diedler J, Sykora M, Juttler E, Steiner T, Hacke W. Intensive care management of acute stroke: general management. *Int J Stroke.* 2009 Oct;**4** (5):365–78.

64. Rivierez M, Landau-Ferey J, Grob R, Grosskopf D, Philippon J. Value of electroencephalogram in prediction and diagnosis of vasospasm after intracranial aneurysm rupture. *Acta Neurochir (Wien).* 1991;**110**(1-2): 17–23.

65. Rathakrishnan R, Gotman J, Dubeau F, Angle M. Using continuous electroencephalography in the management of delayed cerebral ischemia following subarachnoid hemorrhage. *Neurocrit Care.* 2011 Apr;**14**(2):152–61.

66. Implantable tissue ischemia sensor. U.S. Patent US20100312081A1. www.google .ch/patents/US20100312081

67. Zeller JS. EM innovations: new technologies you haven't heard of yet. *Medscape.* 2013 Mar 19.

Chapter 13

Perioperative Monitoring for Congenital Heart Disease Surgery

Shavonne L. Massey and Robert Clancy

Illustrative Case

Case 17 Newborn Heart Surgery: Hypoplastic Left Heart Syndrome

Congenital heart disease (CHD) encompasses a large collection of cardiac malformations discovered at or before birth; it is the single most common form of birth defect. CHD affects roughly 40,000 births in the United States each year, equating to an incidence of 4–50/1000 live births annually. One quarter of affected neonates require corrective surgery shortly after birth [1, 2]. The landscape of newborn heart surgery has substantially changed since the modern era began in the 1970s with the adaptation of adult cardiopulmonary bypass (CPB) circuitry for infants. The initial concern was nothing short of simple survival from these mostly lethal heart defects. After decades of progress, however, the center of focus has now shifted from survival to quality of life following newborn heart surgery (NBHS). Indeed, neurodevelopmental disabilities are now considered the single most common sequela of NBHS. The basis of the lifelong neurological disabilities is multifactorial and complex, but we know that clinical management in the peri-operative period has a significant impact on the infants' long-term outcomes. Consequently, neurological monitoring in the congenital heart disease population is increasing worldwide. With so many infants undergoing NBHS, the field of neuromonitoring for these patients is wide. In this chapter, we first review the neurological effects of hypothermia and the actual conduct of newborn heart surgery. We then will discuss the indications for neuromonitoring and summarize its findings and outcomes in this unique population.

Effects of Hypothermia on the Body and Brain

One of the body's highest homeostatic priorities is the maintenance of its core temperature. This is accomplished by a complex network of sensors and activators, such as muscle shivering and cutaneous vasoconstriction, under the orchestration of the anterior hypothalamus. Normothermia in humans is defined as 36°C to 37.2°C (97°F to 99°F), with temperatures below this defined as hypothermia. Hypothermia is divided into four stages; (1) the range of *clinical* hypothermia is 35°C to 32°C; (2) the range of *surgical* hypothermia is 32°C to 25°C; (3) the range of deep or profound hypothermia is 25°C to 0°C; and (4) the range of frozen or super-cooled hypothermia is 0°C to –8°C. With deepening hypothermia, individuals become progressively amnestic, dysarthric, stuporous, and then frankly comatose with absent brainstem reflexes. At 18°C, cardiac asystole occurs [3, 4]. Table 13.1 summarizes the neurological effects of progressive hypothermia.

As body core temperature lowers, cellular and metabolic functions slow. Accordingly, neuronal metabolism and oxygen consumption decrease along with increasing hypothermia and arrest at –8°C. Hypothermia's resulting reduction in cerebral metabolic activity has been exploited to preserve and protect the central nervous system in impending or actual acute hypoxia-ischemia scenarios. One of the first widespread applications of therapeutic hypothermia was in adult cardiac surgery as a way to lower cerebral metabolic demands intraoperatively and mitigate potential brain injury.

The Conduct of Cardiac Surgery for Serious Forms of Congenital Heart Disease

Modern newborn heart surgery is a technological tour de force. The human heart is roughly the size of a clenched fist. Imagine the tiny heart of a newborn! Imagine further the technical skill needed to delicately operate on such a small organ that's beating 120 times a minute. Since the late 1970s into the early 1980s, "open heart" surgery paradigms have evolved to repair or palliate even the most complex and formerly deadly forms of CHD. A timeline of the conduct of NBHS is shown in Figure 13.1.

Brain cooling is the foundation of neuroprotection during the surgical repair of complex congenital heart disease. Hypothermia reduces cerebral metabolic demands, decreasing metabolic rate and oxygen consumption and thus creating a higher threshold for ischemic brain injury. Patients are typically cooled to a moderate degree of hypothermia (25°C–33°C) when CPB alone is needed for surgery. One advantage is that moderate hypothermia for CPB alone still preserves some degree of cerebrovascular autoregulation. In some complex cases, CPB is instead complemented by deep hypothermic (~18°C) circulatory arrest (DHCA). DHCA allows more time for the surgeon to operate. At this degree of hypothermia, however, cerebral autoregulation is not preserved, and carbon dioxide exchange, mitochondrial function, and cerebral vasculature dynamics are blunted.

The first phase of NBHS begins with the induction of general anesthesia, surface cooling, and local cooling of the head. The baby is then connected to cardiopulmonary bypass. CPB supports circulation and oxygenation to vital organs during cardiac surgery via an *external* circulatory system. This ensures that for the duration of surgery, oxygen and other

Table 13.1 Neurological effects associated with progressive hypothermia

Core body temperature		Neurological and physiological effects	Temperature stage
Degrees Fahrenheit	**Degrees Centigrade**		
97–99	36–37.2	Range of normal body temperatures	Normothermia
95	35	Minimum temperature for ECS† recording by EEG	Clinical Stage Hypothermia
93.2	34	Amnesia; dysarthria	
91.4	33	Ataxia; apathy	
89.6	32	Stupor	
85.2	29	Dilation of pupils	Surgical Stage Hypothermia
78.8	26	Unresponsiveness to pain	
73.4	23	Absent corneal and oculovestibular reflexes	Deep/Profound Stage Hypothermia
66.2	19	Isoelectric EEG	
64.4	18¶	Cardiac asystole	
32	0	Incompatible with life	Frozen/Supercooled Stage Hypothermia

†ECS represents "electrocerebral silence" measured by scalp-recorded EEG. The specialized EEG recording technique required to confirm ECS conservatively requires the presence of a core body temperature of at least 35°C before the diagnosis of brain death can be made.
¶18°C is also the target nasopharyngeal temperature during deep hypothermic circulatory arrest (DHCA) for newborn heart surgery.

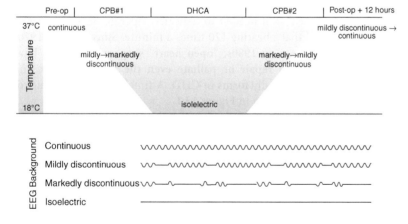

Figure 13.1 Blueprint of newborn heart surgery using cardiopulmonary bypass and deep hypothermic circulatory arrestand the relation to EEG
This illustration shows the phases of NBHS over time (left to right) and as temperature is lowered (top to bottom). Expected EEG findings for each stage are listed for each phase, with examples in the lower panel.
CPB, cardiopulmonary bypass; DHCA, deep hypothermic circulatory arrest.

vital nutrients continue to reach organs, even as the body's own circulatory system is "off line." The temperature of the perfusion solution is then gradually lowered by embedded refrigeration coils.

It is important to keep in mind that brain perfusion via bypass pump carries its own inherent risks. Tissue perfusion is optimal with the natural pulsatile flow of cardiac systole and diastole that is absent during bypass. Catheter size, catheter placement, and selected flow rates can all affect the likelihood of a serious adverse event and therefore must also be chosen with utmost care [5]. Flow rates of 0.5 liters/m² have been shown to adequately support cerebral oxygen consumption and maintain cortical evoked potentials during hypothermia. However, animal data suggest decreased cerebral adenosine triphosphate (ATP) levels even at this standard flow rate [6]. Exposure of the baby's blood to the foreign materials of the CPB circuit induces potent neurotoxic inflammatory cascades. Emboli from air bubbles, clotted blood, and other debris may lead to stroke. Every attempt is made to minimize CPB duration while still allowing enough time for the core of the brain to achieve thermal equilibrium with the rest of the cooled body. In the case of DHCA, once the body and brain temperatures are reduced to deep hypothermic levels (~18°C), the heart is stopped and the CPB cannulae are removed. This provides the surgeon with a still and bloodless operative field to effect the most delicate aspects of heart surgery. During DHCA all brainstem reflexes are absent and the EEG itself is isoelectric. The "safe" duration of DHCA is not known with certainty. Durations of up to 30 minutes generally seem to be tolerated without increased risk of neurological morbidity. However, more than 60 minutes may be needed for some especially complex cardiac anatomies; such prolonged DHCA increases the risks of brain injury.

At the completion of DHCA, the infant is recannulated onto CPB, cardiac action is restarted, and the patient is gradually rewarmed. In the immediate post-cardiac surgery period, the brain and body are extremely stressed from their recent ischemia-reperfusion experience and the lingering effects of anesthesia and hypothermia. Around 12 hours post-operatively, cardiac output reaches its nadir from the myocardial depression induced by its own ischemia-reperfusion injury; it is not surprising to see some EEG abnormalities reflecting that cerebral dysfunction during this period of low cardiac output state after surgery.

A newer low-flow bypass strategy, *antegrade cerebral perfusion* (ACP), includes perfusion of the cerebral vasculature via the carotid artery, while minimizing blood flow to the somatic vasculature and other organs. During ACP, core body temperatures are maintained at 20°C–25°C and continuous cerebral flow rates are lowered to 50 mL/kg, which has been shown to support cerebral perfusion during hypothermia [7]. As this is a newer technique, outcome data are limited; however, a major concern is that ACP prolongs the overall pump exposure time.

One key uncertainty with hypothermic strategies for NBHS is accurately measuring the true brain temperature. Core body temperatures are measured by nasopharyngeal (NP) probes and assumed to be uniform throughout the brain. The deep core brain structures are not directly sampled; it is unclear if an 18°C NP temperature translates to the identical cerebral temperature. It is known that temperature gradients exist between the cooler cortical regions and warmer basal ganglia regions [8], and the exact length of time for the initial CPB cooling to achieve thermal brain equilibrium with the body is uncertain. Overly rapid cooling implies that deep core brain temperatures might not have adequate time to fully equilibrate with the lower body temperatures. At the same time, excessively prolonged CPB cooling unnecessarily increases the brain's exposure to the inherent risks of CPB itself.

Effects of Therapeutic Hypothermia on Neuromonitoring

It is widely appreciated now that a significant morbidity following CHD and NBHS is ongoing neurodevelopmental disability. It is unknown to what degree this is caused by early differences in brain development, including in utero insults, unavoidable stressors inherent to NBHS, and/or additional early life medical factors. There are data that some neurological problems clearly exist in this population before NBHS. The mean head circumferences of babies with serious forms of

CHDs are significantly smaller at birth than their non-CHD counterparts. Pre-operative MRIs of these patients also demonstrate morphological brain immaturity measured by standardized total maturation scores [9, 10]. The same pre-operative imaging may also show acquired abnormalities such as white matter injury, focal brain injury (i.e., "stroke") and tissue lactic acidosis using MR spectroscopy [11, 12].

Pediatric cardiothoracic surgeons have gone to admirable lengths to identify modifiable anesthetic and surgical variables to improve the neurodevelopmental outcomes of their patients. They have studied outcomes of patients following different surgical techniques, such as CPB alone versus CPB coupled with DHCA. Others compared developmental outcomes depending on how acid-base status is managed during surgery (so-called alpha stat versus PH stat blood gas management). Others investigated how the hematocrit of the CPB perfusate affected tissue perfusion and therefore brain vitality. The use of neuroprotective agents such as erythropoietin is also being explored.

The hours and days following NBHS also contribute to the net neurodevelopmental outcomes. This is where prolonged neuromonitoring has played its largest role. Continuous video electroencephalogram monitoring has emerged as one of the premier tools to measure the brain's response to the stress of newborn heart surgery. There are two main goals of EEG monitoring in newborn heart surgery; (1) evaluation of the EEG background and (2) electrographic seizure detection.

Interpretation of the EEG Background

Due to central nervous system (CNS) immaturity, the clinical neonatal neurological examination is an insensitive marker of cortical function compared to older children and adults. Most clinically observable neonatal brain functions, such as spontaneous respirations, oral feeding, small and large body movements, and primitive reflexes, are not controlled by the cortex, but rather by deep gray motor centers, brainstem centers, and spinal reflexes. Consciousness may be the only true measure of higher cortical functions in the neonate, but this is obscured in the post-operative period by their fragile medical state, pharmacological paralysis, and the use of medications for muscle relaxation, anxiolysis, and pain management. As a result, dysfunction of or damage to the cerebral cortex is often clinically invisible in the neonate assessed just by neurological examination. EEG background offers a noninvasive window into the neonate's functional cerebral cortical health.

One of the earliest studies to examine the EEG effects of hypothermia and cardiac surgery was published in 1966 by Ann Harden and colleagues [13]. Their case series described 23 children, ages 3 to 14 years, who underwent open heart surgery with hypothermic total circulatory arrest. The children were divided into two groups: (i) mild hypothermia (28°C–32°C) and light sedation with a veno-venous extracorporeal circuit without CPB; and (ii) moderate hypothermia (18.5°C–24.3°C) with venous-arterial extracorporeal circuit with CPB. In the first group, EEGs initially showed preservation of their baseline electrical frequencies. When the circulation was stopped without CPB, the faster frequencies were replaced with high voltage slowing within 10–20 seconds, followed by gradual voltage attenuation and a flat tracing about 35 seconds later. The second group followed a different trajectory. Once temperatures dropped below 28°C, the EEG also showed replacement of faster frequency activity with high voltage slowing. In three-quarters of these children, generalized, high-voltage discharges appeared without clinical correlate. Their EEGs never completely attenuated despite hypothermia below 20°C. They attributed this preservation to the continued low flow bypass. When circulation was fully arrested, the EEG slowly attenuated, reaching electrical silence in about 109 seconds. In both groups, the EEGs remained silent for the duration of circulatory arrest. While the sample size was small and did not include neonates, this landmark study argued for the use of deeper levels of hypothermia in the pediatric cardiac surgery population to safeguard cerebral metabolism and neuroprotection, demonstrated by the longer duration between cooling onset and EEG changes that represent.

Stecker and colleagues documented EEG changes in 109 adults during hypothermia before inducing cardiac arrest in thoracic aortic surgical procedures [14]. About 8 minutes after the start of cooling at a mean temperature of 29.6°C (21.5°C–34.2°C), the EEG remained continuous but showed periodic complexes that were unilateral or bilateral (synchronous or asynchronous) in the majority of cases. This was followed by a gradual dampening of the continuous background activity until burst suppression was attained at an average 12.7 minutes from cooling onset (2–28 minutes) and mean temperature 24.4°C (15.7°C–33°C). Subsequently, the EEG progressively attenuated, reaching electrocerebral silence (ECS) at a mean time of 27.5 minutes (range 12–50 minutes) and a mean temperature of 17.8°C (12.5°C–27.2°C). In general, patients with longer times to attain one EEG milestone also had delayed times to subsequent milestones. These investigators also examined potential patient-specific and procedural confounders and consistently found that patients with larger body surface area required longer cooling times. Increased time to reach ECS was also associated with increased hemoglobin concentrations, decreased cooling rate, and lower CO_2 tensions during cooling. Based on the heterogeneity of their results, they argued that it was not possible to specify a single standard duration and level of hypothermia to guarantee ECS in every patient. Rather, the procedure should be tailored to each individual using intra-operative EEG monitoring to confirm that ECS has been achieved.

The description of the expected sequential EEG changes during hypothermic cardiac surgery led to an examination of their predictive value for immediate post-operative outcomes. In 2014, Seltzer and colleagues addressed this question in neonates, using post-operative EEG seizures as the dependent outcome variable in a cohort of patients with heterogeneous cardiac abnormalities and surgical repairs [15]. Seventeen infants age ≤3 months who underwent DHCA with regional cerebral perfusion at a mean temperature of 21.2°C were compared to 15 infants with cardiac surgery who did not undergo DHCA. All patients shared the same initial hypothermic EEG progression with diffuse slowing followed by increasing

discontinuity. In the DHCA group, the discontinuity increased until ECS was achieved with temperatures below 25°C. The 15 patients who did not receive DHCA had temperatures above 25°C and never showed isoelectric tracings. With rewarming, most DHCA infants had a gradual reversal from isoelectric tracings to a burst suppression pattern without epileptiform features. In two others, without DHCA, however, unusual bursts of high amplitude, rhythmic sharp activity were noted, and both went on to show frank electrographic seizures post-operatively. Both also had single ventricle heart lesions which required longer operating times. While the generalizability of this study is limited, the findings raise questions about the potential use of intra-operative EEG monitoring to predict post-operative seizures, mortality, hospital length, and other adverse outcomes. Figure 13.1 demonstrates the sequential EEG changes during the course of newborn heart surgery under DHCA.

The Boston Circulatory Arrest Study (BCAS) was a landmark longitudinal neurodevelopmental study of infants (age ≤3 months) who required repair of D-transposition of the great arteries [6]. Study subjects were randomized to undergo *only* low flow CPB versus briefer periods of CPB combined with DHCA. The initial randomized trial assessed the incidence of adverse neurological signs in the two groups such as seizures during the immediate post-operative period. Patients in both treatment arms received deep hypothermia with temperatures lowered to 18°C. Continuous, full array analog EEGs (i.e., paper chart recordings) were performed before, during, and after surgery. The EEGs were not interpreted in real time and their EEG seizures not discovered until long after surgery. In total, 171 infants were randomized. None had any notable findings on pre-operative EEGs. Compared to the CPB alone group, the CPB + DHCA group had significantly longer times to the return of first EEG activity and the onset of some continuous EEG activity. The durations of DHCA correlated with EEG recovery times. None returned to their full pre-surgical EEG baselines by 48 hours post-surgery. In the 48-hour post-operative period, the incidence of EEG seizures was significantly higher in the CPB + DHCA group compared to CPB alone. Furthermore, longer DHCA times were significantly associated with an increased risk for seizures. The presence of seizures in these patient raised the question whether post-operative EEG seizures were in turn associated with worse subsequent neurodevelopmental outcomes.

In both neonates and older children, EEGs recorded for 48 hours following surgery often show a slower frequency background, often related to the combined depressant effects of anesthetics, sedatives, and analgesics. Figure 13.2 is an example of the effect of sedative medications on a neonatal EEG. Collectively, these medications diminish high-frequency rhythms. One pediatric study showed that the resolution of excessive post-operative slowing only occurred in 25% of patients within 48 hours of surgery [16]. Some did not return to their pre-operative EEG frequencies for 5–10 days. However, EEG slowing *per se* does not reliably predict poorer subsequent neurological outcomes. In general, the expected, typical degree of post-operative EEG slowing still has certain features, which if not present, should alert the clinician to

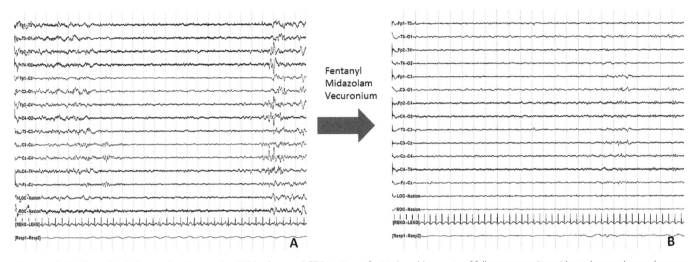

Figure 13.2 Effect of sedation medications on the EEG background. EEG tracings of a 14-day-old neonate of full-term gestation with total anomalous pulmonary venous return (TAPVR) immediately status post-surgical repair with DHCA. The post-surgical EEG background (A) has diffuse excessive beta activity and is excessively discontinuous with prolonged (>6 seconds) and attenuated (<25 μV) inter-burst intervals. Immediately after the patient received boluses of fentanyl, midazolam, and vecuronium, the EEG background (B) temporarily becomes diffusely attenuated (all activity <10 μV) with periods of attenuation lasting up to 40 seconds. EEG displayed at 1 second per vertical time marker, sensitivity 7 μV.

further investigation. Normal slowing is symmetric and bilaterally posteriorly dominant. In neonates, the post-operative EEG may show prolonged suppression, burst suppression, or significant discontinuity. In general, over the first 48 hours of the post-operative period, there should be a gradual improvement of the background from excessively discontinuous to diffusely slow to faster frequency activity. Figure 13.3 shows the expected temporal evolution of the post-operative neonatal EEG following NBHS. More recently, EEG background features have been studied as an early harbinger of decompensation. A single-center observational study included 22 neonates who had cardiac arrest while undergoing EEG following NBHS [17]. All had worsening of the EEG background prior to cardiac arrest, for a median of 3 minutes duration. This raises the question of whether automated early warning systems might use EEG to identify impending decompensation.

Seizure Detection

Seizure detection is the prime goal of EEG monitoring after NBHS. Unaided clinical observation is grossly inadequate to diagnose seizures and quantify their abundance in most neonates. Clinical observation alone both underestimates true seizure occurrence while overdiagnosing non-epileptic movements as seizures in others [18]. Neonates who are critically ill from a variety of acute etiologies have a high occurrence of subclinical (EEG-only) seizures [19, 20]. These consist of unmistakable ictal EEG patterns that fulfill all electrographic criteria for seizures, though the neonate has no outward clinical ictal manifestations. It is theorized that neonates have a higher preponderance of EEG-only seizures due to the inherent immaturity of their central nervous systems. Additionally, in neonates with previously confirmed electroclinical seizures (in which EEG seizures directly trigger simultaneous clinical seizures, such as repetitive clonic jerking of a limb), the use of anti seizure medications (ASM) often results in the

phenomenon of uncoupling. Treatment with ASMs uncouples electroclinical seizures by blocking their clinical manifestations while leaving the EEG seizures unchecked [20]. Finally, the use of neuromuscular blocking agents to achieve deliberate iatrogenic paralysis post-operatively renders visual observation for seizures virtually useless. In all, subclinical seizures have been found to constitute as much as 80% of seizure burden across various neonatal cohorts [21–24]. Clinical diagnosis alone grossly underestimates EEG seizures.

In addition to the high rate of subclinical seizure burden in the neonate, clinical observation can overestimate seizure occurrence in others. Neonates possess a variety of movement patterns that are difficult to interpret, often making it impossible to discriminate epileptic activity from other movements. In a 2009 study, Malone et al. illustrated the enormity of the problem [25]. In their investigation, 137 healthcare providers from 8 different NICUs were asked to make a diagnosis based on 20 videos of infants with paroxysmal movements, shown by EEG to be seizures or not. The average correct score was only 50%. There was poor inter-rater agreement among physicians and nurses, regardless of their levels of experience. There was a dichotomy in correct identification based on seizure semiology. Clonic seizures were correctly identified by 37%–96% of observers. Subtle seizures were correctly identified by only 20%–50% of observers.

Infants born with serious forms of CHDs who require NBHS are subject to the inherent difficulties of seizure diagnosis on clinical grounds alone. There is a high risk of post-operative seizures in this population. Pre-1985 studies reported post-operative *clinical* seizures to occur in up to 50%. However, with clinical advances of the past 30 years, this may not reflect the contemporary CHD population. In older studies, hypocalcemia (sometimes from unrecognized 22q11.2 deletion, frequent among newborns with CHDs) was also fairly common and may have induced seizures. Routine EEG examinations were virtually unheard of in the early eras of

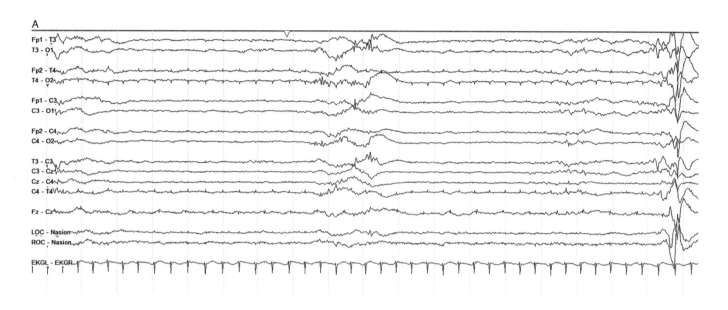

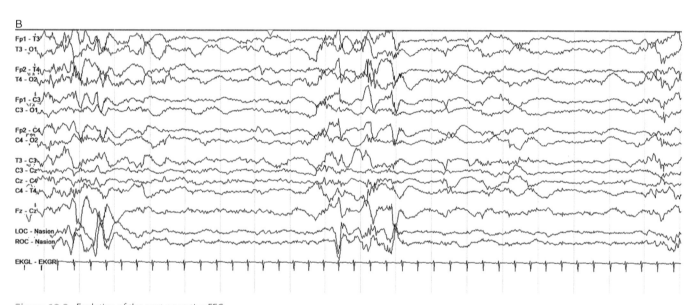

Figure 13.3 Evolution of the post-operative EEG.
EEG tracings of a 7-day-old neonate of full-term gestation with hypoplastic left heart syndrome (HLHS) at (A) 6 hours, (B) 24 hours, and (C) 48 hours post-surgical repair with deep hypothermic circulatory arrest (DHCA). At 6 hours (A), the background is excessively discontinuous with attenuated (<25 μV) and prolonged (>6 seconds) inter-burst intervals. At 24 hours (B), the background remains discontinuous, but bursts are composed of a more diverse mixture of frequencies of moderate amplitude and inter-bursts are less attenuated (>25 μV) and shorter in duration. At 48 hours (C), the background is a continuous symmetric rich admixture of frequencies of moderate amplitudes. EEG displayed at 30 seconds per page, sensitivity 7 μV.

NBHS. Conversely, the common use of benzodiazepines (for anxiolysis and sedation) and neuromuscular blockade makes those early clinical observations highly unreliable to measure the true incidence of post-operative seizures. With the gathering of experience and the technological development of digital EEG, it is now appreciated that subclinical EEG seizures are common in all ICU settings, from neonates to adults. Furthermore, these sick individuals may experience only a few seizures, but many develop electrographic status epilepticus [26]. See Figure 13.4 for examples of electrographic seizures in neonates.

The Boston Circulatory Arrest Study was one of the first to characterize seizure detection by clinical versus EEG diagnosis in the NBHS population specifically. Infants ≤3 months with D-

transposition of the great arteries were randomized into two surgical repair groups using either low-flow CPB alone versus CPB with DHCA [6]. In this cohort, 6% had clinical seizures, while 20% had electrographic seizures post-operatively. Nine of 11 infants with clinical seizures also had EEG seizures. When they occurred, clinical signs always followed the onset of EEG seizures, typically with a prolonged lag time. EEG allowed seizure recognition hours before clinical signs arose. Clinical seizures were more common in the DHCA (11%) than the CPB-alone group (1%) and associated with longer arrest times, typically 35 minutes or more. EEG seizures were also more common in the DHCA (26%) than the CPB-alone group (13%). Seizure burden was high with 139 minutes median total ictal duration. All had seizure onset within

C

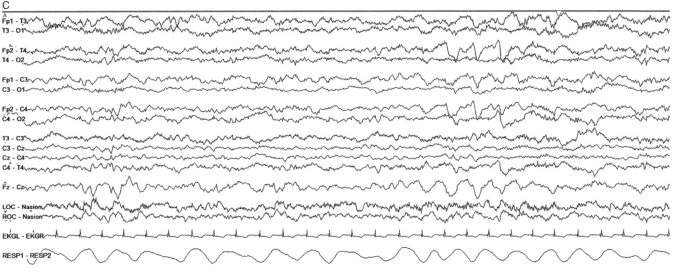

Figure 13.3 (cont.)

A

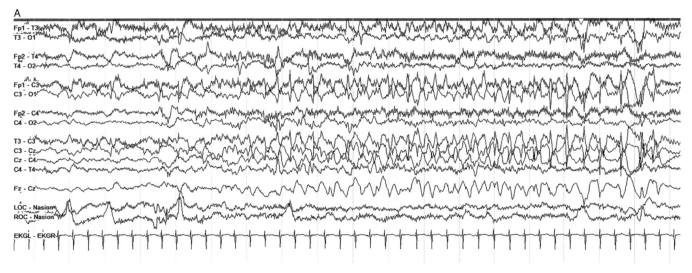

Figure 13.4 Neonatal seizure examples.
A. EEG tracing of a *subclinical seizure* in a 10-day-old neonate of full-term gestation. The seizure begins with rhythmic 1 Hz sharp wave discharges in the right central (C4) region which evolve in amplitude, frequency, and space over 30 seconds. The neonate has no clinical signs during this seizure.
B. EEG tracing of an *electroclinical seizure* in a 1-day-old neonate of full-term gestation. The seizure begins with rhythmic 2–3 Hz sharp wave discharges in the central region, maximal in the left central (C3) region. (1) The sharp wave discharges evolve in amplitude and frequency in the left central region before becoming more diffuse. As the seizure evolves, there is diffuse rhythmic 10 Hz alpha activity (2), and as the seizure concludes, there is further evolution with rhythmic 2 Hz sharp wave discharges maximal in the right temporal (T4) region (3). Following the seizure, there is diffuse attenuation of the EEG background (4). The total seizure duration is 70 seconds. Ten seconds after electrographic onset of the seizure, the infant had rhythmic clonic activity of the right arm. EEGs displayed at sensitivity 7 μV.

the first 36 hours after surgery. While seizure onset did not consistently lateralize, most localized to the frontal and central regions, common watershed regions in the setting of hypoperfusion. Three risk factors for seizures were identified: increased duration of DHCA, the anatomical presence of VSD (as contrasted to those who had an intact ventricular septum), and preoperative acidosis [7].

Complementing this work were studies by the group at Children's Hospital of Philadelphia (CHOP). An early detailed neuropathology study of the type and distribution of acute brain injuries present in those who died after the Stage I Norwood procedure for hypoplastic left heart syndrome

(HLHS) confirmed that hypoxic-ischemic injury to the cortex and subcortical white matter represented the main forms of damage [27]. It was also realized that one specific biochemical mechanism of cell damage was the generation of toxic oxygen free radicals during reperfusion catalyzed by the enzyme xanthine oxidase (XO). Further, allopurinol, a potent inhibitor of XO, suppresses free radical attacks on the brain and heart following reperfusion. This set the stage for a double blinded, randomized, placebo-controlled neurocardiac protection trial [28]. The study subjects were stratified into two risk groups. HLHS infants composed the first group, considered to be at highest risk for death or injury. The second group included all

B1

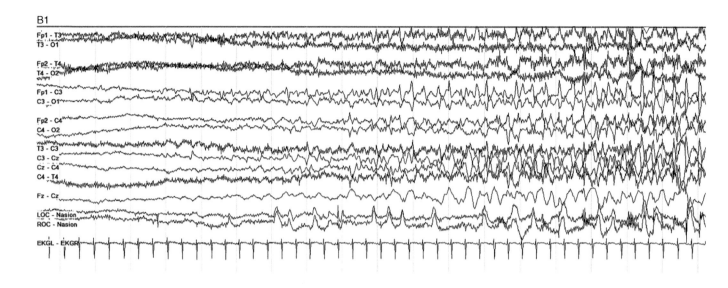

B2

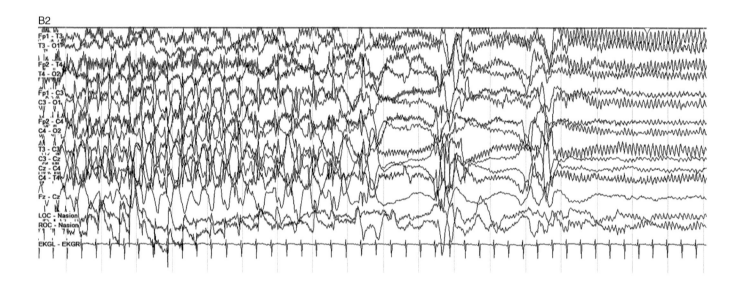

B3

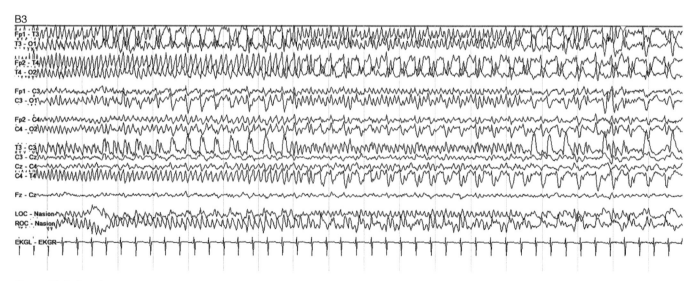

Figure 13.4 (cont.)

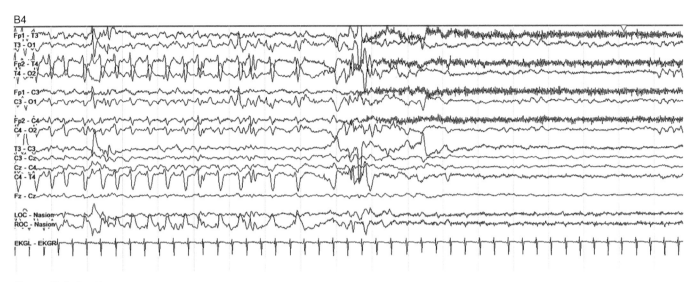

Figure 13.4 (cont.)

other forms of CHDs lumped together (non-HLHS) considered as those with lower risks of death or injury. The efficacy endpoints of the study included post-operative death, clinical seizures, coma, and cardiac arrest. There were no outcome differences between allopurinol and placebo infants in the lower risk, non-HLHS subjects. However, allopurinol use resulted in a significant reduction of cardiac events and seizures in the higher-risk HLHS survivors. Across all study subjects, 17% had clinical seizures, with over 60% starting within 48 hours after surgery. Risk factor analyses later identified significant predictors of post-operative seizures: (i) the presence of suspected genetic conditions, (ii) cardiac anatomy (the presence of an aortic arch obstruction), and (iii) DHCA times ≥60 minutes.

A later cohort included 183 infants under 6 months old who needed heart surgery using CPB and underwent continuous EEG monitoring for 48 hours post-operatively [29, 30]. In this group, DHCA had a median duration of 50 minutes when it was needed, and target core temperatures were around 18°C. When DHCA was not needed, the median temperatures were around 28°C. Electrographic seizures were detected in 11.5%, all of which were subclinical. The median number of EEG seizures per subject was 46. The typical time of EEG seizure onset was 21–22 hours after surgery. Clinical events electronically earmarked by bedside caregivers as possible "seizures" had no correlation with EEG seizures. Univariate predictors of EEG seizures included cardiac anatomy (HLHS or its variants), prostaglandin use, lowest nasopharyngeal temperature, and longer DHCA durations. In multivariate analyses, the single strongest seizure predictor was a DHCA duration exceeding 40 minutes. At the same time, avoidance of DHCA did not eliminate all risk for seizures.

In 2011, the American Clinical Neurophysiology Society (ACNS) published recommendations for continuous EEG monitoring in high-risk newborn populations including NBHS with CPB [31]. A single-center prospective study adhering to this guideline included a total of 161 of 172 eligible neonates with CHD who were monitored for 48 hours post-op over 18 consecutive months. EEG seizures appeared in 8.1% (13 of 161). The seizures were exclusively subclinical in 85% (11 of 13) infants. EEG status epilepticus was seen at some time after surgery in 62% (8 of 13) [23]. The median onset of post-operative seizures was 20 hours. In multivariate analysis, seizures were more common with delayed sternal closure and DHCA durations >40 minutes. EEG background variables did not predict seizures. Mortality was significantly higher in those with seizures (38%) than those without (8%). An accompanying editorial opined that this study set the standard for future neurodevelopmental research in the NBHS population: "it is clearly no longer adequate for investigators reporting outcomes after neonatal cardiac surgery to state that neonates did not have postoperative neurologic complications if they do not use continuous EEG monitoring" [32] Table 13.2 summarizes the results of many reports of seizures after NBHS [6, 23, 27, 28, 33–36].

Neuromonitoring Modalities

Neonatal EEG monitoring serves two main purposes: the detection of seizures and a global characterization of central nervous system health by virtue of EEG background assessment. The 2011 ACNS neonatal guidelines recommend conventional, full array EEG as the *gold standard* of seizure detection [31]. Technical details on the conduct of monitoring including electrode placement, montages, and duration of recordings are included in the guidelines. Monitoring is recommended for at least 24 hours and should continue until no further seizures are detected for 24 hours.

While conventional, full array EEG is considered the technological gold standard of recording, other forms of monitoring are also valuable and merit consideration. Digital trend analyses depict EEG signals transformed over a compressed time scale. These digital displays provide a bird's eye view of many hours of EEG, making long-term trends easier to spot. Non-neurologists can learn to meaningfully interpret trended data without formal

Table 13.2 The evolving incidence of post-operative seizures in the neonatal congenital heart disease population

Series	Era	Subjects (N)	Clinical seizures	EEG seizures	Comment
Scattered case reports	Before 1985		Up to 50%	EEG not performed	
CHOP HLHS autopsy series	1980–1985	50	32% (12/38)	EEG not performed	
BCAS trial *Newburger et al. 1993 [6]*	1988–1992	170	6.4% (11/170)	19.8% (27/136)	TGA only (+VSD or IVS)
Boston α vs. pH stat *du Plessis et al. 1997 [33]*	1992–1996	182	3.3% (6/182)	5.2% (6/116)	TGA, TOF & VSD+
CHOP Allopurinol Trial *Clancy et al. 2001 [28]*	1992–1997	318	22% (15/67) 18% (33/187)	EEG not performed	HLHS vs. Non-HLHS
CHOP apo-E Study *Gaynor et al. 2005 [34]*	2001–2003	183	0%	11.5% (21/183)	Mixed forms of CHD
Baylor CPB with ACP *Andropoulos et al. 2010 [35]*	2005–2008	68	0%	1.5% (1/68)	Continuous benzodiazepine infusion post-surgery
Melbourne, Auckland Norwood-Type operation with ACP *Gunn et al. 2012 [36]*	2005–2008	39	0%	23% intra-op (9/39) 18% post-op (7/39)	aEEG for intra- and post-operative monitoring
CHOP CICU Neonatal QAI *Naim et al. 2015 [23]*	2012–2013	161	1.2% (2/161)	8% (13/161)	All seizures EEG confirmed

EEG, electroencephalogram; CHOP, Children's Hospital of Philadelphia; HLHS, hypoplastic left heart syndrome; BCAS, Boston Circulatory Arrest Study; TGA, transposition of the great arteries; VSD, ventricular septal defect; IVS, intact ventricular system; TOF, tetralogy of Fallot; apoE, apolipoprotein E; CHD, congenital heart disease; CBP, cardiopulmonary bypass; ACP, anterograde cerebral perfusion; aEEG, amplitude-integrated electroencephalogram; CICU, cardiac intensive care unit; QAI, quality assurance initiative.

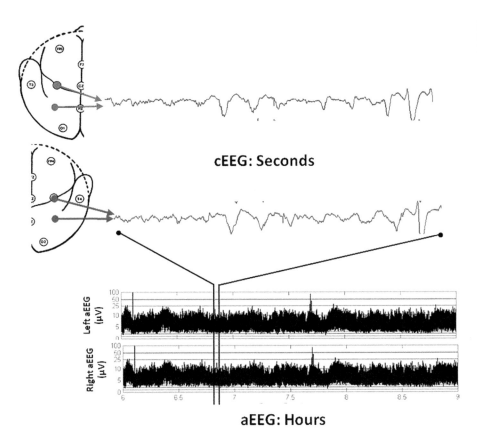

cEEG: Seconds

aEEG: Hours

neurophysiological training. However, these condensed and simplified EEG trend displays have their own perils. Reduced EEG displays do not comprehensively represent the full landscape of the cerebral cortex. The highly compressed time scale also means that brief, but important, EEG events are likely to be missed. Finally, novice interpretation of the complex EEG signal is more likely to be "under-read" or "over-read." Recording artifacts are notorious contaminants of the fragile and faint (microvolt) EEG signals and are difficult to spot without sophisticated knowledge of electrophysiology.

The most commonly used simplified neonatal EEG trending format is amplitude-integrated EEG, or "aEEG." aEEG monitoring typically requires the placement of four recording electrodes. For example, a common montage includes four scalp electrodes placed in the left and right central and parietal regions. The first channel of aEEG is obtained by measuring the electrical difference between the left central and left parietal areas ($C_L \rightarrow P_L$). The second channel records the voltage difference between the right central and right parietal areas ($C_R \rightarrow P_R$). The raw EEG signal from each electrode pair is highly filtered to remove electrical frequencies less than 2 Hz or more than 15 Hz. While conventional EEG displays 1 second of raw EEG per 15 mm, aEEG typically displays 1 hour of EEG compressed into just 6 cm, which comes out to 900 seconds of EEG per 15 mm (see Figure 13.5). As such, the best use of aEEG is for long term assessment of background trends.

Amplitude-integrated EEG is superior to unaided clinical diagnosis of seizures. However, because of the short duration and unpredictable spatial fields of many electrographic seizures, there are sizeable limitations in quantifying seizures by aEEG, as compared to full array EEG. Numerous studies have shown that in a variety of high-risk neonatal populations, aEEG is less accurate for seizure detection than EEG [31, 37–42]. The accuracy of aEEG in seizure detection varies by the experience of the aEEG reader, with more experienced readers having greater accuracy in seizure detection [41, 43]. Amplitude-integrated EEG can be an excellent complementary tool to aid in rapid bedside diagnosis of seizures with later confirmation by continuous EEG monitoring. If continuous EEG is unavailable, aEEG can be the primary method for seizure detection, but confirmation by reviewing the imbedded two channels of raw EEG on the aEEG device is essential [31].

Just as there are differences in seizure detection by EEG and aEEG, there are also disagreements in assessing background abnormalities between the two methods. In one study, 48 hours of continuous EEG was performed after NBHS [44, 45]. These were divided into four 12-hour epochs, and assessments of EEG backgrounds were judged by standard EEG interpretive criteria as "normal" or "mildly," "moderately," or "markedly" abnormal. Those same digital EEGs were mathematically re-processed to create four corresponding 12-hour segments of aEEG backgrounds that were independently judged by standard aEEG interpretive criteria. Paired EEGs and aEEGs were available for 637 epochs recorded from 179 infants. The distribution of EEG backgrounds included 60% normal, 22% mildly abnormal, 13% moderately abnormal, and

5% markedly abnormal. The distribution of aEEG backgrounds was significantly different from EEG and included 22% normal, 73% moderately abnormal, and 5% markedly abnormal. Markedly abnormal aEEGs were relatively good predictors of moderately or markedly abnormal EEGs. However, most moderately abnormal aEEGs were associated with normal or mildly abnormal EEGs. Thus, aEEG often overestimated the severity of EEG background as being moderately abnormal when continuous EEG of the same epoch was interpreted to be normal or only mildly abnormal.

Treatment of Seizures in the Newborn Heart Surgery Population

No randomized, placebo-controlled efficacy trial has ever been conducted to establish the efficacy of medications used to treat neonatal seizures [46]. However, Painter et al prospectively compared EEG seizure responses in 59 drug-naive neonates randomly assigned to receive either intravenous phenobarbital or phenytoin [47]. In those initially assigned to phenobarbital treatment, only 43% stopped having EEG seizure, while 45% of those given phenytoin responded. When seizures persisted after the initial medication assignment, the other study medication was administered as second-line treatment. Of the initial treatment phenobarbital failures, 27% responded to phenytoin, the second drug. Of the initial treatment phenytoin failures, 38% went on to respond to phenobarbital. In total, 59% of neonates who received phenobarbital alone, phenytoin alone or a combination of both responded. In another systematic drug treatment study without a placebo control, Boylan et al. investigated EEG seizure response to a randomized choice of a second-line drug [48]. Twenty-two infants met study criteria and received phenobarbital as their first-line drug. There were 11 nonresponders who were then randomized to receive either a second-line benzodiazepine or lignocaine. None responded to benzodiazepines whereas lignocaine had a 60% response rate, defined as a ≥80% seizure reduction. In contrast, other non-controlled trial studies showed more favorable responses to benzodiazepines [49–51]. Despite a lack of efficacy data, levetiracetam and topiramate have also gained favor for use in neonatal seizures [52–56]. The most recently published randomized trial of neonatal seizure treatment, NeoLev2, assessed the efficacy of intravenous phenobarbital 20mg/kg compared to intravenous levetiracetam 40mg/kg for first-line therapy.[75] The study included neonates with seizures from a heterogenous group of etiologies, though none of the neonates had CHD. Of the 53 neonates who received levetiracetam initially, 28.3% achieved seizure freedom and of the 30 neonates who received phenobarbital initially, 80% achieved seizure freedom for 24 hours after ASM administration. This head-to-head comparison of levetiracetam versus phenobarbital demonstrated a clear superiority of phenobarbital for treating neonatal seizures at the doses utilized.

The lack of high-quality efficacy data about anti-seizure medications applies equally to the NBHS population. Their treatment may be further confounded by additional considerations such as these patients' tenuous cardiorespiratory profiles and uncertain drug elimination via renal and hepatic clearance. Baseline hypotension is relatively common postoperatively from cardiac dysfunction due to the myocardial hypoxia-ischemia encountered during CPB with DHCA. The main concern from phenobarbital is additional myocardial depression [57]. To mitigate this risk, some practitioners divide the recommended 20 mg/kg phenobarbital loading dose into smaller 5 mg/kg boluses given over a longer time. The effect of this dosing strategy is not known. Phenytoin is rarely used first line to treat seizures following NBHS because of the potential risk of cardiovascular collapse. Hypotension and sinus bradycardia and sinoatrial or atrioventricular block can occur if given rapidly. Phenytoin must be slowly administered intravenously at a rate not faster than 1.0 mg/kg/minute. Further, neonates who have undergone CHD surgical repair are at risk of baseline arrhythmia if the cardiac conduction pathways were severed or damaged during intervention, increasing the concern for both arrhythmia and cardiac collapse with phenytoin administration in this group. Maintaining adequate phenytoin blood levels is also notoriously difficult in neonates [58].

Observational data from our institution of ASM administered for EEG seizures after NBHS were recently reviewed [59]. Of the 53 neonates who were treated with ASMs over a 6-year period, 58% received phenobarbital first, with 58% of those achieving seizure freedom. Another 42% received first-line levetiracetam, with 55% achieving seizure freedom. Decisions on when and how to treat seizure recurrence were left to the treating physician. For second-line ASDs, 10 received levetiracetam and 7 received phenobarbital, with 41% of those neonates achieving seizure freedom after second ASM.

The high incidence of seizures using CPB and DHCA has prompted some centers to explore alternative NBHS methods such as high flow CPB coupled with anterograde cerebral perfusion (ACP) [35], and in this setting, the effect of different sedation strategies and their effect on seizures has been noted. A total of 68 neonates undergoing hypothermic (<30°C) CPB for at least 60 minutes were studied. No patient with 2-ventricle CHD anatomy (e.g., VSD) had seizures. Only 1.5% of 1-ventricle patients (e.g., HLHS) had seizures, a much lower incidence than other comparable cohorts (see Table 13.2). The authors concluded that the seizure decrease was not due to cerebral oxygenation differences. Ninety-four percent of the cohort had been preemptively given a post-operative benzodiazepine for sedation purposes; this may explain some or all of their lower seizure burden.

Neurological Outcomes in the NBHS Population

It is now recognized that chronic neurodevelopmental disorders are the most common morbidities in NBHS survivors. These increased risks are related to all stages of their disease: pre-, intra-, and post-operative factors. The challenge is to identify which risks are amenable to therapeutic intervention. Post-operative seizures are near the top of that short list.

Pre-operative Risk of CNS Injury in CHD

The fetal brain enjoys preferential perfusion, with a quarter of all cardiac output directed there by the third trimester. During states of diminished cardiac output, fetal circulation reflexively spares the brain by shunting to cerebral blood flow (CBF) at the expense of other, less vital organs. An example of such "head sparing" is intrauterine growth retardation in which the head circumference is preserved at the expense of height and weight. However, beyond certain thresholds of decreased cardiac output, CBF is also restricted and ultimately blunts brain growth. This has been shown in single-ventricle CHDs such as HLHS in which head circumferences at birth commonly fall into the small or microcephalic range. Pre-operative brain MRIs also show structural brain maturation delays of 4–5 weeks at term [10]. Pre-operative MRIs have also shown ischemic white matter injury (periventricular leukomalacia) in around 20%. Finally, pre-operative MR spectroscopy shows deep white matter lactate peaks. These observations collectively suggest that CHDs seriously restrict CBF and brain maturation long before the baby's birth [10, 12, 60–64]. Pre-operative MRI abnormalities in CHD, including injury and delayed brain development, have been associated with abnormal network function as measured by EEG connectivity. Early brain development is abnormal both in structure and function [65].

Intra-operative Risks

Cerebral blood flow is significantly distressed during NBHS. Brain tissue perfusion is optimal with the pulsatile blood flow of the natural cycles of cardiac systole and diastole. Continuous, non-pulsatile blood flow using the mechanical roller pumps of CPB does not match nature well. Emboli from clotted blood, air bubbles and other detritus within the bypass pump may obstruct cerebral vessels. During DHCA, all cerebral blood flow is completely stopped under the relative protection of deep hypothermia. This may be well tolerated briefly, but as noted earlier, seizures increase significantly with the longer DHCA times needed to repair the most complex forms of CHDs. Systemic inflammatory responses are also triggered by the infants' blood contacting the foreign materials of the CPB tubing and membranes. Taken as a whole, the intra-operative period poses significant risks to the newborn brain. Studies have suggested an increased risk of post-operative brain injury for neonates with evidence of pre-existing brain immaturity [66]. A small case series found that a longer isoelectric state during DHCA was associated with lower developmental scores at follow-up, raising the question of whether intra-operative EEG to minimize isoelectric states during NBHS might be an opportunity for intervention [67]. Further study is needed to replicate these findings across a larger population.

Post-operative Risks

As discussed above, post-operative seizures are common and usually undetected without EEG monitoring. EEG seizures are significantly associated with increased mortality [23]. In the EEG monitoring subset of the CHOP apoE polymorphisms and neurodevelopmental outcomes study, 11.5% of 183 subjects had post-operative seizures [29, 30]. Of these, 114 survivors returned at 1 year for neurological examinations and measurements of their mental developmental index (MDI) and psychomotor developmental index (PDI) of the Bayley Scales of Infant Development [68]. A significantly higher risk of abnormal neurological examinations appeared in those with post-operative seizures (73% versus 41%, p=0.027). Frontal-onset seizures also predicted lower MDI (cognitive) but not PDI scores. The cohort returned again at 4 years to measure cognition, language, attention, impulsivity, executive function, behavior problems, academic achievement, and visual and fine motor skills [69]. Those with post-operative EEG seizures had significantly more deficits in executive function and social behaviors.

Survivors of the BCAS trial also underwent serial neurodevelopmental examinations at 1 year, 2.5 years, 4 years, 8 years, and in adolescence, providing one of the best longitudinal studies of this population to date. At 1-year follow-up, infants with seizures performed worse on their PDI assessments (p=0.02), with a trend of longer total seizure duration correlating with lower PDI scores (p=0.09) [70]. They also scored significantly lower on assessments of eye-hand coordination, object relations, and vocalization, and were more likely to have an abnormal neurological examination (p=0.008). Seizures were also significantly associated with more MRI abnormalities (p=0.002). By age 2.5 years, 113 returned for assessment using the Minnesota Child Development Inventory [70]. Those with seizures scored significantly poorer in general development, expressive language, and personal-social skills. The trend of poorer outcomes after seizures persisted after adjustment for surgical group stratification. At 4-year follow-up, 185 members of the original cohort were reassessed with neurological examination, audiological testing, speech evaluation, and developmental testing with the Wechsler Preschool and Primary Scale of Intelligence-Revised [71]. Overall, full-scale, verbal and performance IQs were significantly lower than normal (p<0.001). Post-operative seizures significantly increased the risk of lower IQ scores and abnormal neurological outcomes. Their neurodevelopmental deficits persisted at 8-year follow-up. They suffered academically, with 33% needing remedial academic support and 10% repeating a grade. By age 16 years, 139 returned for their final follow-up [72]. The frequent use of special services, including grade retention, tutoring, special education, occupational therapy, and psychosocial services, was seen in 65%. The presence of seizures was the only medical variable significantly associated with poorer math and reading scores, memory, executive function, and visual-spatial scores. Longer DHCA times predicted worse visual-spatial scores.

In addition to primary cerebral impact during surgery, the myocardium itself also experiences an ischemia-reperfusion injury from CPB with DHCA impacting the risk for mortality and more systemic deficits. Cardiac output significantly sags in the first 12 to 24 hours after surgery. The cerebral vasculature also tries to adjust to systemic blood flow, and pressure changes after circulation is restored [16]. Post-operative heart failure and frank cardiac arrest occur in about one-third which may require CPR, ionotropic support, and sometimes extracorporeal membrane oxygenation (ECMO). A mortality rate of 9% is seen within 30 days of surgery. Higher death rates are associated with body weight, Aristotle basic score, CPB time, aortic cross-clamp time, DHCA time, and single ventricle pathology [73].

Improving Care for the NBHS Population

The optimal parameters of the medical management for NBHS have never been formally established by randomized controlled clinical trials. For example, despite precise temperature regulation within the operating room during cardiac surgery, scant attention has been paid to temperature management post-operatively. Measurements of serum glucose levels immediately after surgery show huge variability. The tricky art of balancing systemic, pulmonary, and cerebral blood flows varies from one center to the next. The widespread use of CNS-depressant medications to induce surgical anesthesia, sedation, pain relief, and anxiolysis varies widely but could also influence neurological outcomes by their synaptic suppression, which can trigger neuronal apoptosis. Steroid administration may reduce neuronal stem cell populations. Standardized protocols for the rapid detection and effective treatment of EEG seizures are also needed.

A recent literature review assessed the limited studies that evaluate available neuromonitoring and neuroprotective modalities used in NBHS [74]. Many studies were retrospective or simple case series. Some were prospective but with very small sample sizes. It concluded that there was insufficient evidence to demonstrate that EEG monitoring improved outcomes, but highlighted the need for future, prospective, well-designed studies to assess the utility of EEG monitoring and its impact on neurodevelopmental outcomes in the NBHS population.

References

1. Hoffman JI, Kaplan S. The incidence of congenital heart disease. *J Am Coll Cardiol*. 2002;**39**(12):1890–900.

2. National Center on Birth Defects and Developmental Disabilities, Centers for Disease Control and Prevention. Congenital heart defects. 2015. www.cdc.gov/ncbddd/heartdefects/data.html

3. Rosomoff HL. Pathophysiology of the central nervous system during hypothermia. *Acta Neurochir Suppl*. 1964;**14**(Suppl 13):11–22.

4. Nakagawa TA, Ashawal S, Mathur M, et al. Guidelines for the determination of brain death in infants and children: an update of the 1987 Task Force recommendations. *Crit Care Med*. 2011;**39**(9):2139–55.

5. Follis MW. Neurologic/myocardial protection during pediatric cardiac surgery. *Medscape*. 2015. http://emedicine.medscape.com/article/902765-overview

6. Newburger JW, Jones RA, Wernovsky G, et al. A comparison of the perioperative neurologic effects of hypothermic circulatory arrest versus low-flow cardiopulmonary bypass in infant heart surgery. *N Engl J Med*. 1993;**329**(15):1057–64.

7. Helmers SL, Wypij D, Constantinou JE, et al. Perioperative electroencephalographic seizures in infants undergoing repair of complex congenital cardiac defects. *Electroencephalogr Clin Neurophysiol*. 1997;**102**(1):27–36.

8. Wang H, Wang B, Normoyle KP, et al. Brain temperature and its fundamental properties: a review for clinical neuroscientists. *Front Neurosci*. 2014; **8**: 307.

9. Vossough A, Limperopoulos C, Putt ME, et al. Development and validation of a semiquantitative brain maturation score on fetal MR images: initial results. *Radiology*. 2013;**268** (1):200–7.

10. Licht DJ, Shera DM, Clancy RR, et al. Brain maturation is delayed in infants with complex congenital heart defects. *J Thorac Cardiovasc Surg*. 2009;**137** (3):529–36; discussion 536–7.

11. Abdel Raheem MM, Mohamed WA. Impact of congenital heart disease on brain development in newborn infants. *Ann Pediatr Cardiol*. 2012;**5**(1):21–6.

12. Miller SP, McQuillen PS, Hamrick S, et al. Abnormal brain development in newborns with congenital heart disease. *N Engl J Med*. 2007;**357**(19): 1928–38.

13. Harden A, Pampiglione G, Waterston DJ. Circulatory arrest during hypothermia in cardiac surgery: an E.E. G. study in children. *Br Med J*. 1966;**2** (5522):1105–8.

14. Stecker MM, Cheung AT, Pochettino A, et al. Deep hypothermic circulatory arrest: II. Changes in electroencephalogram and evoked potentials during rewarming. *Ann Thorac Surg*. 2001;**71**(1):22–8.

15. Seltzer LE, Swartz M, Kwon JM, et al. Intraoperative electroencephalography predicts postoperative seizures in infants with congenital heart disease. *Pediatr Neurol*. 2014;**50**(4):313–7.

16. Schmitt B, Finckh B, Christen S, et al. Electroencephalographic changes after pediatric cardiac surgery with cardiopulmonary bypass: is slow wave activity unfavorable? *Pediatr Res*. 2005; **58**(4):771–8.

17. Massey SL, Abend NS, Gaynor JW, et al. Electroencephalographic patterns preceding cardiac arrest in neonates following cardiac surgery. *Resuscitation*. 2019;**144**:67–74.

18. Murray DM, Boylan B, Ali I, et al. Defining the gap between electrographic seizure burden, clinical expression and staff recognition of neonatal seizures. *Arch Dis Child Fetal Neonatal Ed*. 2008;**93** (3):F187–91.

19. Scher MS. Neonatal seizures and brain damage. *Pediatr Neurol*. 2003;**29** (5):381–90.

20. Scher MS, Alvin J, Gaus L, Minnigh B, Painter MJ. Uncoupling of EEG-clinical neonatal seizures after antiepileptic drug use. *Pediatr Neurol*. 2003;**28** (4):277–80.

21. Glass HC, Shellhaas RA, Wusthoff CJ, et al. Contemporary profile of seizures in neonates: a prospective cohort study. *J Pediatr*. 2016;**174**:98–103.

22. Connell J, Oozeer R, De Vries, L, et al. Clinical and EEG response to anticonvulsants in neonatal seizures. *Arch Dis Child*. 1989;**64**(4 Spec No):459–64.

23. Naim MY, Gaynor JW, Chen J, et al. Subclinical seizures identified by postoperative electroencephalographic monitoring are common after neonatal cardiac surgery. *J Thorac Cardiovasc Surg*. 2015;**150**(1):169–78; discussion 178–80.

24. Hahn JS, Vaucher Y, Bejar R, Coen RW. Electroencephalographic and neuroimaging findings in neonates undergoing extracorporeal membrane oxygenation. *Neuropediatrics.* 1993;**24**(1):19–24.

25. Malone A, Ryan CA, Fitzgerald A, et al. Interobserver agreement in neonatal seizure identification. *Epilepsia.* 2009;**50**(9):2097–101.

26. Abend NS, Dlugos DJ, Clancy RR. A review of long-term EEG monitoring in critically ill children with hypoxic-ischemic encephalopathy, congenital heart disease, ECMO, and stroke. *J Clin Neurophysiol.* 2013;**30**(2):134–42.

27. Glauser TA, Rorke LB, Weinberg PM, Clancy RR. Acquired neuropathologic lesions associated with the hypoplastic left heart syndrome. *Pediatrics.* 1990;**85**(6):991–1000.

28. Clancy RR, McGaurn SA, Goin JE, et al. Allopurinol neurocardiac protection trial in infants undergoing heart surgery using deep hypothermic circulatory arrest. *Pediatrics.* 2001**108**(1):61–70.

29. Clancy RR, McGaurn SA, Wernovsky G, et al. Risk of seizures in survivors of newborn heart surgery using deep hypothermic circulatory arrest. *Pediatrics.* 2003;**111**(3):592–601.

30. Clancy RR, Sharif U, Ichord R, et al. Electrographic neonatal seizures after infant heart surgery. *Epilepsia.* 2005;**46**(1):84–90.

31. Shellhaas RA, Chang T, Tsuchida T, et al. The American Clinical Neurophysiology Society's Guideline on Continuous Electroencephalography Monitoring in Neonates. *J Clin Neurophysiol.* 2011;**28**(6):611–17.

32. Backer CL, Marino BS. Protecting the neonatal brain: finding, treating, and preventing seizures. *J Thorac Cardiovasc Surg.* 2015;**150**(1):6–7.

33. du Plessis AJ, Jonas RA, Wypij D, et al. Perioperative effects of alpha-stat versus pH-stat strategies for deep hypothermic cardiopulmonary bypass in infants. *J Thorac Cardiovasc Surg.* 1997;**114**(6):991–1000; discussion 1000–1.

34. Gaynor JW, Nicolson SC, Jarvik GP, et al. Increasing duration of deep hypothermic circulatory arrest is associated with an increased incidence of postoperative electroencephalographic seizures. *J Thorac Cardiovasc Surg.* 2005;**130**(5):1278–86.

35. Andropoulos DB, Mizrahi EM, Hrachovy RA, et al. Electroencephalographic seizures after neonatal cardiac surgery with high-flow cardiopulmonary bypass. *Anesth Analg.* 2010;**110**(6):1680–5.

36. Gunn JK, Beca J, Penny DJ, et al. Amplitude-integrated electroencephalography and brain injury in infants undergoing Norwood-type operations. *Ann Thorac Surg.* 2012;**93**(1):170–6.

37. Frenkel N, Friger M, Meledin I, et al. Neonatal seizure recognition–comparative study of continuous-amplitude integrated EEG versus short conventional EEG recordings. *Clin Neurophysiol.* 2011;**122**(6):1091–7.

38. Rennie JM, Chorley G, Boylan GB, et al. Non-expert use of the cerebral function monitor for neonatal seizure detection. *Arch Dis Child Fetal Neonatal Ed.* 2004;**89**(1):F37–40.

39. Shah DK, Mackay MT, Lavery S, et al. Accuracy of bedside electroencephalographic monitoring in comparison with simultaneous continuous conventional electroencephalography for seizure detection in term infants. *Pediatrics.* 2008;**121**(6):1146–54.

40. Shellhaas RA, Clancy RR. Characterization of neonatal seizures by conventional EEG and single-channel EEG. *Clin Neurophysiol.* 2007;**118**(10):2156–61.

41. Shellhaas RA, Soaita AI, Clancy RR. Sensitivity of amplitude-integrated electroencephalography for neonatal seizure detection. *Pediatrics.* 2007;**120**(4):770–7.

42. Shellhaas RA, Gallagher PR, Clancy RR. Assessment of neonatal electroencephalography (EEG) background by conventional and two amplitude-integrated EEG classification systems. *J Pediatr.* 2008;**153**(3):369–74.

43. Boylan G, Burgoyne L, Moore C, O'Flaherty B, Rennie JM. An international survey of EEG use in the neonatal intensive care unit. *Acta Paediatr.* 2010;**99**(8):1150–5.

44. Clancy RR, Bergqvist AGC, Dlugos DJ, Nordli DR, Jr. Normal pediatric EEG: neonates and children. In Ebersole JS, Nordli D, Jr., editors. *Current Practice of Clinical Electroencephalography.* Philadelphia: Wolters Kluwer Health; 2014, pp. 125–212.

45. Clancy RR, Dicker L, Cho S, et al. Agreement between long-term neonatal background classification by conventional and amplitude-integrated EEG. *J Clin Neurophysiol.* 2011;**28**(1):1–9.

46. Clancy RR. Summary proceedings from the neurology group on neonatal seizures. *Pediatrics.* 2006;**117**(3 Pt 2): S23–7.

47. Painter MJ, Scher MS, Stein AD, et al. Phenobarbital compared with phenytoin for the treatment of neonatal seizures. *N Engl J Med.* 1999;**341**(7):485–9.

48. Boylan GB, Rennie JM, Chorley G, et al. Second-line anticonvulsant treatment of neonatal seizures: a video-EEG monitoring study. *Neurology.* 2004;**62**(3):486–8.

49. Shany E, Benzaqen O, Watemberg N. Comparison of continuous drip of midazolam or lidocaine in the treatment of intractable neonatal seizures. *J Child Neurol.* 2007;**22**(3):255–9.

50. Castro Conde JR, Hernández Borges A, Doménech Martinez E, et al. Midazolam in neonatal seizures with no response to phenobarbital. *Neurology.* 2005;**64**(5):876–9.

51. Sirsi D, Nangia S, LaMothe J, et al. Successful management of refractory neonatal seizures with midazolam. *J Child Neurol.* 2008;**23**(6):706–9.

52. Abend NS, Gutierrez-Colina AM, Monk HM, et al. Levetiracetam for treatment of neonatal seizures. *J Child Neurol.* 2011;**26**(4):465–70.

53. Khan O, Chang E, Cipriani C, et al. Use of intravenous levetiracetam for management of acute seizures in neonates. *Pediatr Neurol.* 2011;**44**(4):265–9.

54. Khan O, Cipriani C, Wright C, et al. Role of intravenous levetiracetam for acute seizure management in preterm neonates. *Pediatr Neurol.* 2013;**49**(5):340–3.

55. Glass HC, Poulin C, Shevell MI. Topiramate for the treatment of neonatal seizures. *Pediatr Neurol.* 2011; **44**(6):439–42.

56. Riesgo, R., Winckler MI, Ohlweiler L, et al. Treatment of refractory neonatal seizures with topiramate. *Neuropediatrics.* 2012;**43**(6):353–6.

57. Booth D, Evans DJ. Anticonvulsants for neonates with seizures. *Cochrane Database Syst Rev.* 2004(4): CD004218.

58. Sicca F, Contaldo A, Rey E, Dulac O. Phenytoin administration in the newborn and infant. *Brain Dev.* 2000;**22**(1):35–40.

59. Thibault C, Naim MY, Abend NS, et al. A retrospective comparison of phenobarbital and levetiracetam for the treatment of seizures following cardiac surgery in neonates. *Epilepsia.* 2020;**61**(4):627–635.

60. McQuillen PS, Goff DA, Licht DJ. Effects of congenital heart disease on brain development. *Prog Pediatr Cardiol.* 2010;**29**(2):79–85.

61. Clancy RR. The neurology of hypoplastic left heart syndrome. In Rychik JW, Wernovsky G, editors. *Hypoplastic Left Heart Syndrome.* New York:Springer;2003, pp. 251–72.

62. Fountain DM, Schaer M, Mutlu AK, et al. Congenital heart disease is associated with reduced cortical and hippocampal volume in patients with 22q11.2 deletion syndrome. *Cortex.* 2014;**57**:128–42.

63. Mulkey SB, OU X, Ramakrishnaiah RH, et al. White matter injury in newborns with congenital heart disease: a diffusion tensor imaging study. *Pediatr Neurol.* 2014;**51**(3):377–83.

64. Cheong JL, Thompson DK, Spittle AJ, et al. Brain volumes at term-equivalent age are associated with 2-year neurodevelopment in moderate and late preterm children. *J Pediatr.* 2016;**174**:91–7.

65. Birca A, Vakorin FA, Porayette P, et al. Interplay of brain structure and function in neonatal congenital heart disease. *Ann Clin Transl Neurol.* 2016;**3**(9):708–22.

66. Andropoulos DB, Hunter JV, Nelson DP, et al. Brain immaturity is associated with brain injury before and after neonatal cardiac surgery with high-flow bypass and cerebral oxygenation monitoring. *J Thorac Cardiovasc Surg.* 2010;**139**(3):543–56.

67. Seltzer L, Swartz MF, Kwon J, et al. Neurodevelopmental outcomes after neonatal cardiac surgery: Role of cortical isoelectric activity. *J Thorac Cardiovasc Surg.* 2016;**151**(4):1137–42.

68. Gaynor JW, Jarvik GP, Bernbaum J, et al. The relationship of postoperative electrographic seizures to neurodevelopmental outcome at 1 year of age after neonatal and infant cardiac surgery. *J Thorac Cardiovasc Surg.* 2006;**131**(1):181–9.

69. Gaynor JW, Jarvik GP, Gerdes M, et al. Postoperative electroencephalographic seizures are associated with deficits in executive function and social behaviors at 4 years of age following cardiac surgery in infancy. *J Thorac Cardiovasc Surg.* 2013;**146**(1):132–7.

70. Rappaport LA, Wypij D, Bellinger DC, et al. Relation of seizures after cardiac surgery in early infancy to neurodevelopmental outcome. Boston Circulatory Arrest Study Group. *Circulation.* 1998;**97**(8):773–9.

71. Bellinger DC, Wypij D, Kuban KC, et al. Developmental and neurological status of children at 4 years of age after heart surgery with hypothermic circulatory arrest or low-flow cardiopulmonary bypass. *Circulation.* 1999;**100**(5):526–32.

72. Bellinger DC, Wypij D, Rivkin MJ, et al. Adolescents with d-transposition of the great arteries corrected with the arterial switch procedure: neuropsychological assessment and structural brain imaging. *Circulation.* 2011;**124**(12):1361–9.

73. Kansy A, Tobota A, Maruszewski P, Maruxzewski B. Analysis of 14,843 neonatal congenital heart surgical procedures in the European Association for Cardiothoracic Surgery Congenital Database. *Ann Thorac Surg.* 2010;**89**(4):1255–9.

74. Hirsch JC, Jacobs ML, Andropoulos D, et al. Protecting the infant brain during cardiac surgery: a systematic review. *Ann Thorac Surg.* 2012;**94**(4):1365–73; discussion 1373.

75. Sharpe C, Reiner GE, Davis SL, Nespeca M, Gold JJ, Rasmussen M, Kuperman R, Harbert MJ, Michelson D, Joe P, Wang S, Rismanchi N, Le NM, Mower A, Kim J, Battin MR, Lane B, Honold J, Knodel E, Arnell K, Bridge R, Lee L, Ernstrom K, Raman R, Haas RH; NEOLEV2 INVESTIGATORS. Levetiracetam Versus Phenobarbital for Neonatal Seizures: A Randomized Controlled Trial. Pediatrics. 2020 Jun;145(6):e20193182. doi: 10.1542/peds.2019-3182. Epub 2020 May 8. Erratum in: Pediatrics. 2021 Jan;147(1): PMID: 32385134; PMCID: PMC7263056.

EEG Monitoring in Neonates and Children Undergoing Extracorporeal Membrane Oxygenation

Jainn-Jim Lin, Sarah Welsh, Alexis A. Topjian, and Nicholas S. Abend

Illustrative Case

Case 18 Extracorporeal Membrane Oxygenation

Key Points

- Seizures are common in neonates and children undergoing ECMO.
- The majority of seizures during ECMO are subclinical and can only be diagnosed through continuous EEG monitoring.

Introduction

Extracorporeal membrane oxygenation (ECMO) is a temporary cardiopulmonary support for neonates and children with potentially reversible cardiopulmonary disorders. Patients requiring ECMO support are at risk for brain injury due to pre-ECMO medical conditions, ECMO cannula placement in the carotid artery and internal jugular vessels, and complications arising during ECMO [1–9]. Acute brain injury may result in acute symptomatic seizures [10]. Clinical and electrographic seizures have been reported in 5%–30% of neonates and children undergoing ECMO. Because sedation and/or paralysis are often utilized during ECMO support, identification of neurological complications, including acute symptomatic seizures, may not be possible based on clinical observation alone. Thus, recent consensus statements have recommended increasing use of continuous EEG monitoring (cEEG) during ECMO in neonates [11] and children [12, 13] based on the theory that electrographic seizure identification and management may mitigate secondary brain injury and improve neurodevelopmental outcomes. This chapter reviews the available data regarding seizure incidence, risk factors, and outcomes in neonates and children requiring ECMO support.

Seizure Incidence

Clinical and electrographic seizures have been reported in 5%–30% of neonates and children requiring ECMO support. Most of the early studies included nonconsecutive cohorts without standardized use of cEEG to identify electrographic-only (subclinical, nonconvulsive) seizures. Thus, a 2015 systematic literature review regarding the use and effectiveness of neuromonitoring methods during ECMO identified only seven studies that addressed EEG, including two studies with 1–2 channel amplitude-integrated EEG and five studies with intermittent conventional EEG [14]. However, more recent studies have used cEEG in consecutive cohorts of children and have generally identified a higher incidence of seizures. A quality improvement study utilized cEEG in a nearly consecutive cohort of 99 neonates and children undergoing ECMO. Electrographic seizures occurred in 18% of subjects, of which 61% had electrographic status epilepticus. Seizures were exclusively EEG-only in 83% of patients, while 17% had both EEG-only and electroclinical seizures. The median duration from cEEG initiation to the initial electrographic seizure was 15 hours. Seizures occurred in 28% of patients in the cardiac intensive care unit, 9% of patients in the neonatal intensive care unit, and 8% of patients in the pediatric intensive care unit [15]. Another study utilized 72-hours of cEEG of 70 neonates and pediatric patients undergoing ECMO and identified seizures in 23% of patients. Among those with seizures, over half had nonconvulsive seizures, and only half had seizures in the first 24 hours of recording [16]. Another study used cEEG for the most of the ECMO duration in 66 nearly consecutive neonates and children requiring ECMO and identified seizures in 17% of patients, including 45% with status epilepticus and 72% with exclusively EEG-only seizures [17]. A large study of 201 pediatric patients who underwent cEEG during the initial 24 hours of ECMO identified electrographic seizures in 16% occurring a median of 3.2 hours after cEEG initiation [18]. A study of cEEG in 19 children undergoing ECMO support that reported 21% of subjects had electrographic seizures. Among those with seizures, 50% had electrographic status epilepticus, and 75% of subjects had exclusively EEG-only seizures [8].

Lower seizure rates were identified in cohorts monitored exclusively with amplitude-integrated electroencephalography or brief conventional EEGs. One series of amplitude-integrated electroencephalography monitoring in 26 neonates undergoing ECMO for the first 5 days identified 11% of subjects as having electrographic seizures, including 8% of subjects with exclusively EEG-only seizures [19]. An early study of EEG in 36 neonates requiring ECMO support reported nonconvulsive seizures in 17% of patients, including 11% with nonconvulsive status epilepticus [20]. A study of serial, routine EEG studies in 145 neonates undergoing ECMO support identified electrographic seizures in 8% of patients [21].

Several studies have investigated seizure incidence without the use of cEEG, and they generally report slightly lower seizure incidences than the studies described above. The Extracorporeal Life Support Organization Registry included 26,529 children and reported clinical seizures in 8% of patients, including electrographic seizures in 2% of patients, though most subjects did not undergo cEEG. That study also excluded patients with cardiopulmonary arrest. Seizures were reported in 9% of neonates with respiratory conditions, 8% of neonates with cardiac conditions, 6% of pediatric patients with respiratory conditions, 11% of pediatric patients aged 1 month to 1 year with cardiac conditions, and 7% of pediatric patients older than 1 year with cardiac conditions [4]. An earlier registry study that included only patients with cardiac etiologies reported acute clinical seizures in 8% of neonates, 10% of children aged 31 days to 1 year, and 6% of children aged 1–16 years [22]. Higher seizure rates were reported in an older single-center study of 50 infants receiving ECMO support, with reported clinical seizures in 30% [23]. A study utilizing the United States Nationwide Inpatient Sample evaluated 23,951 patients who underwent ECMO and identified neurological complications in 11%, including seizures in 4% of patients, although again the majority of patients did not undergo cEEG. Seizures were not associated with longer lengths of stay, discharge to long-term care facilities, or mortality [24].

Together, these studies using continuous conventional EEG or aEEG monitoring indicate that seizures occur in about 10%–25% of patients requiring ECMO support, that patients with seizures often experience a high seizure exposure, and that most seizures can only be identified using EEG monitoring. Since many patients with seizures have exclusively EEG-only seizures, clinical observation alone is likely insufficient to identify patients experiencing seizures. Thus, consensus reports and guidelines by the American Clinical Neurophysiology Society advocate for the use of cEEG to identify acute symptomatic seizures in these patients. The neonatal guideline describes ECMO as a "clinical scenario conferring a high risk for neonatal seizures" and thus indicates continuous EEG monitoring should be considered [11]. The adult and pediatric consensus statement does not specifically discuss ECMO, but recommends cEEG in patients with conditions which may be present in patients requiring ECMO such as "requiring pharmacological and at risk for seizures" and "patients with acute supratentorial brain injury with altered mental status " [12].

Seizure Risk Factors

Identifying risk factors for seizures could help optimize utilization of limited cEEG resources by focusing use on the patients most likely to experience seizures. Especially for patients who might require more than one day of cEEG, the pre-test probability of seizure has a substantial impact on the cost-effectiveness of cEEG strategies [25, 26]. Table 14.1 summarizes the risk factors that have been associated with seizures in neonates and children undergoing ECMO. Reported risk factors include younger age, including neonates [4] and children under 1 year old [24], patients with low cardiac output syndrome [15], the presence of epileptiform discharges [8], and ipsilateral lesions on neuroimaging [18]. In one study, seizures occurred in 21% of 85 patients who received veno-arterial ECMO support and 0% of 14 patients who received veno-venous ECMO support, although this difference was not significantly different (p=0.06). Similarly, seizures did not occur in any of the 16 patients with a normal EEG background or any of the 9

patients with an attenuated-featureless EEG background, but seizures occurred in 24% of 68 patients with a slow-disorganized EEG background and 33% of 6 patients with an excessively discontinuous or burst suppression EEG background [15]. In one study, electrographic seizures always occurred ipsilateral to neuroimaging injury, but only about one-third with neuroimaging injury experienced electrographic seizures [18]. Similarly, in one study electrographic seizures were associated with cerebral edema evident on neuroimaging [17]. Several investigators did not identify associations between seizures and clinical features, such as vital signs and hemodynamic data preceding ECMO, pre-ECMO diagnoses, ECMO indication (respiratory, cardiac or extracorporeal cardiopulmonary resuscitation), ECMO mode (veno-arterial or venovenous), and ECMO duration [4, 8, 15, 23]. These discrepancies may be attributed to the different populations studied and the small number of subjects included in many of these studies. Larger prospective cohort studies with cEEG in all patients for an extended duration might allow development of seizure prediction models that could help optimize utilization of limited cEEG resources.

Seizures and Outcome

The causal impact of seizures on outcome among children undergoing ECMO support remains uncertain. While it is possible that acute symptomatic seizures cause secondary brain injury, which in turn worsens outcomes, seizures might also be primarily biomarkers of more severe underlying brain injury. Several studies have reported that seizures are associated with higher mortality and less favorable neurodevelopmental outcomes among survivors including developmental delay, lower IQ, and higher rates of cerebral palsy and language disorders [4, 15, 16, 20, 21, 23, 27, 28]. However, other investigations have not identified associations between seizures and outcomes [5, 8, 24]. Larger studies with more standardized outcome assessments are needed to determine whether the presence of clinical and/or electrographic seizures remains associated with mortality and neurodevelopmental morbidity after adjusting for variables reflecting critical illness and brain injury severity. Similarly, further study is needed to determine to what degree optimized seizure identification and management improves patient outcomes.

Technical Issues

Continuous EEG monitoring in neonates and children undergoing ECMO support can be complex since these patients are often medically unstable, and they are surrounded by an enormous amount of equipment. Involvement of experienced EEG Technologists is essential. Acetone, often used to remove collodion-affixed EEG electrodes, could damage the plastic tubing of the ECMO apparatus; careful use of acetone is required and many centers use paste (rather than collodion) for EEG monitoring in these patients [29]. Consideration of electrode type may be important. Use of conductive plastic electrodes

Table 14.1 Summary of seizure incidence, risk factors, and outcome in newborns and children undergoing ECMO

Reference	Population study design	Number of patients/ subjects	Key inclusion/ exclusion criteria	Seizure incidence	Seizure risk factors	Seizures and outcome
Campbell et al. (1991)	Single center Retrospective	50	Neonates	Clinical: 30%	-	Seizures associated with cerebral palsy or developmental delay at 2 years of age
Streletz et al. (1992)	Single center Retrospective	145	Neonates	Electrographic seizures: 8%	-	Seizures associated with an increased risk of mortality and short-term adverse outcomes
Hahn et al. (1993)	Single center Retrospective	36	Neonates	Electrographic seizure in 17% Electrographic status epilepticus: 11%	-	Electrographic seizures or status epilepticus increased risk of death or severe outcome
Bennett et al. (2002)	Single center Prospective	-	Neonates with severe respiratory failure	-	-	Seizures associated with an increased relative risk (2.25) of disabilities at 4 years of age
Parish et al. (2004)	Single center Prospective	162	Neonates	-	-	Seizures associated with lower intelligence quotient scores and higher rates of cerebral palsy and language disorders
Horan et al. (2007)	Single center Prospective **Used continuous aEEG**	26	Neonates	Electrographic seizures: 11% EEG-only seizures: 8%	-	-
Haines et al. (2009)	ESLO Registry Study Retrospective	7 597	Neonates and children. Included only cardiac cases.	Clinical seizures: Newborn: 8.1% Children (1 m~1 y): 10% Children (1~16 y): 5.5%	-	-

Table 14.1 (cont.)

Reference	Population study design	Number of patients/ subjects	Key inclusion/ exclusion criteria	Seizure incidence	Seizure risk factors	Seizures and outcome
Hervey-Jumper et al. (2011)	ESLO Registry Study Retrospective	26 529	Neonates and children. Excluded cardiac arrest.	Clinical seizures: 8% Electrographic seizures: 2% Age/Etiology sub-analysis: Newborn: respiratory: 9% Cardiac: 8% Children: Respiratory: 6% Cardiac (1 m~1 y): 11% Cardiac (>1 y): 7.4%	Neonates at higher risk for seizures	Seizures associated with decreased survival
Polito et al. (2013)	ESLO Registry Study Retrospective	7 190	Neonates	Clinical Seizures: 7%	–	–
Piantino et al. (2013)	Single center Retrospective **Some continuous EEG monitoring**	19	Children	Electrographic seizures: 21% Electrographic status epilepticus: 11% EEG-only seizures: 16%	Interictal discharges	Seizures not associated with increased mortality
Chrysostomou et al. (2013)	Single center Retrospective	69	Children and neonates. Included only cardiac cases.	Clinical or electrographic seizures: 6%	–	Seizures not associated with worse neurodevelopmental outcomes
Nasr and Rabinstein (2015)	Nationwide Inpatient Sample Retrospective	12 906	Neonates and children.	Clinical seizures: 5% Newborn: 8% Children (1 m–1 y): 10% Children (1–16 y): 6%	Aged between 1 m and 1 y, cardiac arrest, nonrespiratory distress syndrome	Seizures not associated with mortality

Study	Design	N	Population	Seizure incidence	Risk factors	Outcome
Lin et al. (2017)	Single center Prospective **Continuous EEG monitoring**	99	Neonates and children.	Electrographic seizure: 18% Electrographic status epilepticus: 11% EEG-only seizures: 15%	Low cardiac output prior to ECMO	Seizure associated with higher mortality and worse discharge outcomes
Okochi et al. (2018)	Single center retrospective **Continuous EEG monitoring**	70	Neonates and children	Electrographic seizure: 23% Electrographic status epilepticus: 7%	Low platelet count prior to ECMO Low pH prior to ECMO	Seizures associated with reduced survival to hospital discharge
Yuliati et al. (2020)	Single center Retrospective **Continuous EEG monitoring**	66	Neonates and children	Electrographic seizure: 17% Electrographic status epilepticus: 8% EEG-only seizures: 13%	Edema on imaging	Seizures associated with edema on imaging which was associated with worse outcome
Sansevere et al. (2020)	Single center Retrospective **Continuous EEG monitoring**	201	Children	Electrographic seizures: 16%	Occurring ipsilateral to imaging abnormalities	Seizures associated with ipsilateral injury on neuroimaging

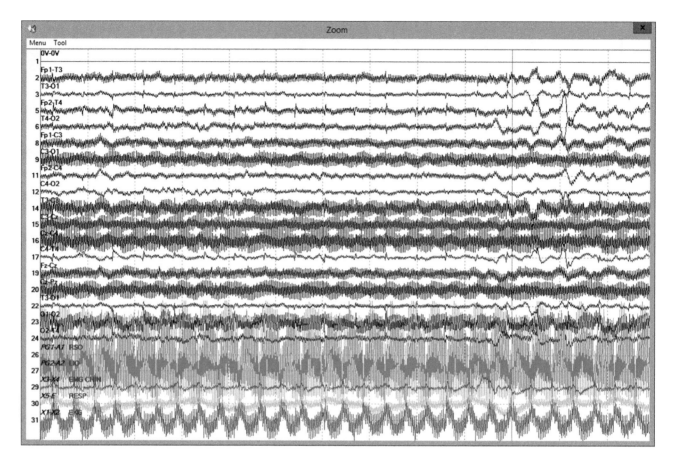

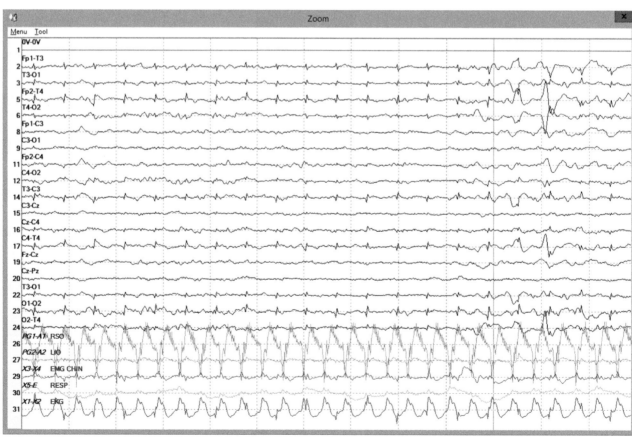

Figure 14.1 Example of artifact in EEG during ECMO.
This EEG was recorded in a 1-day-old term-born baby with congenital heart disease who required ECMO soon after birth. Without filtering for external 60 Hz electrical artifact (top), the recording is largely uninterpretable. With 60 Hz filter applied (bottom), there remains EKG artifact visible in multiple channels in addition to ECMO artifact visible in the extracerebral channels. Recording is 15 seconds per screen, Sens 7 μV, Tc 0.1 sec.

in place of conventional gold electrodes has been associated with reduced artifact and greater confidence in EEG interpretation accuracy [30]. These plastic electrodes may also allow performance of computerized tomography [31] (which can be performed at bedside at some institutions) without need for removal and reattachment of electrodes in these unstable patients. Interpretation may be challenging for EEG recorded during ECMO given frequent resulting artifact (see Figure 14.1). EEG terminology which may guide standardized reporting of cEEG in patients undergoing ECMO support has been provided by the American Clinical Neurophysiology Society for neonates [32] and older patients [33].

Summary

Seizures are common in neonates and children undergoing ECMO. Studies that used cEEG have identified a higher incidence of seizures than studies relying on clinical identification. Since many patients requiring ECMO may not manifest clinically evident seizures, clinical observation along may fail to identify electrographic seizures. Further research is needed to better determine the risk factors for electrographic seizures, establish optimal management strategies, and then determine whether optimized seizure identification and management ultimately improves patient outcomes.

References

1. Cengiz P, Seidel K, Rycus PT, Brogan TV, Roberts JS. Central nervous system complications during pediatric extracorporeal life support: incidence and risk factors. *Crit Care Med.* 2005;**33** (12):2817–24.

2. Short BL. The effect of extracorporeal life support on the brain: a focus on ECMO. *Semin Perinatol.* 2005;**29**(1):45–50.

3. Karimova A, Brown K, Ridout D, et al. Neonatal extracorporeal membrane oxygenation: practice patterns and predictors of outcome in the UK. *Arch Dis Child Fetal Neonatal Ed.* 2009;**94**(2):F129–32.

4. Hervey-Jumper SL, Annich GM, Yancon AR, et al. Neurological complications of extracorporeal membrane oxygenation in children. *J Neurosurg Pediatr.* 2011;**7** (4):338–44.

5. Chrysostomou C, Maul T, Callahan PM, et al. Neurodevelopmental outcomes after pediatric cardiac ECMO support. *Front Pediatr.* 2013;**1**:47.

6. de Mol AC, Liem KD, van Heijst AF. Cerebral aspects of neonatal extracorporeal membrane oxygenation: a review. *Neonatology.* 2013;**104**(2):95–103.

7. Mehta A, Ibsen LM. Neurologic complications and neurodevelopmental outcome with extracorporeal life support. *World J Crit Care Med.* 2013;**2**(4):40–7.

8. Piantino JA, Wainwright MS,. Grimason M, et al. Nonconvulsive seizures are common in children treated with extracorporeal cardiac life support. *Pediatr Crit Care Med.* 2013;**14**(6):601–9.

9. Polito A, Barrett CS, Wypij D, et al. Neurologic complications in neonates supported with extracorporeal membrane oxygenation. An analysis of ELSO registry data. *Intensive Care Med.* 2013;**39**(9):1594–601.

10. Beghi E, Carpio A, Forsgren L., et al. Recommendation for a definition of acute symptomatic seizure. *Epilepsia.* 2010;**51**(4):671–5.

11. Shellhaas RA, Chang T, Tsuchida T, et al. The American Clinical Neurophysiology Society's guideline on continuous electroencephalography monitoring in neonates. *J Clin Neurophysiol.* 2011;**28** (6):611–17.

12. Herman ST, Abend NS, Bleck TP, et al., and E. E. G. T. F. o. t. A. C. N. S. Critical Care Continuous. Consensus statement on continuous EEG in critically ill adults and children, part I: indications. *J Clin Neurophysiol.* 2015a;**32**(2):87–95.

13. Herman ST, Abend, NS, Bleck, TP, et al. Consensus statement on continuous EEG in critically ill adults and children, part II: personnel, technical specifications, and clinical practice. *J Clin Neurophysiol.* 2015b;**32**(2):96–108.

14. Bembea MM, Felling R, Anton B. Salorio CF, Johnston MV. Neuromonitoring during extracorporeal membrane oxygenation: a systematic review of the literature. *Pediatr Crit Care Med.* 2015;**16**(6):558–64.

15. Lin JJ, Banwell BL, Berg RA, et al. Electrographic seizures in children and neonates undergoing extracorporeal membrane oxygenation. *Pediatr Crit Care Med.* 2017;**18**(3):249–57.

16. Okochi S, Shakoor A, Barton S, et al. Prevalence of seizures in pediatric extracorporeal membrane oxygenation patients as measured by continuous electroencephalography. *Pediatr Crit Care Med.* 2018;**19**(12):1162–7.

17. Yuliati A, Federman M, Rao, LM, et al. Prevalence of seizures and risk factors for mortality in a continuous cohort of pediatric extracorporeal membrane oxygenation patients. *Pediatr Crit Care Med.* 2020;**21**(11):949–58.

18. Sansevere AJ, DiBacco ML, Akhondi-Asl A, et al. EEG features of brain injury during extracorporeal membrane oxygenation in children. *Neurology.* 2020;**95**(1):e1372–e1380.

19. Horan M, Azzopardi D, Edwards AD, Firmin RK, Field D. Lack of influence of mild hypothermia on amplitude integrated-electroencephalography in neonates receiving extracorporeal membrane oxygenation. *Early Hum Dev.* 2007;**83**(2):69–75.

20. Hahn JS, Vaucher Y, Bejar R, Coen RW. Electroencephalographic and neuroimaging findings in neonates undergoing extracorporeal membrane oxygenation. *Neuropediatrics.* 1993;**24** (1):19–24.

21. Streletz LJ, Bej MD, Graziani LJ, et al. Utility of serial EEGs in neonates during extracorporeal membrane oxygenation. *Pediatr Neurol.* 1992;**8** (3):190–6.

22. Haines NM, Rycus PT, Zwischenberger JB, Bartlett RH, Undar A. Extracorporeal Life Support Registry Report 2008: neonatal and pediatric cardiac cases. *ASAIO J.* 2009;**55**(1):111–16.

23. Campbell LR, Bunyapen C, Gangarosa ME, Cohen M, Kanto Jr., WP. Significance of seizures associated with extracorporeal membrane oxygenation. *J Pediatr.* 1991;**119**(5):789–92.

24. Nasr D. M, Rabinstein AA. Neurologic complications of extracorporeal membrane oxygenation. *J Clin Neurol.* 2015;**11**(4):383–9.

25. Abend NS, Topjian AA, Williams S. Could EEG monitoring in critically ill children be a cost-effective neuroprotective strategy? *J Clin Neurophysiol.* 2015a;**32**(6):486–94.

26. Abend NS, Topjian AA, Williams S. How much does it cost to identify a critically ill child experiencing

electrographic seizures? *J Clin Neurophysiol.* 2015b;**32**(3):257–64.

27. Bennett CC, Johnson A, Field DJ. A comparison of clinical variables that predict adverse outcome in term infants with severe respiratory failure randomised to a policy of extracorporeal membrane oxygenation or to conventional neonatal intensive care. *J Perinat Med.* 2002;**30**(3):225–30.

28. Parish AP, Bunyapen C, Cohen MJ, Garrison T, Bhatia J. Seizures as a predictor of long-term neurodevelopmental outcome in survivors of neonatal extracorporeal membrane oxygenation (ECMO). *J Child Neurol.* 2004;**19**(12):930–4.

29. Fitzgerald MP, Donnelly M, Vala L, Allen-Napoli L, Abend NS. Collodion remover can degrade plastic-containing medical devices commonly used in the intensive care unit. *Neurodiagn J.* 2019;**59**(3):163–8.

30. Matsumoto JH, McArthur DL, Szeliga CW, et al. Conductive plastic electrodes reduce EEG artifact during pediatric ECMO therapy. *J Clin Neurophysiol.* 2016;**33**(5):426–30.

31. Abend NS, Dlugos DJ, Zhu X, Schwartz ES. Utility of CT-compatible EEG electrodes in critically ill children. *Pediatr Radiol.* 2015;**45**(5):714–18.

32. Tsuchida TN, Wusthoff CJ, Shellhaas RA, et al.; C. American Clinical Neurophysiology Society Critical Care Monitoring. American Clinical Neurophysiology Society standardized EEG terminology and categorization for the description of continuous EEG monitoring in neonates: report of the American Clinical Neurophysiology Society critical care monitoring committee. *J Clin Neurophysiol.* 2013;**30**(2):161–73.

33. Hirsch LJ, LaRoche SM, Gaspard N, et al. American Clinical Neurophysiology Society's Standardized Critical Care EEG Terminology: 2012 version. *J Clin Neurophysiol.* 2013;**30**(1):1–27.

Chapter 15

Neuromonitoring after Cardiac Arrest

Genevieve Du Pont-Thibodeau, Nicholas S. Abend, and Alexis A. Topjian

Illustrative Case

Case 19 Cardiac Arrest

Key Points

- Neuromonitoring can guide patient management and aid in prognostication following cardiac arrest.
- EEG background patterns may be useful in outcome prognostication for some patients within 24 hours of cardiac arrest.
- Seizures are common in children after cardiac arrest, and seizures are most often subclinical.
- The greatest risk for seizures is in the first 24 hours after return of spontaneous circulation (ROSC) and during rewarming from hypothermia.
- Hypothermia may impact the interpretation and optimal timing of neuromonitoring data used for prognostication.
- Experts recommend a multimodal approach to prognostication.

Introduction

Every year in the United States, more than 8000 children experience a cardiac arrest (CA) [1]. Survival from in-hospital cardiac arrest (IHCA) has improved substantially from ~10% in the 1980s to ~45% in more recent years [2, 3]. Approximately 60%–78% of children who experience an IHCA will have return of spontaneous circulation (ROSC), of which 45%–49% will survive to discharge and 75%–89% will have a favorable neurological outcome [2, 4, 5]. Out-of-hospital cardiac arrest (OHCA) survival rates have also improved for select age groups but still remain low at 2%–9%, with many patients experiencing subsequent severe neurological morbidity [6–8]. However, among children who survive OHCA to hospital admission, approximately 25%–38% will survive to discharge, and 62% of survivors will have a favorable neurological outcome [3, 9]. Those patients who survive with neurological disability are usually severely affected [10]. Recent characterization of long-term CA survivors shows that many children have worse cognition and executive function, worse overall health status, and lower quality of life than children their age [11, 12].

The period following ROSC is a critical time during which the identification and management of neurological injury may lead to increased survival and improved long-term functional outcomes [13]. Methods to improve outcomes have focused on (1) identification and management of ongoing brain injury to prevent or minimize secondary brain injury and improve outcomes, and (2) neurological prognostication to help clinicians and families determine when to withdraw technological support.

While prognostication historically focused on the use of pre-CA and CA characteristics, experts now advocate for a multimodal approach combining patient and arrest characteristics, the clinical examination, biomarkers, neuroimaging, electroencephalography (EEG), and somatosensory evoked potentials (SSEPs) [14]. This type of combined approach, particularly when variables reflecting brain function are included, is generally more accurate than prognostication based on any single variable. Furthermore, the use of therapeutic hypothermia and sedating medications can confound the reliability of some neurological assessments; these are important to consider when interpreting examination signs and functional test results for prognostication. Careful and thoughtful interpretation of these modalities is essential to avoid premature withdrawal of technological support in patients who could have a favorable recovery, or overly aggressive resuscitation in patients that will have a severe outcome such as a persistent vegetative state.

The pathophysiology of post-CA brain injury is complex and is characterized by vascular injury, excitotoxicity, altered calcium homeostasis, free radical production, and cell death [13]. Loss of cerebral vascular autoregulation as well as periods of hypoxia, hypotension, fever, hyperglycemia, and seizures can also further worsen neurological injury [13, 15]. Treatment focused on cerebral resuscitation involving avoidance of hypotension, hyperoxia, hypercarbia and hypocarbia, glucose derangements, and hyperpyrexia may impact outcomes [16]. EEG monitoring can be useful to identify seizures, which may also worsen underlying hypoxic-ischemic brain injury.

Physicians are faced with the challenges of judiciously titrating post-resuscitation therapies to optimize brain recovery in the face of limited understanding of an individual patient's brain physiology and extent of injury. Neuroprotection is an essential but challenging aspect of post-resuscitation care; many physiological parameters can alter the fragile balance between oxygen delivery and demand. Neuromonitoring can help physicians better understand the brain's evolving pathophysiology so that individualized therapies can be implemented to optimize neurological outcome.

There are several neuromonitoring tools that can help physicians better understand brain pathophysiology and contribute to both management and prognostication. Conventional continuous EEG (cEEG) monitoring as well as quantitative EEG (QEEG) analysis methods can provide insight to the severity of encephalopathy and the presence of

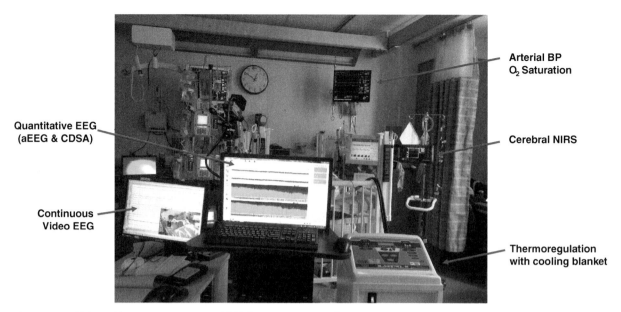

Figure 15.1 Multimodal neuromonitoring in a child following resuscitation from cardiac arrest.

electrographic seizures and status epilepticus. Somatosensory evoked potentials (SSEPs) have been identified as the most reliable prognostication tool in comatose adults, but fewer data are available in children. Recently, the role of near-infrared spectroscopy (NIRS), a measurement of a regional oxygen saturation (rSO_2), has been used as a surrogate for brain oxygen saturation and extraction. No single neuromonitoring tool is able to provide a complete assessment of brain function; however, when these tools are used in conjunction, clinicians may be able to understand the complex and ongoing pathophysiology of the post-CA brain (Figure 15.1).

In this chapter, we will discuss cEEG monitoring, quantitative EEG methods for seizure identification, and EEG background interpretation. We will discuss SSEPs and NIRS and their respective roles in neurological management and prognostication. We will also address how therapeutic hypothermia (TH) and medication exposure can change the reliability of some of these neuromonitoring tools.

Electroencephalography (EEG)

Seizures

Epidemiology

Studies have found that 15%–79% of children who achieve ROSC after CA will develop acute symptomatic seizures in the hours to days following their initial hypoxic-ischemic brain injury [17, 18]. This is similar to the seizure prevalence in adults following CA, reported in 10%–59% of patients [19]. The majority of seizures following CA are electrographic-only (i.e., nonconvulsive, subclinical). Since they do not have any identifiable clinical correlate, identification requires cEEG monitoring [20, 21]. In some patients the clinical manifestations may be masked by paralytic administration, but in many patients the seizures have no clinical manifestations even in the absence of any paralytic medication administration. In a prospective study of 19 children monitored with cEEG for 72 hours post-CA, 47% experienced electrographic seizures, of which 67% were EEG-only and 78% were electrographically generalized [22]. The seizure burden is often high in children who experience seizures. Status epilepticus (SE), including convulsive or nonconvulsive SE (NCSE), occurred in 32%.

Timing of Seizure Onset

Continuous EEG monitoring is the gold standard technique used to identify electrographic seizures and status epilepticus. In one study, 87% of electrographic seizures in critically ill children occurred within the first 24 hours following ROSC [23]. In a study of 19 children undergoing 24 hours of TH, one patient developed seizures during the first 12 hours of TH, 4 patients had seizure onset in the subsequent 12 hours of TH, and 4 patients developed seizures during the rewarming phase (Figure 15.2) [22]. More recently, in a study of 128 children initiated on cEEG monitoring within the first 24 hours following ROSC, only 16% experienced seizures while undergoing monitoring [17]. In adults treated with TH, seizures often occur in the first 24 hours post-CA or during the rewarming phase [24]. However, adults typically undergo TH for up to 24 hours and rewarming over 6 hours, thereby completing their temperature treatment period more rapidly than children managed with TH [25–27]. As a result of these data, recent guidelines and consensus statements have recommended cEEG monitoring in all patients with hypoxic-ischemic brain injury to identify seizures for at least the first 24 hours following ROSC, or longer in certain clinical scenarios such as in patients treated with TH [14, 19, 28]. EEG monitoring should be started early following ROSC, and monitored for at least 24 hours or through rewarming if TH is utilized.

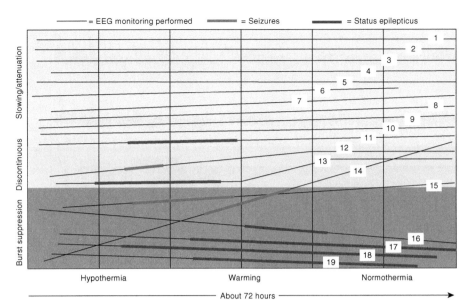

Figure 15.2 Seizure occurrence in a cohort following pediatric cardiac arrest. Each line represents EEG characteristics for individual subjects who underwent cEEG monitoring during hypothermia, rewarming, and normothermia. Seizures were most common during rewarming, and among subjects with a burst suppression or discontinuous EEG background. Reproduced with permission from [22].

Quantitative EEG (QEEG) for Seizure Identification

Although cEEG monitoring is the gold standard to detect seizures, it is resource intense: it requires EEG equipment, EEG Technologist availability to apply electrodes and trouble-shoot artifact issues, and electroencephalographer expertise for interpretation. Even when these resources are available, cEEG monitoring interpretation is time consuming since each page or screen of EEG must be reviewed one at a time. Thus, there is limited access to cEEG in most North American pediatric intensive care units [29]. Based on data from a survey of large North American pediatric institutions, 21% do not have 24/7 EEG technologist availability [30]. Even when these resources are available, interpretation is often periodic (about 2–3 times per day) and not continuous, potentially leading to delays in seizure identification.

QEEG techniques such as aEEG and color density spectral array (CDSA) may allow more efficient review by electroencephalographers and may enable non-EEG trained clinicians to identify seizures and assess the EEG background [31].

Amplitude-integrated EEG is a processed, filtered, and time-compressed EEG display that presents amplitude (y-axis) data over time (x-axis). It displays peak-to-peak amplitude values of filtered and rectified EEG. CDSA uses Fourier transformation to present EEG power (amplitude^2/Hz) (color) and frequency (y-axis) over time (x-axis). Both modalities have the advantage of displaying several hours of compressed EEG data in a single image [32–34]. The time compression used by these techniques may allow more rapid review of large volumes of cEEG data; however, because of the time compression, short seizures could be also be missed (Figures 15.3 and 15.4).

QEEG has been studied for seizure identification by both neurologists and intensivists. Most investigations have studied etiologically heterogeneous cohorts. While neurologists have focused on using this modality for screening many hours of EEG for seizures efficiently, intensivists have focused on detecting seizures more rapidly at bedside. Several studies have

evaluated QEEG techniques in heterogeneous cohorts of critically ill children. In one study, 3 electroencephalographers reviewed 27 CDSA and aEEG tracings. The median sensitivity for seizure identification was 83% using CDSA and 82% using aEEG. However, for individual tracings the sensitivity varied from 0% to 100%, indicating excellent performance for some patients and poor performance for other patients, likely related to individual seizure characteristics. False positives (event identified as a seizure which was not a seizure based on conventional EEG review) occurred about every 17–20 hours [35]. In a second study, 8 electroencephalographers reviewed 84 CDSA images. Sensitivity for seizure identification was 65%, specificity was 95%, and only about half of seizures were identified by 6 or more of the raters [36]. A study of CSDA and envelope trend EEG review by electroencephalographers found that seizure identification was impacted by both modifiable factors (interpreter experience, display size, and quantitative EEG method) and non-modifiable factors inherent to the EEG pattern (maximum spike amplitude, seizure duration, seizure frequency, and seizure duration) [37].

Studies of neurologist interpreted CDSA, following two-hour training sessions, showed seizure identification sensitivities of 83% and 89% [35, 38, 39]. A study using a shorter training session had lower sensitivity for seizure identification (65%–75%) [36]. Despite the variable reliability for seizure identification, review of QEEG may decrease the amount of time required for data interpretation. Despite these early data, optimal QEEG trends have not been identified. Further, cEEG monitoring should be reviewed in conjunction to QEEG to minimize the risk of false seizure identification [39, 40] to avoid unnecessary exposure to anti-seizure medications.

The role of QEEG for bedside interpretation for seizure detection is still in its infancy. However, early data suggest that these tools may be viable for screening of seizures for non-EEG trained providers. One study in children specifically addressed QEEG for seizure identification after CA by

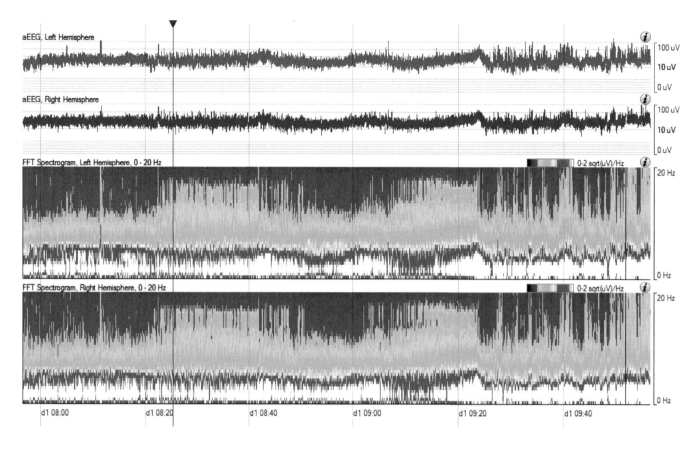

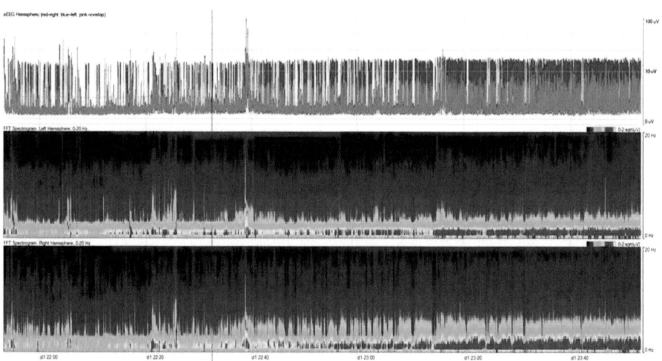

Figure 15.3 Background patterns on QEEG.
Top panel is aEEG of right [blue] and left [red] hemispheric average brain activity. Bottom two panels are CDSA of right and left hemispheric average brain activity. (a) Continuous background with diffuse slowing, (b) burst suppression, (c) attenuated background.

non-neurology-trained providers [34]. Twenty critical care physicians and 19 critical care nurses with a brief training session regarding CDSA were asked to determine whether

each of 200 CDSA images contained electrographic seizures. Their sensitivity for seizure detection was 70% (indicating that some electrographic seizures were not identified), and the

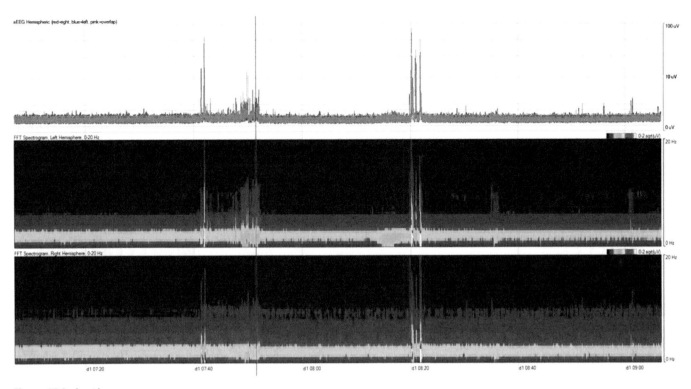

Figure 15.3 (cont.)

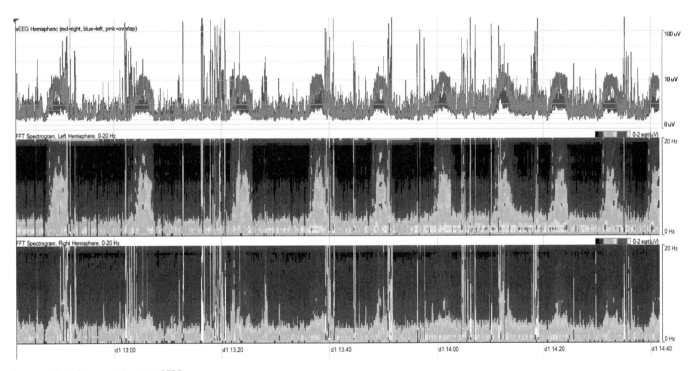

Figure 15.4 Seizure patterns on QEEG.
Top panel is aEEG of right [blue] and left [red] hemispheric average brain activity. Bottom two panels are CDSA of right and left hemispheric average brain activity. (a) Recurrent seizures, (b) persistent and sustained seizures with intermittent return to baseline, (c) sustained status epilepticus.

specificity for seizure detections was 68% (indicating that some images categorized as containing EEG seizures did not contain seizures based on conventional EEG review).

Evaluation of QEEG in adult neuroscience ICUs had sensitivities of ≥80% when evaluated by physicians and bedside nurses after a 15-minute training session [41, 42]. Notably,

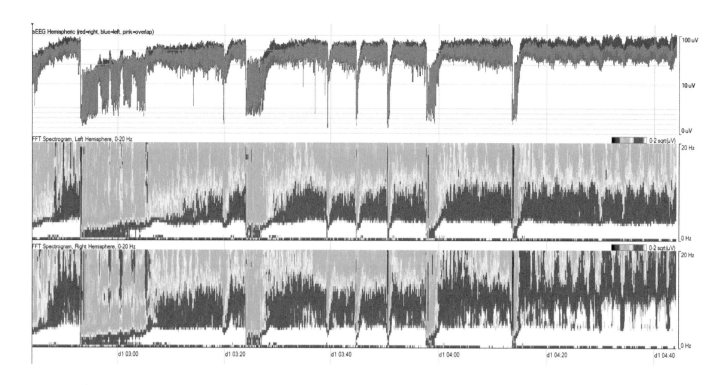

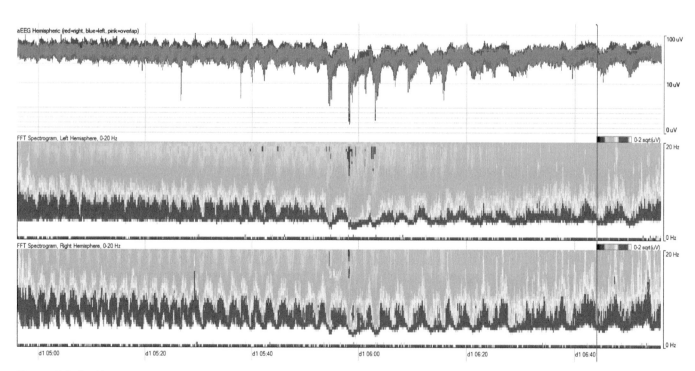

Figure 15.4 (cont.)

there was no difference between specialty and seizure identification rates, indicating the techniques may achieve similar results when used by electroencephalographers and critical care clinicians. Amplitude-integrated EEG has been extensively evaluated in newborns with hypoxic-ischemic encephalopathy with reported seizure detection rates of 22%–80%, and interpretation is usually performed by bedside neonatologists and neonatal nurses [33, 43–49]. Similarly, QEEG techniques may enable critical care clinicians to identify nonconvulsive seizures more rapidly than by periodic cEEG and might allow independent use in centers with limited cEEG monitoring resources. It remains to be seen whether utilization of these modalities leads to more rapid seizure identification, earlier treatment, and improved outcomes, but they may be an important part of future bedside multimodal monitoring.

Seizures and Outcome

It remains unclear whether seizures post-CA are merely biomarkers of more extensive hypoxic-ischemic injury or whether the seizures lead to secondary brain injury which might worsen outcome. The "excitotoxic" theory of seizures explains that increases in pre-synaptic glutamate activate post-synaptic N-methyl-D-aspartate (NMDA) receptors, leading to cellular calcium influx and initiating a cascade of intracellular processes that result in free radical production, DNA damage, and cell death [50, 51]. Because it is difficult to determine whether there is a causal relationship between seizures and outcomes, most clinicians aim to treat seizures. Few studies have investigated the impact of anti-seizure medications on outcome in the CA population. Some series have reported favorable recovery with aggressive seizure treatment in a select group of patients (i.e., preserved brainstem reflexes, present cortical response on SSEPs, and a reactive EEG) [52–54]. Further, adults with post-CA nonconvulsive seizures and reactive EEG backgrounds treated with anti-seizure medications have been reported with favorable neurological outcomes [55–57]. Aggressive treatment of seizures may prevent secondary brain injury and thus less favorable neurological outcomes [58]. In adults, seizure duration and time to detection are associated with mortality, and delay in seizure recognition and treatment can lead to refractory seizure control and need for increased therapy [28, 58–60]. Interestingly, neonatal human data indicate that early and aggressive treatment of nonconvulsive seizures following hypoxic-ischemic injury decreases MRI abnormalities and improves outcome [61]. In contrast, a study of post-CA adults reported that the routine use of cEEG improved seizure detection but did not impact outcome [62].

Given these conflicting data, most clinicians aim to identify and treat seizures, while recognizing that aggressive therapies may not change outcome and carry a risk for adverse events such as hypotension, hypoxia, and respiratory depression [63–65]. Future studies are needed to delineate prognostic factors that may impact whether seizure treatment improves neurological outcomes.

Historically, the development of seizures and status epilepticus in children and adults post-CA has been associated with a unfavorable neurological outcome [66]. In particular, myoclonic status epilepticus has been considered a harbinger for unfavorable outcomes, often leading to withdrawal of technological support when identified. However, with increased cEEG utilization, it has become easier to detect electrographic seizures and status epilepticus without clinical correlates which might be impacting the brain without signifying as unfavorable an outcome. The prognostic significance of seizures and myoclonus warrant further scrutiny.

Substantially more data are available in adults than children. Comatose adults treated with TH who experienced status epilepticus had a 92% positive predictive value for unfavorable outcome [67]. Further, in several single center studies of comatose adults post-CA treated with TH, 94% of patients with epileptiform activity and all patients with electrographic seizures had unfavorable neurological outcome or death [24, 68]. However, there are also reports of adults with status epilepticus who survived with only moderate impairment or returned to baseline [54].

In the subset of critically ill children who had seizures, some studies have reported that in children who had CA, electrographic seizures were not associated with worse outcome, while status epilepticus was associated with unfavorable outcome [17, 69]. Despite this, a recent retrospective observational study of 73 children managed with and without TH following cardiac arrest found that all patients with seizures in the first hour of monitoring had unfavorable outcomes [70].

The presence of epileptiform activity as defined by sporadic epileptiform discharges, periodic discharges, or seizures does not appear to improve prognostic accuracy when compared to EEG background patterns alone [71]. A study of 111 comatose patients post-CA continuously monitored with EEG demonstrated that status epilepticus was common (27%) and occurred over two types of backgrounds. All patients with status epilepticus developing over a background of burst suppression had an unfavorable outcome, while 20% of patients with status epilepticus but a continuous EEG background had a full neurological recovery [66]. Similar results have been observed in patients with status epilepticus with background reactivity [54]. Clinicians should be wary that status epilepticus is not a sole predictor of outcome in patients, but must be considered in the context of other information. EEG background patterns may provide better prognostic value than seizure activity alone, discussed further below.

Myoclonic seizures and non-epileptic myoclonus pose particular challenges in cEEG monitoring interpretation after CA. Myoclonus is a brief, involuntary twitching of a muscle or a group of muscles. Myoclonus without EEG correlate is common in adults following cardiac arrest; it is far less common in children after cardiac arrest. Myoclonic seizures are episodes of clinical myoclonus that are of cortical origin, and are time-locked to an EEG correlate. Prior to cEEG monitoring, post-arrest myoclonus had been difficult to fully characterize [72]. Status myoclonus was considered a very ominous sign. However, use of cEEG monitoring allows closer inspection of affected patients. In some cases, short-acting neuromuscular blockade has been used to remove the myogenic artifact in myoclonus to clarify whether EEG seizures are present [73]. Status myoclonus refers to generalized myoclonus in comatose patients lasting more than 30 minutes, either with or without associated epileptiform activity. Certain subtypes of clinical myoclonus, such as myoclonus status epilepticus within the first 24 hours after primary circulatory arrest in adults [74, 75] or synchronous, stereotyped status myoclonus, have been shown to carry poor prognosis [76]. However, even in these cases, outcome is not universally dismal. Recovery has been reported following both myoclonus and myoclonic seizures after CA, [77]. In a cohort of 401 adults after CA, 16% developed early myoclonus. None of those with an EEG background of burst suppression associated with myoclonic jerks or with subcortical myoclonus survived with a favorable outcome. On the other hand, half of patients with a continuous background and associated myoclonic jerks survived and all had a favorable outcome [78], suggesting it is not the myoclonus but the EEG pattern that is most important. Less is known regarding the prognostic significance of myoclonus following pediatric CA, making it all the more important to be cautious in assigning prognostic significance to the finding [75, 78, 79].

EEG Background

Background Classification Using EEG

EEG background patterns have been evaluated as potential predictors of neurological outcome in children post-CA. As early as the 1960s, Pampiglione described that patients with continuous EEG backgrounds and no epileptiform activity had a favorable outcome, while one patient with burst suppression and generalized periodic epileptiform discharges died [80]. Since then, multiple classification systems grouping EEG backgrounds into predictive categories have been developed to help physicians with prognostication [81–84]. Malignant background as identified by American Clinical Neurophysiology Society (ACNS) EEG terminology has been shown to reliably predict poor outcome in adults after return to normothermia, whereas a benign EEG was highly predictive of good outcome [85]. Malignant EEG patterns associated with unfavorable neurological outcomes have included generalized epileptiform discharges [86], lack of reactivity [86, 87], severe attenuation [88], excessive discontinuity [86], and burst suppression [89]. More benign EEG patterns associated with more favorable neurological outcomes include EEG reactivity [90], normal sleep patterns [43, 90, 91], and rapid EEG improvement [92]. In 2006, the American Academy of Neurology (AAN) concluded that a flat background, burst suppression pattern, and generalized epileptiform discharges over a flat background were strongly associated with an unfavorable outcome in adults following CA [74].

Data in pediatric CA are consistent with adult findings. Good inter-rater agreement has been demonstrated in application of ACNS Standardized Critical Care EEG Terminology to EEG recorded in children following CA supporting use of this categorization system [93]. In a small retrospective study of 34 children post-CA, discontinuous and isoelectric EEG patterns had a positive predictive value of 90% for unfavorable neurological outcome, while the negative predictive value of a continuous normal voltage EEG for unfavorable neurological outcome was 91% [81]. A recent study of 128 children after CA who were not treated with hypothermia had EEG backgrounds interpreted from reports within the first 24 hours following ROSC [17]. Background category was normal in four subjects (3%), slow-disorganized in 58 subjects (45%), discontinuous-burst suppression in 24 subjects (19%), and attenuated-flat in 42 subjects (33%). Forty-six subjects (36%) had a reactive EEG. Absence of reactivity (p<0.001) and seizures (p=0.04) were associated with worse EEG background category. After controlling for covariates, for each incrementally worse background score the odds of death

were 3.63 (95% CI, 2.18–6.0; p<0.001) and the odds of unfavorable neurological outcome were 4.38 (95% CI, 2.51–7.17; p=0.001). Another recent pediatric CA study evaluated 73 children who underwent cEEG monitoring and scored the EEG for background features and seizures at 1 and 24 hours after cEEG initiation, and cEEG monitoring end. Multivariate analysis revealed duration of CA cardiac arrest less than 20 minutes or cEEG background activity within 12 hours of ROSC was associated with favorable short-term neurological outcome [94]. A prospective study of 89 infants and children resuscitated following CA applied standardized EEG scoring to identify features that most accurately predicted short-term outcomes [95]. The most predictive model incorporated findings of background (normal, slow-disorganized, discontinuous or burst suppression, or attenuated-flat), presence of sleep transients, and reactivity/variability. The resulting model demonstrated specificity for unfavorable neurological outcome of 95%. These data suggest that, similar to neonatal studies, early EEG background features following pediatric CA may be able to stratify brain injury severity [17, 96]. Similarly, background continuity has been shown to be an important component of prognostication in adults after CA. In 60 adults treated with TH and monitored with cEEG, continuous patterns (continuous, diffuse slow electroencephalogram rhythms) were present in 43% of patients with favorable outcome, whereas they were never seen in patients with unfavorable outcome. Moreover, isoelectric or low-voltage patterns 24 hours after ROSC predicted unfavorable outcome with a sensitivity of 40%, almost two times higher than the bilateral absence of somatosensory evoked potential responses [97].

Absence of EEG background reactivity to external stimuli may also predict unfavorable outcome, although this requires further validation [55]. EEG reactivity relies on the integrity of the ascending reticular activating system and is strongly associated with awakening [98]. Multiple studies have found that absence of EEG reactivity is associated with unfavorable outcome in patients treated with TH [54–56, 99]. Further prospective studies are warranted to increase the reliability of this finding.

The interaction of background features and seizure activity may impact prognosis. Although seizures may present late in some patients, the first 30-minute cEEG background interpretation appears to correlate with the later onset of seizures and can be of value in resource-limited settings. Seizures more often occur in patients with an EEG background that is excessively discontinuous, burst suppression, or attenuated [17, 22].

Limitations of cEEG monitoring for prognosis are inconsistent between studies [83, 100] and lack of inter-rater agreement for EEG interpretation in critically ill adults, particularly in studies using nonstandard terminology [24, 101–105]. However, interpretation of cEEG background has high inter-rater reliability in children with hypoxic-ischemic encephalopathy [93, 101].

More recent work has examined the prognostic value of QEEG following pediatric CA. One small series of 30 children (median age 10 months) retrospectively examined aEEG monitoring after CA [106]. The authors reported that aEEG backgrounds that showed an inactive trace or burst suppression have a specificity of 94% for poor neurological outcome. This was consistent with findings from a larger single-center study of 87 consecutive children with QEEG following CA [107]. In that study, eight QEEG features were analyzed in relation to outcome: spectral density of each channel; normalized band power in alpha, beta, theta, delta, and gamma wave frequencies; line length; and regularity function scores. A model composed of these features in combination had a sensitivity of 0.84 in predicting patients with favorable outcomes and a specificity of 0.75 in predicting patients with unfavorable outcomes. Further study is needed to validate prognostic accuracy of QEEG following pediatric CA.

Impact of Hypothermia and Sedating Medications on EEG

The use of TH and sedating medications may impact accuracy of EEG for prognostication. The AAN recommendations from 2006 were defined prior to the high utilization of induced TH for the treatment of CA [74]. During deep hypothermic circulatory arrest, the EEG background becomes discontinuous and isoelectric [108, 109]. These EEG changes have not been observed in adults and neonates treated with mild TH (33.5°C–36°C) [110, 111] Recent studies have also demonstrated that EEG patterns seen during mild TH have the same prognostic significance as those seen during normothermia [112]. A study of 35 children treated with TH and undergoing cEEG monitoring found that patients with unreactive tracings, discontinuity, burst suppression, or lack of cerebral activity were more likely to have an unfavorable prognosis than those with a continuous and reactive EEG despite temperature [112].

It is important to recognize the potential impact of sedative medications that can alter EEG tracings [113]. Sedative medications are frequently administered post-CA, especially when TH is implemented to decrease metabolic demand, for patient comfort, and to prevent shivering. TH can slow drug metabolism, particularly in patients with impaired hepatic and renal clearance due to hypoxic-ischemic organ injury, which may prolong the effects of sedatives [114–117]. Sedatives have been shown to impact prognostication of patients after CA treated with TH such that prognosis is overly pessimistic [118]. As a result, International Liaison Committee on Resuscitation (ILCOR) recommends that neuroprognostication not occur until after 72 hours from ROSC in patients who are treated with TH, and even later in patients in whom assessment may have confounding with TH and sedation [119]. EEG interpretation for prognostication should be performed with caution, and sometimes postponed until benzodiazepines or barbiturates are no longer confounding the EEG data. Prospective studies are warranted to evaluate the direct impact of these medications on EEG interpretation and prognostication [74].

Somatosensory Evoked Potentials

Somatosensory evoked potentials (SSEPs) are a series of electrical potentials generated by electrical stimulation of a peripheral nerve to assess sensory pathways at peripheral, spinal, subcortical, and cortical levels. Cortical SSEPs are elicited by repetitive stimulation of the median nerve and measure the integrity of the afferent sensory pathway over the primary somatosensory cortex. Accurate interpretation of cortical SSEPs requires the integrity of both the peripheral nerves and the cervical cord. Abnormal SSEPs are defined by the absence of an obligate waveform or by the prolongation of a component beyond 2.5 or 3 SD of the normal range [120]. An absent negative 20 (N20) response refers to a lack of response 20 milliseconds after stimulation of the median nerve at the level of the primary somatosensory cortex, which, if lost bilaterally, can indicate global loss of cortical function [120].

Somatosensory evoked potentials can be used as markers of neurological outcome in patients with hypoxic-ischemic encephalopathy [121–123]. Neuropathology reports of post-CA patients with absent bilateral cortical SSEPs show evidence of widespread ischemia and/or cortical necrosis [120, 124]. SSEPs have been of particular interest for prognostication because their reliability does not appear to be altered by sedatives, neuromuscular blockade, or mild hypothermia [120, 125].

Prognosis

The absence of cortical SSEPs in adults post-CA has been associated with vegetative state [123] and brain death [120, 121]. A systematic review suggested that absence of cortical SSEPs in patients with hypoxic-ischemic encephalopathy older than 10 years of age was the most useful tool to predict unfavorable neurological outcome with a specificity of nearly 100% [126]. A prospective trial including 32 ICUs demonstrated that in 301 of 305 patients unconscious at 72 hours, 45% had at least one recording showing bilateral absence of N20 and that all had a unfavorable outcomes (95% CI of false positive rate 0 to 3%) [127]. In 2006, the AAN published guidelines to assist bedside clinicians with neuroprognostication following adult CA that stipulated that absent SSEPs at day 3 after CPR (category B) along with absent corneal reflexes, absent pupillary light response, absent motor response to pain, and serum neuron specific enolase cut-points could predict unfavorable neurological outcome [74]. Bilaterally absent N20 responses was identified as the most reliable single predictor of unfavorable outcome with a false positive rate of 0.7%. Conversely, the presence of cortical SSEPs alone could not reliably be used as a marker of predicted favorable neurological outcome. The presence of SSEPs without other positive predictive markers conferred a sensitivity of only 46% at predicting favorable neurological outcome [74].

Despite absent SSEPs predicting unfavorable neurological outcome, reports of survivors have raised concerns regarding their reliability [120, 128–133]. Absent SSEPs with favorable neurological outcome have mainly, but not exclusively, been described in children when SSEPs were performed in the first 24–48 hours post-CA [120, 124, 134, 135]. Absence of SSEPs in CA-arrest patients should be used as one component of multi-modal prognostication approaches.

Impact of Therapeutic Hypothermia

The introduction of TH in the management of patients post-CA has changed the reliability of SSEP as a prognostic marker [74, 129]. A retrospective study of 112 comatose patients post-CA treated with TH found that 97% of patients with bilateral absent N20 SSEPs had an unfavorable outcome, while 2 patients with absent or minimally detectable N20 SSEPs 3 days after CA eventually recovered consciousness [129]. Conversely, a prospective randomized controlled trial of 60 patients post-CA treated with TH who demonstrated absent N20 predicted unfavorable neurological outcome in 100% of both hypothermic and normothermic patients [125]. Two recent meta-analyses found that the reliability of SSEPs was the same for patients treated with or without hypothermia, with similar false positive rates as those reported by the AAN in 2006 [74, 136, 137]. Golan et al. suggested that the accuracy increased in patients treated with TH when measured beyond the first 72 hours after CA [137] while Sandroni et al. suggested that SSEPs were reliable even during TH [138]. Reliability of SSEPs performed in the first 24 hours post-CA and during hypothermia has been inconsistent [135, 139]. Measurements of SSEPs beyond the first 24 hours post-CA and after rewarming appears safest to avoid false positives, especially in the context of TH [120, 135, 137, 139].

Much like EEG, interpretation of SSEPs requires training and confirmation of inter-rater reliability for classification of cortical SSEP as bilaterally absent or present [140, 141]. Although SSEPs are likely the most reliable prognostic neurological biomarker available to bedside clinicians, and the least likely to be altered by sedation or TH, experts advocate for a multimodal approach to neuroprognostication that should include, but not exclusively, SSEPs [119].

Near-Infrared Spectroscopy (NIRS)

Near-infrared spectroscopy (NIRS) is a noninvasive, easily applicable cerebral monitoring tool that provides real-time continuous data on tissue oxygenation saturation. NIRS was first introduced in the 1970s [142] and has recently gained interest in intra- and post-CA neurological monitoring. NIRS light penetrates tissues, including bone, to a depth of a few centimeters [143]. By using different wavelengths, it measures the relative proportion of oxyhemoglobin and deoxyhemoglobin in the blood, both of which have different absorbance capacities, providing an estimate of oxygen saturation [144]. Because it does not require pulsatile flow, it is an attractive cerebral monitoring tool during CA [144]. In practice, a cerebral NIRS sensor is applied to the forehead and allows noninvasive continuous monitoring of the regional oxygen saturation (rSO_2) of the superficial cerebral cortex. Given that the majority of the blood volume in the brain is venous, it provides an estimate of venous oxygen saturation and brain oxygen extraction [144]. NIRS correlates well with cerebral venous saturation measured at the jugular bulb level [145–148] and with central venous saturation measured in the superior vena cava [147–150].

Intra-cardiac Arrest Monitoring

Near-infrared spectroscopy monitoring during resuscitation is feasible and certain rSO_2 values are positively correlated with achieving ROSC [151–157]. Small studies have demonstrated that higher mean rSO_2 during CPR of patients in pulseless electrical activity (PEA) or asystole strongly correlated with ROSC ($42.7\pm10.7\%$ vs. $31.7\pm12.8\%$, p<0.0001) [155, 158]. These differences were not found in patients with ventricular fibrillation (VF) / ventricular tachycardia (VT). More recently, in a large adult multicenter trial, rSO_2 values $\geq65\%$ during CA were 99% sensitive for ROSC [159]. Furthermore, Ito et al. found that higher rSO_2 values on hospital admission were associated with a better 90-day neurological outcome (mean [$\pm SD$] $55.6\pm20.8\%$ vs. $19.7\pm11.0\%$, p<0.001) [160].

Higher rSO_2 likely correlate with higher coronary perfusion pressure [161], and coronary perfusion pressure correlates with cerebral perfusion pressure, both of which are associated with increased rates of ROSC [162]. Moreover, NIRS correlates with depth of chest compressions [163] and overall quality of CPR [152, 164–168]. Future studies of the role of NIRS for guided resuscitation during CPR are needed in both children and adults.

Post-cardiac Arrest Monitoring

Near-infrared spectroscopy has also been investigated as a potential prognostic tool for patients after ROSC. Recent studies have yielded conflicting results. Ahn et al. demonstrated that higher average rSO_2 values during the first 24 hours post–adult CA were associated with increased survival but not after 24 hours post-CA [152]. Storm et al. measured rSO_2 on 60 adults following ROSC and demonstrated an rSO_2 threshold of 50% within the first 40 hours yielded 70% specificity and 86% sensitivity for unfavorable outcome [169]. Another study of adults post-CA patients treated with TH could not find a difference in rSO_2 values between survivors and non-survivors [170]. To date no pediatric CA NIRS trials have been published.

Regional cerebral oxygen saturation is a complicated measurement impacted by multiple factors and should be interpreted with caution. Low rSO_2 values during or after CA can represent low cerebral blood flow and low cerebral oxygenation that may result from a no flow/low flow state or the post–cardiac arrest syndrome [13]. Cerebral hypoperfusion can be caused by myocardial dysfunction[13], hyperthermia [171], and hyperventilation [172, 173]. Low NIRS values may be due to increased oxygen consumption due to seizures.

Future Directions

Multimodal cerebral monitoring following CA for both the titration of therapies and prognostication is a developing field. As mortality has decreased, the focus on minimizing morbidity has come to the forefront and a one-size-fits-all approach to assessment and treatments is quickly becoming antiquated. In the future, a combination of direct cerebral multimodal monitoring early after CA may allow clinicians to determine the severity of brain injury with the goal of allowing clinicians to determine the impact of their treatments in real time and carry out individualized management strategies [174, 175]. Also promising is early work showing early EEG patterns that precede CA in neonates after cardiac repair surgery [176]; the use of EEG as a biomarker for impending CA warrants further exploration.

Conclusion

Brain injury is a leading cause of morbidity in CA survivors, yet physicians have limited information on the state of the brain for targeted neuroprotection and when assisting families with potential end-of-life decisions. Monitoring tools such as cEEG, QEEG, NIRS, and SSEPs may help with both management and prognostication by identifying seizures, encephalopathy severity, hypoperfusion states, and brain function.

References

1. Abend NS, Mani R, Tschuda TN, et al. EEG monitoring during therapeutic hypothermia in neonates, children, and adults. *Am J Electroneurodiagnostic Technol*. 2011;51(3):141–64.

2. Girotra S, Spertus JA, Li Y, et al. Survival trends in pediatric in-hospital cardiac arrests: an analysis from Get With the Guidelines-Resuscitation. *Circ Cardiovasc Qual Outcomes*. 2013;6(1):42–9.

3. Topjian AA, Berg RA, Nadkarni VM. Pediatric cardiopulmonary resuscitation: advances in science, techniques, and outcomes. *Pediatrics*. 2008;122(5):1086–98.

4. Meert KL, Donaldson A, Nadkarni V, et al. Multicenter cohort study of in-hospital pediatric cardiac arrest. *Pediatr Crit Care Med*. 2009;10(5):544–53.

5. Berg RA, Nadkarni VM, Clark AE, et al. Incidence and outcomes of cardiopulmonary resuscitation in PICUs. *Crit Care Med*. 2016;44(4):798–808.

6. Topjian AA, Nadkarni VM, Berg RA. Cardiopulmonary resuscitation in children. *Curr Opin Crit Care*. 2009;15(3):203–8.

7. Donoghue AJ, Nadkarni V, Berg RA, et al. Out-of-hospital pediatric cardiac arrest: an epidemiologic review and assessment of current knowledge. *Ann Emerg Med*. 2005;46(6):512–22.

8. Atkins DL, Everson-Stewart S, Sears GK, et al. Epidemiology and outcomes from out-of-hospital cardiac arrest in children: the Resuscitation Outcomes Consortium Epistry-Cardiac Arrest. *Circulation*. 2009;119(11):1484–91.

9. Moler FW, Donaldson AE, Meert K, et al. Multicenter cohort study of out-of-hospital pediatric cardiac arrest. *Crit Care Med*. 2011;39(1):141–9.

10. Slomine BS, Silverstein FS, Christensen JR, et al. Neurobehavioral outcomes in children after out-of-hospital cardiac arrest. *Pediatrics*. 2016;137(4):e20153412.

11. van Zellem L, Buysse C, Madderom M, et al. Long-term neuropsychological outcomes in children and adolescents after cardiac arrest. *Intensive Care Med*. 2015;41(6):1057–66.

12. van Zellem L, Utens EM, Legerstee JS, et al. Cardiac arrest in children: long-term health status and health-related quality of life. *Pediatr Crit Care Med*. 2015;16(8):693–702.

13. Neumar RW, Nolan JP, Adrie C, et al. Post-cardiac arrest syndrome: epidemiology, pathophysiology, treatment, and prognostication. A consensus statement from the International Liaison Committee on Resuscitation (American Heart Association, Australian and New Zealand Council on Resuscitation, European Resuscitation Council, Heart and Stroke Foundation of Canada, InterAmerican Heart Foundation, Resuscitation Council of Asia, and the Resuscitation Council of Southern Africa); the American Heart Association Emergency Cardiovascular Care Committee; the Council on Cardiovascular Surgery and Anesthesia; the Council on Cardiopulmonary, Perioperative, and Critical Care; the Council on Clinical Cardiology; and the Stroke Council. *Circulation* 2008;118(23):2452–83.

14. Topjian AA, Raymond TT, Atkins D, et al. Part 4: pediatric basic and advanced life support: 2020 American Heart Association Guidelines for Cardiopulmonary Resuscitation and Emergency Cardiovascular Care. *Circulation*. 2020;142(16 Suppl 2):S469–S523.

15. Bembea MM, Nadkarni VM, Diener-West M, et al. American Heart Association National Registry of Cardiopulmonary Resuscitation I: temperature patterns in the early postresuscitation period after pediatric inhospital cardiac arrest. *Pediatr Crit Care Med*. 2010;11(6):723–30.

16. Topjian AA, de Caen A, Wainwright MS, et al. Pediatric post-cardiac arrest care: a scientific statement from the American Heart Association. *Circulation*. 2019;140(6):e194–e233.

17. Topjian AA, Sanchez SM, Shults J, et al. Early electroencephalographic background features predict outcomes in children resuscitated from cardiac arrest. *Pediatr Crit Care Med*. 2016;17(6):547–57.

18. Williams K, Jarrar R, Buchhalter J. Continuous video-EEG monitoring in pediatric intensive care units. *Epilepsia*. 2011;52(6):1130–6.

19. Herman ST, Abend NS, Bleck TP, et al. Consensus statement on continuous EEG in critically ill adults and children, part I: indications. *J Clin Neurophysiol*. 2015;32(2):87–95.

20. Jette N, Claassen J, Emerson RG, Hirsch LJ. Frequency and predictors of nonconvulsive seizures during continuous electroencephalographic monitoring in critically ill children. *Arch Neurol*. 2006;63(12):1750–5.

21. Abend NS, Marsh E. Convulsive and nonconvulsive status epilepticus in children. *Curr Treat Options Neurol*. 2009;11(4):262–72.

22. Abend NS, Topjian A, Ichord R, et al. Electroencephalographic monitoring during hypothermia after pediatric cardiac arrest. *Neurology*. 2009;72(22):1931–40.

23. Abend NS, Gutierrez-Colina AM, Topjian AA, et al. Non-convulsive seizures are common in critically ill

children. *Neurology*. 2011;**76** (12):1071–7.

24. Mani R, Schmitt SE, Mazer M, Putt ME, Gaieski DF. The frequency and timing of epileptiform activity on continuous electroencephalogram in comatose post-cardiac arrest syndrome patients treated with therapeutic hypothermia. *Resuscitation*. 2012;**83**(7):840–7.

25. Hypothermia after Cardiac Arrest Study Group. Mild therapeutic hypothermia to improve the neurologic outcome after cardiac arrest. *N Engl J Med*. 2002;**346**(8):549–56.

26. Bernard SA, Gray TW, Buist MD, et al. Treatment of comatose survivors of out-of-hospital cardiac arrest with induced hypothermia. *N Engl J Med*. 2002;**346**(8):557–63.

27. Nielsen N, Wetterslev J, Cronberg T, et al. Targeted temperature management at 33 degrees C versus 36 degrees C after cardiac arrest. *N Engl J Med*. 2013;**369** (23):2197–206.

28. Brophy GM, Bell R, Claassen J, et al. Guidelines for the evaluation and management of status epilepticus. *Neurocrit Care*. 2012;**17**(1):3–23.

29. Abend NS, Dlugos DJ, Hahn CD, Hirsch LJ, Herman ST. Use of EEG monitoring and management of non-convulsive seizures in critically ill patients: a survey of neurologists. *Neurocrit Care*. 2010;**12** (3):382–9.

30. Sanchez SM, Carpenter J, Chapman KE, et al. Pediatric ICU EEG monitoring: current resources and practice in the United States and Canada. *J Clin Neurophysiol*. 2013;**30** (2):156–60.

31. Scheuer ML, Wilson SB. Data analysis for continuous EEG monitoring in the ICU: seeing the forest and the trees. *J Clin Neurophysiol*. 2004;**21**(5):353–78.

32. Shah NA, Wusthoff CJ. How to use: amplitude-integrated EEG (aEEG). *Arch Dis Child Educ Pract Ed*. 2015;**100** (2):75–81.

33. Mathur AM, Morris LD, Teteh F, Inder TE, Zempel J. Utility of prolonged bedside amplitude-integrated encephalogram in encephalopathic infants. *Am J Perinatol*. 2008;**25** (10):611–15.

34. Topjian AA, Fry M, Jawad AF, et al. Detection of electrographic seizures by critical care providers using color density spectral array after cardiac arrest is feasible. *Pediatr Crit Care Med*. 2015;**16**(5):461–7.

35. Stewart CP, Otsubo H, Ochi A, et al. Seizure identification in the ICU using quantitative EEG displays. *Neurology*. 2010;**75**(17):1501–18.

36. Pensirikul AD, Beslow LA, Kessler SK, et al. Density spectral array for seizure identification in critically ill children. *J Clin Neurophysiol*. 2013;**30**(4):371–5.

37. Akman CI, Micic V, Thompson A, Riviello JJ, Jr. Seizure detection using digital trend analysis: Factors affecting utility. *Epilepsy Res*. 2011;**93**(1):66–72.

38. Williamson CA, Wahlster S, Shafi MM, Westover MB. Sensitivity of compressed spectral arrays for detecting seizures in acutely ill adults. *Neurocrit Care*. 2014;**20**(1):32–9.

39. Moura LM, Shafi MM, Ng M, et al. Spectrogram screening of adult EEGs is sensitive and efficient. *Neurology* 2014;**83**(1):56–64.

40. Haider HA, Esteller R, Hahn CD, et al. Sensitivity of quantitative EEG for seizure identification in the intensive care unit. *Neurology* 2016;**87**(9):935–44.

41. Swisher CB, White CR, Mace BE, et al. Diagnostic accuracy of electrographic seizure detection by neurophysiologists and non-neurophysiologists in the adult ICU using a panel of quantitative EEG trends. *J Clin Neurophysiol*. 2015;**32**(4):324–30.

42. Dericioglu N, Yetim E, Bas DF, et al. Non-expert use of quantitative EEG displays for seizure identification in the adult neuro-intensive care unit. *Epilepsy Res*. 2015;**109**:48–56.

43. Evans E, Koh S, Lerner J, Sankar R, Garg M. Accuracy of amplitude integrated EEG in a neonatal cohort. *Arch Dis Child Fetal Neonatal Ed*. 2010;**95**(3):F169-73.

44. Shah DK, Mackay MT, Lavery S, et al. Accuracy of bedside electroencephalographic monitoring in comparison with simultaneous continuous conventional electroencephalography for seizure detection in term infants. *Pediatrics*. 2008;**121**(6):1146–54.

45. Tao JD, Mathur AM. Using amplitude-integrated EEG in neonatal intensive care. *J Perinatol*. 2010;**30** Suppl:S73–81.

46. Toet MC, van der Meij W, de Vries LS, Uiterwaal CS, van Huffelen KC. Comparison between simultaneously recorded amplitude integrated electroencephalogram (cerebral function monitor) and standard electroencephalogram in neonates. *Pediatrics*. 2002;**109**(5):772–9.

47. Glass HC, Kan J, Bonifacio SL, Ferriero DM. Neonatal seizures: treatment practices among term and preterm infants. *Pediatr. Neurol*. 2012;**46** (2):111–15.

48. Shah NA, Van Meurs KP, Davis AS. Amplitude-integrated electroencephalography: a survey of practices in the United States. *Am J Perinatol*. 2015;**32**(8):755–60.

49. Shellhaas RA, Soaita AI, Clancy RR. Sensitivity of amplitude-integrated electroencephalography for neonatal seizure detection. *Pediatrics*. 2007;**120** (4):770–7.

50. Fujikawa DG. Prolonged seizures and cellular injury: understanding the connection. *Epilepsy Behav*. 2005;**7** (Suppl 3):S3–11.

51. Abend NS, Dlugos DJ, Clancy RR. A review of long-term EEG monitoring in critically ill children with hypoxic-ischemic encephalopathy, congenital heart disease, ECMO, and stroke. *J Clin Neurophysiol*. 2013;**30**(2):134–42.

52. Hovland A, Nielsen EW, Kluver J, Salvesen R. EEG should be performed during induced hypothermia. *Resuscitation*. 2006;**68**(1):143–6.

53. Westhall E, Rundgren M, Lilja G, Friberg H, Cronberg T. Postanoxic status epilepticus can be identified and treatment guided successfully by continuous electroencephalography. *Ther Hypothermia Temp Manag*. 2013;**3** (2):84–7.

54. Rossetti AO, Oddo M, Liaudet L, Kaplan PW. Predictors of awakening from postanoxic status epilepticus after therapeutic hypothermia. *Neurology*. 2009;**72**(8):744–9.

55. Rossetti AO, Oddo M, Logroscino G, Kaplan PW. Prognostication after cardiac arrest and hypothermia: a prospective study. *Ann Neurol*. 2010;**67** (3):301–7.

56. Rossetti AO, Urbano LA, Delodder F, Kaplan PW, Oddo M. Prognostic value of continuous EEG monitoring during therapeutic hypothermia after cardiac arrest. *Critical Care*. 2010;**14**(5):R173.

57. Rundgren M, Westhall E, Cronberg T, Rosen I, Friberg H. Continuous amplitude-integrated electroencephalogram predicts outcome in hypothermia-treated cardiac arrest patients. *Crit Care Med*. 2010;**38**(9):1838–44.

58. Young GB, Jordan KG, Doig GS. An assessment of nonconvulsive seizures in the intensive care unit using continuous

EEG monitoring: an investigation of variables associated with mortality. *Neurology.* 1996;**47**(1):83–9.

59. Lewena S, Young S. When benzodiazepines fail: how effective is second line therapy for status epilepticus in children? *Emerg Med Australas.* 2006;**18**(1):45–50.

60. Hayashi K, Osawa M, Aihara M, et al. Efficacy of intravenous midazolam for status epilepticus in childhood. *Pediatr Neurol.* 2007;**36**(6):366–72.

61. van Rooij LG, Toet MC, van Huffelen AC, et al. Effect of treatment of subclinical neonatal seizures detected with aEEG: randomized, controlled trial. *Pediatrics.* 2010;**125**(2):e358–66.

62. Crepeau AZ, Fugate JE, Mandrekar J, et al. Value analysis of continuous EEG in patients during therapeutic hypothermia after cardiac arrest. *Resuscitation.* 2014;**85**(6):785–9.

63. Kaplan PW. No, some types of nonconvulsive status epilepticus cause little permanent neurologic sequelae (or: "the cure may be worse than the disease"). *Neurophysiol Clin.* 2000;**30**(6):377–82.

64. Freeman JM. Beware: the misuse of technology and the law of unintended consequences. *Neurotherapeutics.* 2007;**4**(3):549–54.

65. Abend NS, Dlugos DJ: Treatment of refractory status epilepticus: literature review and a proposed protocol. *Pediatric neurology* 2008, **38**(6):377–390.

66. Rundgren M, Rosen I, Friberg H. Amplitude-integrated EEG (aEEG) predicts outcome after cardiac arrest and induced hypothermia. *Intensive Care Med.* 2006;**32**(6):836–42.

67. Oh SH, Park KN, Shon YM, et al. Continuous amplitude-integrated electroencephalographic monitoring is a useful prognostic tool for hypothermia-treated cardiac arrest patients. *Circulation.* 2015;**132**(12):1094–1103.

68. Knight WA, Hart KW, Adeoye OM, et al. The incidence of seizures in patients undergoing therapeutic hypothermia after resuscitation from cardiac arrest. *Epilepsy Res.* 2013;**106**(3):396–402.

69. Wagenman KL, Blake TP, Sanchez SM, et al. Electrographic status epilepticus and long-term outcome in critically ill children. *Neurology.* 2014;**82**(5):396–404.

70. Ostendorf AP, Hartman ME, Friess SH. Early electroencephalographic findings correlate with neurologic outcome in children following cardiac arrest. *Pediatr Crit Care Med.* 2016;**17**(7):667–76.

71. Lamartine Monteiro M, Taccone FS, Depondt C, et al. The prognostic value of 48-h continuous EEG during therapeutic hypothermia after cardiac arrest. *Neurocrit Care.* 2015;**24**(2):153–62.

72. Bouwes A, van Poppelen D, Koelman JH, et al. Acute posthypoxic myoclonus after cardiopulmonary resuscitation. *BMC Neurol.* 2012;**12**: 63.

73. Newey CR, Hornik A, Guerch M, et al. The benefit of neuromuscular blockade in patients with postanoxic myoclonus otherwise obscuring continuous electroencephalography (CEEG). *Crit Care Res Pract.* 2017;**2017**:2504058.

74. Wijdicks EF, Hijdra A, Young GB, Bassetti CL, Wiebe S. Practice parameter: prediction of outcome in comatose survivors after cardiopulmonary resuscitation (an evidence-based review): report of the Quality Standards Subcommittee of the American Academy of Neurology. *Neurology.* 2006;**67**(2):203–10.

75. Wijdicks EF, Parisi JE, Sharbrough FW. Prognostic value of myoclonus status in comatose survivors of cardiac arrest. *Ann Neurol.* 1994;**35**(2):239–43.

76. Mikhaeil-Demo Y, Gavvala JR, Bellinski, II, et al. Clinical classification of post anoxic myoclonic status. *Resuscitation.* 2017;**119**:76–80.

77. Lucas JM, Cocchi MN, Salciccioli J, et al. Neurologic recovery after therapeutic hypothermia in patients with post-cardiac arrest myoclonus. *Resuscitation.* 2012;**83**(2):265–9.

78. Elmer J, Rittenberger JC, Faro J, et al.; Pittsburgh Post-Cardiac Arrest S. Clinically distinct electroencephalographic phenotypes of early myoclonus after cardiac arrest. *Ann Neurol.* 2016;**80**(2):175–84.

79. Seder DB, Sunde K, Rubertsson S, et al. Neurologic outcomes and postresuscitation care of patients with myoclonus following cardiac arrest. *Crit Care Med.* 2015;**43**(5):965–72.

80. Pampiglione G. Electroencephalographic studies after cardiorespiratory resuscitation. *Proc R Soc Med.* 1962;**55**:653–7.

81. Nishisaki A, Sullivan J, 3rd, Steger B, et al. Retrospective analysis of the prognostic value of electroencephalography patterns obtained in pediatric in-hospital cardiac arrest survivors during three years. *Pediatr Crit Care Med.* 2007;**8**(1):10–17.

82. Synek VM. Value of a revised EEG coma scale for prognosis after cerebral anoxia and diffuse head injury. *Clin Electroencephalogr.* 1990;**21**(1):25–30.

83. Hockaday JM, Potts F, Epstein E, Bonazzi A, Schwab RS. Electroencephalographic changes in acute cerebral anoxia from cardiac or respiratory arrest. *Electroencephalogr Clin Neurophysiol.* 1965;**18**:575–86.

84. Young GB, Doig G, Ragazzoni A. Anoxic-ischemic encephalopathy: clinical and electrophysiological associations with outcome. *Neurocrit Care.* 2005;**2**(2):159–64.

85. Westhall E, Rossetti AO, van Rootselaar AF, et al. Standardized EEG interpretation accurately predicts prognosis after cardiac arrest. *Neurology.* 2016;**86**(16):1482–90.

86. Mandel R, Martinot A, Delepoulle F, et al. Prediction of outcome after hypoxic-ischemic encephalopathy: a prospective clinical and electrophysiologic study. *J Pediatr.* 2002;**141**(1):45–50.

87. Ramachandrannair R, Sharma R, Weiss SK, Cortez MA. Reactive EEG patterns in pediatric coma. *Pediatr Neurol.* 2005;**33**(5):345–9.

88. Tasker RC, Boyd S, Harden A, Matthew DJ. Monitoring in non-traumatic coma. Part II: electroencephalography. *Arch Dis Child.* 1988;**63**(8):895–9.

89. Pampiglione G, Harden A. Resuscitation after cardiocirculatory arrest. Prognostic evaluation of early electroencephalographic findings. *Lancet.* 1968;**1**(7555):1261–5.

90. Cheliout-Heraut F, Sale-Franque F, Hubert P, Bataille J. [Cerebral anoxia in near-drowning of children. The prognostic value of EEG] In French. *Neurophysiol Clin.* 1991;**21**(2):121–32.

91. Ducharme-Crevier L, Press CA, Kurz JE, et al. Early presence of sleep spindles on electroencephalography is associated with good outcome after pediatric cardiac arrest. *Pediatr Crit Care Med.* 2017;**18**(5):452–60.

92. Pampiglione G, Chaloner J, Harden A, O'Brien J. Transitory ischemia/anoxia in young children and the prediction of quality of survival. *Ann N Y Acad Sci.* 1978;**315**:281–92.

93. Abend NS, Massey SL, Fitzgerald M, et al. Interrater agreement of EEG interpretation after pediatric cardiac arrest using standardized critical care EEG terminology. *J Clin Neurophysiol.* 2017;**34**(6):534–41.

94. Ostendorf AP, Hartman ME, Friess SH. Early electroencephalographic findings correlate with neurologic outcome in children following cardiac arrest. *Pediatr Crit Care Med.* 2016;**17**(7):667–76.

95. Fung FW, Topjian AA, Xiao R, Abend NS. Early EEG features for outcome prediction after cardiac arrest in children. *J Clin Neurophysiol.* 2019;**36**(5):349–57.

96. Toet MC, Hellstrom-Westas L, Groenendaal F, Eken P, de Vries LS. Amplitude integrated EEG 3 and 6 hours after birth in full term neonates with hypoxic-ischaemic encephalopathy. *Arch Dis Child Fetal Neonatal Ed.* 1999;**81**(1):F19–23.

97. Cloostermans MC, van Meulen FB, Eertman CJ, Hom HW, van Putten MJ. Continuous electroencephalography monitoring for early prediction of neurological outcome in postanoxic patients after cardiac arrest: a prospective cohort study. *Crit Care Med.* 2012;**40**(10):2867–75.

98. Synek VM, Shaw NA. Epileptiform discharges in presence of continuous background activity in anoxic coma. *Clin Electroencephalogr.* 1989;**20**(2):141–6.

99. Rossetti AO, Carrera E, Oddo M. Early EEG correlates of neuronal injury after brain anoxia. *Neurology.* 2012;**78**(11):796–802.

100. Synek VM. Revised EEG coma scale in diffuse acute head injuries in adults. *Clin Exp Neurol.* 1990;**27**:99–111.

101. Abend NS, Gutierrez-Colina A, Zhao H, et al. Interobserver reproducibility of electroencephalogram interpretation in critically ill children. *J Clin Neurophysiol.* 2011;**28**(1):15–19.

102. Husain AM. Electroencephalographic assessment of coma. *J Clin Neurophysiol.* 2006;**23**(3):208–20.

103. Gerber PA, Chapman KE, Chung SS, et al. Interobserver agreement in the interpretation of EEG patterns in critically ill adults. *J Clin Neurophysiol.* 2008;**25**(5):241–9.

104. Hirsch LJ, Brenner RP, Drislane FW, et al. The ACNS subcommittee on research terminology for continuous EEG monitoring: proposed standardized terminology for rhythmic and periodic EEG patterns encountered in critically ill patients. *J Clin Neurophysiol.* 2005;**22**(2):128–35.

105. Ronner HE, Ponten SC, Stam CJ, Uitdehaag BM. Inter-observer variability of the EEG diagnosis of seizures in comatose patients. *Seizure.* 2009;**18**(4):257–63.

106. Bourgoin P, Barrault V, Joram N, et al. The prognostic value of early amplitude-integrated electroencephalography monitoring after pediatric cardiac arrest. *Pediatr Crit Care Med.* 2020;**21**(3):248–55.

107. Lee S, Zhao X, Davis KA, et al. Quantitative EEG predicts outcomes in children after cardiac arrest. *Neurology.* 2019;**92**(20):e2329–e2338.

108. Stecker MM, Cheung AT, Pochettino A, et al. Deep hypothermic circulatory arrest: I. Effects of cooling on electroencephalogram and evoked potentials. *Ann Thorac Surg.* 2001;**71**(1):14–21.

109. Levy WJ. Quantitative analysis of EEG changes during hypothermia. *Anesthesiology.* 1984;**60**(4):291–7.

110. Horan M, Azzopardi D, Edwards AD, Firmin RK, Field D. Lack of influence of mild hypothermia on amplitude integrated-electroencephalography in neonates receiving extracorporeal membrane oxygenation. *Early Hum Dev.* 2007;**83**(2):69–75.

111. Kochs E. Electrophysiological monitoring and mild hypothermia. *J Neurosurg Anesthesiol.* 1995;**7**(3):222–8.

112. Kessler SK, Topjian AA, Gutierrez-Colina AM, et al. Short-term outcome prediction by electroencephalographic features in children treated with therapeutic hypothermia after cardiac arrest. *Neurocrit Care.* 2011;**14**(1):37–43.

113. Veselis RA, Reinsel R, Marino P, Sommer S, Carlon GC. The effects of midazolam on the EEG during sedation of critically ill patients. *Anaesthesia.* 1993;**48**(6):463–70.

114. Tortorici MA, Kochanek PM, Poloyac SM. Effects of hypothermia on drug disposition, metabolism, and response: a focus of hypothermia-mediated alterations on the cytochrome P450 enzyme system. *Crit Care Med.* 2007;**35**(9):2196–2204.

115. Sessler DI. Complications and treatment of mild hypothermia. *Anesthesiology.* 2001;**95**(2):531–43.

116. Arpino PA, Greer DM. Practical pharmacologic aspects of therapeutic hypothermia after cardiac arrest. *Pharmacotherapy.* 2008;**28**(1):102–11.

117. Fritz HG, Holzmayr M, Walter B, et al. The effect of mild hypothermia on plasma fentanyl concentration and biotransformation in juvenile pigs. *Anesth Analg.* 2005;**100**(4):996–1002.

118. Samaniego EA, Mlynash M, Caulfield AF, Eyngorn I, Wijman CA. Sedation confounds outcome prediction in cardiac arrest survivors treated with hypothermia. *Neurocrit Care.* 2011;**15**(1):113–19.

119. Callaway CW, Soar J, Aibiki M, et al. Part 4: Advanced Life Support: 2015 International Consensus on Cardiopulmonary Resuscitation and Emergency Cardiovascular Care Science with Treatment Recommendations. *Circulation.* 2015;**132**(16 Suppl 1):S84–145.

120. Kane N, Oware A. Somatosensory evoked potentials aid prediction after hypoxic-ischaemic brain injury. *Pract Neurol.* 2015;**15**(5):352–60.

121. Goldie WD, Chiappa KH, Young RR, Brooks EB. Brainstem auditory and short-latency somatosensory evoked responses in brain death. *Neurology.* 1981;**31**(3):248–56.

122. Trojaborg W, Jorgensen EO. Evoked cortical potentials in patients with "isoelectric" EEGs. *Electroencephalogr Clin Neurophysiol.* 1973;**35**(3):301–9.

123. Zegers de Beyl D, Brunko E. Prediction of chronic vegetative state with somatosensory evoked potentials. *Neurology.* 1986;**36**(1):134.

124. Rothstein TL. The role of evoked potentials in anoxic-ischemic coma and severe brain trauma. *J Clin Neurophysiol.* 2000;**17**(5):486–97.

125. Tiainen M, Kovala TT, Takkunen OS, Roine RO. Somatosensory and brainstem auditory evoked potentials in cardiac arrest patients treated with hypothermia. *Crit Care Med.* 2005;**33**(8):1736–40.

126. Zandbergen EG, de Haan RJ, Stoutenbeek CP, Koelman JH, Hijdra A. Systematic review of early prediction of poor outcome in anoxic-ischaemic coma. *Lancet.* 1998;**352**(9143):1808–12.

127. Zandbergen EG, Hijdra A, Koelman JH, et al. Prediction of poor outcome within the first 3 days of postanoxic coma. *Neurology.* 2006;**66**(1):62–8.

128. Howell K, Grill E, Klein AM, Straube A, Bender A. Rehabilitation outcome of anoxic-ischaemic encephalopathy survivors with prolonged disorders of consciousness. *Resuscitation.* 2013;**84**(10):1409–15.

129. Leithner C, Ploner CJ, Hasper D, Storm C. Does hypothermia influence the predictive value of bilateral absent N20 after cardiac arrest? *Neurology.* 2010;**74**(12):965–9.

130. Bender A, Howell K, Frey M, et al. Bilateral loss of cortical SSEP responses is compatible with good outcome after cardiac arrest. *J Neurol.* 2012;**259**(11):2481–3.

131. Pfeiffer G, Pfeifer R, Isenmann S. Cerebral hypoxia, missing cortical somatosensory evoked potentials and recovery of consciousness. *BMC Neurol.* 2014;**14**:82.

132. Arch AE, Chiappa K, Greer DM. False positive absent somatosensory evoked potentials in cardiac arrest with therapeutic hypothermia. *Resuscitation.* 2014;**85**(6):e97–98.

133. Bouwes A, Binnekade JM, Zandstra DF, et al. Somatosensory evoked potentials during mild hypothermia after cardiopulmonary resuscitation. *Neurology.* 2009;**73**(18):1457–61.

134. Carter BG, Butt W. Review of the use of somatosensory evoked potentials in the prediction of outcome after severe brain injury. *Crit Care Med.* 2001;**29**(1):178–86.

135. Robinson LR, Micklesen PJ, Tirschwell DL, Lew HL. Predictive value of somatosensory evoked potentials for awakening from coma. *Crit Care Med.* 2003;**31**(3):960–7.

136. Kamps MJ, Horn J, Oddo M, et al. Prognostication of neurologic outcome in cardiac arrest patients after mild therapeutic hypothermia: a meta-analysis of the current literature. *Intensive Care Med.* 2013;**39**(10):1671–82.

137. Golan E, Barrett K, Alali AS, et al. Predicting neurologic outcome after targeted temperature management for cardiac arrest: systematic review and meta-analysis. *Crit Care Med.* 2014;**42**(8):1919–30.

138. Sandroni C, Cavallaro F, Callaway CW, et al. Predictors of poor neurological outcome in adult comatose survivors of cardiac arrest: a systematic review and meta-analysis. Part 2: patients treated with therapeutic hypothermia. *Resuscitation.* 2013;**84**(10):1324–38.

139. Bouwes A, Binnekade JM, Kuiper MA, et al. Prognosis of coma after therapeutic hypothermia: a prospective cohort study. *Ann Neurol.* 2012;**71**(2):206–12.

140. Pfeifer R, Weitzel S, Gunther A, et al. Investigation of the inter-observer variability effect on the prognostic value of somatosensory evoked potentials of the median nerve (SSEP) in cardiac arrest survivors using an SSEP classification. *Resuscitation.* 2013;**84**(10):1375–81.

141. Zandbergen EG, Hijdra A, de Haan RJ, et al. Interobserver variation in the interpretation of SSEPs in anoxic-ischaemic coma. *Clin Neurophysiol.* 2006;**117**(7):1529–35.

142. Jobsis FF. Noninvasive, infrared monitoring of cerebral and myocardial oxygen sufficiency and circulatory parameters. *Science.* 1977;**198**(4323):1264–7.

143. Scheeren TW, Schober P, Schwarte LA. Monitoring tissue oxygenation by near infrared spectroscopy (NIRS): background and current applications. *J Clin Monit Comput.* 2012;**26**(4):279–87.

144. Tobias JD. Cerebral oxygenation monitoring: near-infrared spectroscopy. *Expert Rev Med Devices.* 2006;**3**(2):235–43.

145. Watzman HM, Kurth CD, Montenegro LM, et al. Arterial and venous contributions to near-infrared cerebral oximetry. *Anesthesiology.* 2000;**93**(4):947–53.

146. Abdul-Khaliq H, Troitzsch D, Berger F, Lange PE. [Regional transcranial oximetry with near infrared spectroscopy (NIRS) in comparison with measuring oxygen saturation in the jugular bulb in infants and children for monitoring cerebral oxygenation]. *Biomed Tech (Berl).* 2000;**45**(11):328–32.

147. Nagdyman N, Ewert P, Peters B, et al. Comparison of different near-infrared spectroscopic cerebral oxygenation indices with central venous and jugular venous oxygenation saturation in children. *Paediatr Anaesth.* 2008;**18**(2):160–6.

148. Nagdyman N, Fleck T, Schubert S, et al. Comparison between cerebral tissue oxygenation index measured by near-infrared spectroscopy and venous jugular bulb saturation in children. *Intensive Care Med.* 2005;**31**(6):846–50.

149. Bhutta AT, Ford JW, Parker JG, et al. Noninvasive cerebral oximeter as a surrogate for mixed venous saturation in children. *Pediatr Cardiol.* 2007;**28**(1):34–41.

150. Ranucci M, Isgro G, De la Torre T, et al. Near-infrared spectroscopy correlates with continuous superior vena cava oxygen saturation in pediatric cardiac surgery patients. *Paediatr Anaesth.* 2008;**18**(12):1163–9.

151. Sanfilippo F, Serena G, Corredor C, et al. Cerebral oximetry and return of spontaneous circulation after cardiac arrest: a systematic review and meta-analysis. *Resuscitation.* 2015;**94**:67–72.

152. Parnia S, Nasir A, Ahn A, et al. A feasibility study of cerebral oximetry during in-hospital mechanical and manual cardiopulmonary resuscitation. *Crit Care Med.* 2014;**42**(4):930–3.

153. Genbrugge C, Dens J, Meex I, et al. Regional cerebral oximetry during cardiopulmonary resuscitation: useful or useless? *J Emerg Med.* 2015;**50**(1):198–207.

154. Newman DH, Callaway CW, Greenwald IB, Freed J. Cerebral oximetry in out-of-hospital cardiac arrest: standard CPR rarely provides detectable hemoglobin-oxygen saturation to the frontal cortex. *Resuscitation.* 2004;**63**(2):189–94.

155. Singer AJ, Ahn A, Inigo-Santiago LA, et al. Cerebral oximetry levels during CPR are associated with return of spontaneous circulation following cardiac arrest: an observational study. *Emerg Med J.* 2015;**32**(5):353–6.

156. Parnia S, Nasir A, Shah C, et al. A feasibility study evaluating the role of cerebral oximetry in predicting return of spontaneous circulation in cardiac arrest. *Resuscitation.* 2012;**83**(8):982–5.

157. Meex I, De Deyne C, Dens J, et al. Feasibility of absolute cerebral tissue oxygen saturation during cardiopulmonary resuscitation. *Crit Care.* 2013;**17**(2):R36.

158. Ahn A, Nasir A, Malik H, D'Orazi F, Parnia S. A pilot study examining the role of regional cerebral oxygen saturation monitoring as a marker of return of spontaneous circulation in shockable (VF/VT) and non-shockable (PEA/Asystole) causes of

cardiac arrest. *Resuscitation*. 2013;**84**(12):1713–16.

159. Parnia S, Yang J, Nguyen R, et al. Cerebral oximetry during cardiac arrest: a multicenter study of neurologic outcomes and survival. *Crit Care Med*. 2016;**44**(9):1663–74.

160. Ito N, Nishiyama K, Callaway CW, et al. Noninvasive regional cerebral oxygen saturation for neurological prognostication of patients with out-of-hospital cardiac arrest: a prospective multicenter observational study. *Resuscitation*. 2014;**85**(6):778–84.

161. Paradis NA, Martin GB, Rivers EP, et al. Coronary perfusion pressure and the return of spontaneous circulation in human cardiopulmonary resuscitation. *JAMA*. 1990;**263**(8):1106–13.

162. Yannopoulos D, McKnite S, Aufderheide TP, et al. Effects of incomplete chest wall decompression during cardiopulmonary resuscitation on coronary and cerebral perfusion pressures in a porcine model of cardiac arrest. *Resuscitation*. 2005;**64**(3):363–72.

163. Koyama Y, Wada T, Lohman BD, et al. A new method to detect cerebral blood flow waveform in synchrony with chest compression by near-infrared spectroscopy during CPR. *Am J Emerg Med*. 2013;**31**(10):1504–8.

164. Kamarainen A, Sainio M, Olkkola KT, et al. Quality controlled manual chest compressions and cerebral oxygenation during in-hospital cardiac arrest. *Resuscitation*. 2012;**83**(1):138–42.

165. Paarmann H, Heringlake M, Sier H, Schon J. The association of non-invasive cerebral and mixed venous oxygen saturation during cardiopulmonary resuscitation. *Interact Cardiovasc Thorac Surg*. 2010;**11**(3):371–3.

166. Mayr NP, Martin K, Kurz J, Tassani P. Monitoring of cerebral oxygen saturation during closed-chest and open-chest CPR. *Resuscitation*. 2011;**82**(5):635–6.

167. Martens PR, Dhaese HL, Van den Brande FG, Van Laecke SM. External cardiac massage improved cerebral tissue oxygenation shown by near-infrared spectroscopy during transcatheter aortic valve implantation. *Resuscitation*. 2010;**81**(11):1590–1.

168. Pilkington SN, Hett DA, Pierce JM, Smith DC. Auditory evoked responses and near infrared spectroscopy during cardiac arrest. *Br J Anaesth*. 1995;**74**(6):717–19.

169. Storm C, Leithner C, Krannich A, et al. Regional cerebral oxygen saturation after cardiac arrest in 60 patients – a prospective outcome study. *Resuscitation*. 2014;**85**(8):1037–41.

170. Meex I, Dens J, Jans F, et al. Cerebral tissue oxygen saturation during therapeutic hypothermia in post-cardiac arrest patients. *Resuscitation*. 2013;**84**(6):788–93.

171. Shum-Tim D, Nagashima M, Shinoka T, et al. Postischemic hyperthermia exacerbates neurologic injury after deep hypothermic circulatory arrest. *J Thorac Cardiovasc Surg*. 1998;**116**(5):780–92.

172. Pynnonen L, Falkenbach P, Kamarainen A, et al. Therapeutic hypothermia after cardiac arrest – cerebral perfusion and metabolism during upper and lower threshold normocapnia. *Resuscitation*. 2011;**82**(9):1174–9.

173. Mayr NP, Martin K, Hausleiter J, Tassani P. Measuring cerebral oxygenation helps optimizing post-resuscitation therapy. *Resuscitation*. 2011;**82**(8):1110–11.

174. Hoffman GM, Brosig CL, Mussatto KA, Tweddell JS, Ghanayem NS. Perioperative cerebral oxygen saturation in neonates with hypoplastic left heart syndrome and childhood neurodevelopmental outcome. *J Thorac Cardiovasc Surg*. 2013;**146**(5):1153–64.

175. Deschamps A, Lambert J, Couture P, et al. Reversal of decreases in cerebral saturation in high-risk cardiac surgery. *J Cardiothorac Vasc Anesth*. 2013;**27**(6):1260–16.

176. Massey SL, Abend NS, Gaynor JW, et al. Electroencephalographic patterns preceding cardiac arrest in neonates following cardiac surgery. *Resuscitation*. 2019;**144**:67–74.

Pitfalls in aEEG Interpretation

Diane Wilson

Clinical Presentation

An infant was born via normal spontaneous vaginal delivery at 39 weeks' gestation to a healthy primigravid woman following an uneventful pregnancy. Rupture of membranes occurred 48 hours prior to delivery and antibiotics were started promptly. Group B *Streptococcus* status was unknown at the time of delivery. Following delivery, the infant was vigorous with good tone, a normal heart rate, and regular respiratory effort. Apgar scores were 8 at 1 minute and 8 at 5 minutes. The baby appeared well and went to stay in the mother's room. At 27 hours of age the baby had 3 episodes over a 10-minute period of right-sided arm and leg flexion and left-sided arm and leg extension. The infant was transferred to the NICU, where aEEG monitoring was commenced upon arrival.

Discussion

Infants who present with clinically suspected seizures are good candidates for aEEG monitoring, which can be applied promptly by bedside caregivers to help guide early intervention. When aEEG findings are inconsistent with the clinical findings, or the corresponding raw EEG does not demonstrate a clear rhythmic pattern in the setting of suspected seizure, it is important for the bedside staff to use troubleshooting techniques to ensure good aEEG signal quality. In this case, the right-sided electrodes were placed too close together, causing artifact. Once the leads were replaced, the aEEG tracing became more reliable and revealed the infant's electroclinical seizures.

Key Neuromonitoring Findings

Baseline elevations were noted on the right-sided aEEG tracing; however, the corresponding raw EEG did not show a rhythmic pattern, instead showing an inconclusive pattern (Figure C1.1). Because of this unusual pattern, the nurse checked the electrode placement and found that the electrodes were touching each other and did not appear to be placed symmetrically on the infant's head. Once the electrodes were repositioned, the right-sided aEEG tracing continued to demonstrate an elevation in the baseline and upper margin (Figure C1.2). This elevation was now clearly associated with a rhythmic pattern on the corresponding raw EEG, which evolved in frequency and amplitude during the course of the epoch, indicative of an electrographic seizure. This

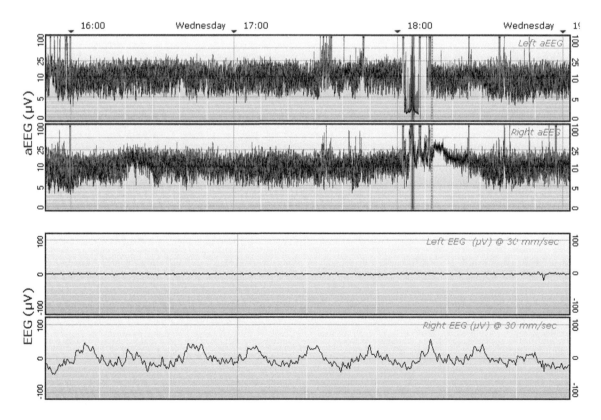

Figure C1.1 Two-channel (C3-P3, C4-P4) aEEG tracing (upper panel) showing left-sided attenuation and intermittent right-sided baseline elevations at the time of the red cursor. The corresponding raw EEG tracing (lower panel) showed an attenuated tracing on the left and apparent artifact on the right.

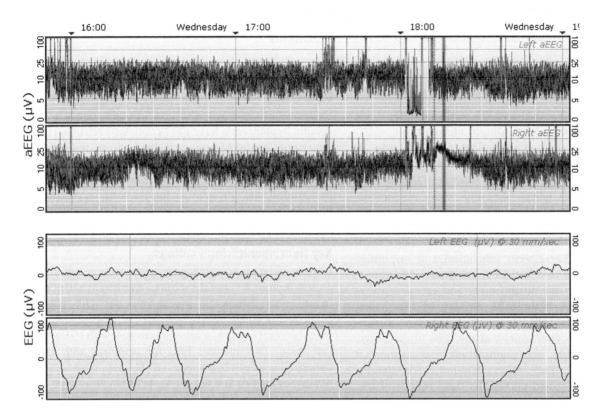

Figure C1.2 Two-channel (C3-P3, C4-P4) aEEG tracing (upper panel) after electrode repositioning at the dashed green line, showing persistent elevation of the lower and upper aEEG margins on the right, correlating with a rhythmic, evolving pattern on the corresponding raw EEG tracing (lower panel), indicative of an electrographic seizure.

electrographic seizure coincided with tonic extension of the left arm and leg. The infant received a loading dose of phenobarbital, after which the clinical and electrographic seizure stopped. A brain MRI subsequently showed a large right-sided intraventricular hemorrhage. Following the MRI, the infant underwent conventional continuous EEG monitoring, which detected no further electrographic seizures.

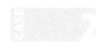

Neonatal Hypoxic-Ischemic Encephalopathy

Erin Fedak Romanowski and Renée A. Shellhaas

Clinical Presentation

A 3240 g boy was born at 41 and 2/7 weeks gestational age via emergency cesarean section due to uterine rupture. His Apgar scores were 0, 3, 4, and 7 at 1, 5, 10, and 20 minutes, respectively. His arterial cord blood gas pH was 6.87 with a base deficit of −17.5. He was transferred to a Level IV NICU where he underwent therapeutic hypothermia. Continuous video EEG monitoring was performed as per the NICU protocol (Figure C2.1). EEG demonstrated numerous seizures on the second day of life (Figure C2.2). These were subclinical and responded to phenobarbital. His interictal EEG was moderately abnormal because of excessive discontinuity and excessive negative sharp waves. A brain MRI on day of life 7 was interpreted as normal. His examination improved significantly during his hospital course; at the time of discharge, his only abnormality on examination was somewhat increased tone in the lower extremities bilaterally. Phenobarbital was weaned during the third month of life. Developmental assessment at age 18 months was normal.

Discussion

Since half of newborns with HIE who are treated with therapeutic hypothermia have EEG-confirmed seizures [1, 2], the American Clinical Neurophysiology Society Guideline recommends continuous video-EEG monitoring throughout cooling and rewarming [3]. The time to normalization of the EEG background has prognostic implications; neonates whose EEG backgrounds normalize within 48 hours after birth are the most likely to have favorable outcomes.

Key Neuromonitoring Findings

Hypoxic-ischemic encephalopathy is the most common cause of acute symptomatic neonatal seizures. As many as half of neonates treated with therapeutic hypothermia for HIE have EEG-confirmed seizures, as was the case for this patient. As with other neonatal seizures, seizures in neonates with HIE are usually subclinical. The interictal EEG for newborns with HIE who undergo therapeutic hypothermia is often suppressed and discontinuous on the first and second day of life, but this improves over the third and fourth days of life (Figures C2.1–C2.3).

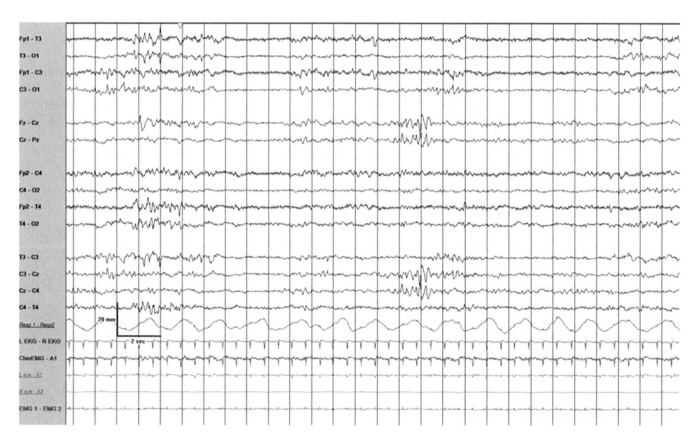

Figure C2.1 Day of life 1. Low-voltage, discontinuous EEG background with excessive negative sharp waves (especially at Cz) and a paucity of normal graphoelements.

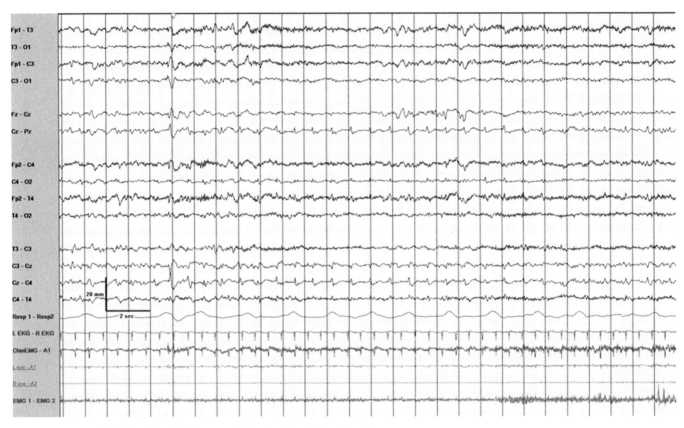

Figure C2.2   Day of life 2. A subclinical seizure recorded at Cz with a field to C4 and Pz.

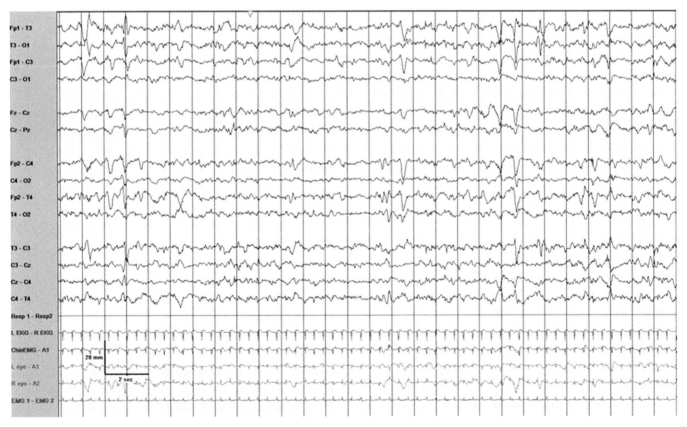

Figure C2.3   Day of life 3. Normal amplitude background activity, with a mixture of fast and slow frequencies; excessive negative sharp waves are still present.

References

1. Glass HC, et al. Risk factors for EEG seizures in neonates treated with hypothermia: a multi-center cohort study. *Neurology.* 2014;**82**:1–6.

2. Glass HC, et al. Contemporary profile of seizures in neonates: a prospective cohort study. *J Pediatr.* 2016;**174**:98–103.

3. Shellhaas RA, et al. The American Clinical Neurophysiology Society's Guideline on continuous electroencephalography monitoring in neonates. *J Clin Neurophysiol.* 2011;**28**: 611–17.

Perinatal Stroke

Elena Pavlidis, Andreea Pavel, and Geraldine B. Boylan

Clinical Presentation

A female infant was born to a 37-year-old G3P2 at term (40+5 weeks) by ventouse (vacuum) delivery in a local hospital. Apgar scores were 8 and 10 at 1st and 5th minute, respectively. Family and maternal histories were negative. A history of reduced fetal movements was reported at 28 and 36+6 weeks of gestation. At 44 hours after birth, rhythmic movements of the baby's right upper and lower limbs were noticed. She was transferred to the NICU and treated with two loading doses of phenobarbital (20 + 10 mg/kg). Due to the persistence of unilateral clonic movements, a loading dose of phenytoin (18 mg/kg) was subsequently administered. Electrolytes and glucose were normal. A full septic screen was performed and therapy with antibiotics and antivirals were started. Cerebral ultrasound scan was unremarkable. The infant was then transferred to a tertiary level NICU for continuous EEG monitoring at 53 hours of age. On admission, she was stable; clonic movements had not recurred. Neurological examination showed axial hypotonia and hyporeflexia. Antibiotic and antiviral treatments were continued until the septic screen results were reported as negative. Continuous video EEG monitoring showed preserved sleep–wake cycling with background activity characterized by focal interictal epileptiform discharges over the left centro-temporal regions (Figure C3.1). Four hours after the EEG started (at 58.5 hours of age), she experienced a 10-minute focal electrographic-only seizure over the left

central region (Figure C3.2). Phenobarbital was continued. Brain MRI showed an extensive ischemic stroke involving the left hemisphere (Figure C3.3).

Discussion

The incidence of perinatal ischemic stroke is 1/2800 – 1/5000 live births [1]. It is usually underestimated because in infants it is often asymptomatic. In infants showing clinical manifestations, as in this case, focal recurrent clonic and/or tonic seizures presenting mainly within the first 3 days of life are the most common sign [1, 2]. As in the present case, the majority of strokes occur unilaterally, usually involving the left hemisphere and the middle cerebral artery territory [2].

Key Neuromonitoring Findings

In perinatal arterial ischemic stroke, the EEG often shows diffuse excessive background discontinuity, but with larger strokes, EEG may show an asymmetry of the background activity with suppression over the infarcted side. Unilateral bursts of theta activity with sharp waves or spikes intermixed and focal sharp waves can also be present over the infarcted region [3, 4] Sleep–wake cycling is generally present, but may be disturbed over the infarcted side [4] Focal seizures with sharp waves, spikes or polyspikes are common over the central region [4].

References

1. Chabrier S, Husson B, Dinomais M, Landrieu P, Nguyen TheTich S. New insights (and new interrogations) in perinatal arterial ischemic stroke. *Thromb Res.* 2011;**127** (1):13–22.

2. Lee J, Croen LA, Lindan C, et al. Predictors of outcome in perinatal arterial stroke: a population-based study. *Ann Neurol.* 2005 Aug;**58**(2):303–8.

3. Walsh BH, Low E, Bogue CO, Murray DM, Boylan GB. Early continuous video electroencephalography in neonatal

stroke. *Dev Med Child Neurol.* 2011 Jan;**53**(1):89–92.

4. Low E, Mathieson SR, Stevenson NJ, et al. Early postnatal EEG features of perinatal arterial ischaemic stroke with seizures. *PLoS ONE.* 2014 Jul 22;**9**(7): e100973.

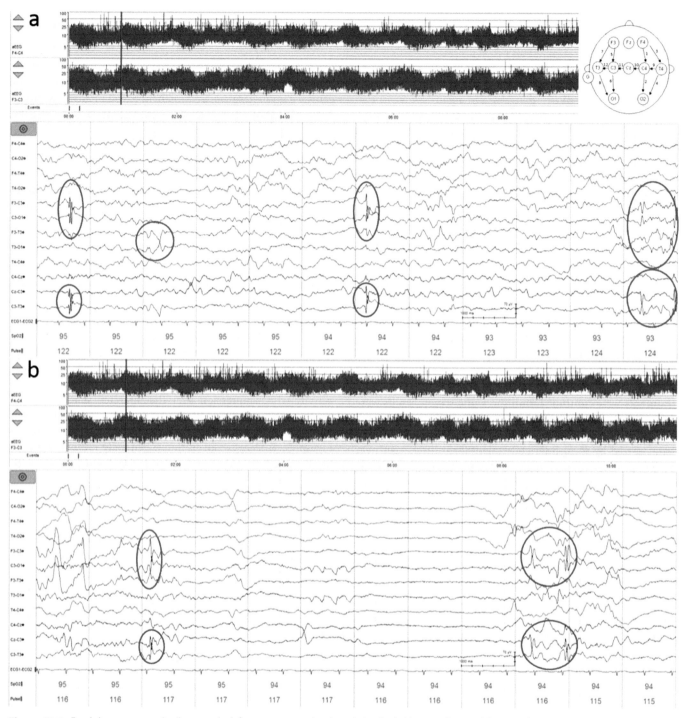

Figure C3.1 Focal sharp waves and spikes over the left centro-temporal regions during both (a) active sleep and (b) quiet sleep, during which there is excessive background discontinuity for conceptional age (inter-burst interval amplitude ≤25 μV). The corresponding time-point on the aEEG is indicated with a red line. (Sensitivity: 70 μV/cm; high-frequency filter: 70 Hz; low-frequency filter: 0.5 Hz; time base: 30 mm/sec.)

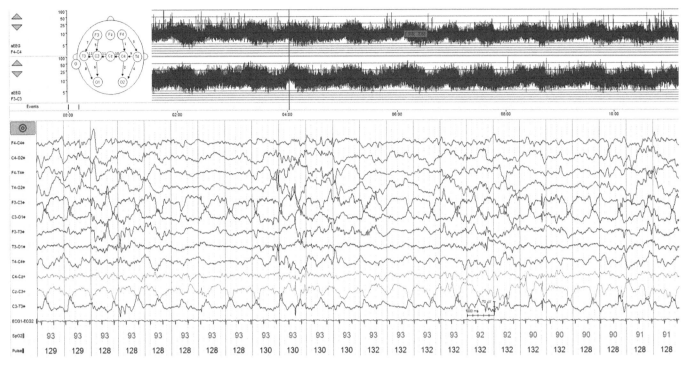

Figure C3.2 Ten-minute seizure, characterized by rhythmic sharply contoured delta activity intermixed with sharp waves and spikes localized over the left central region. The corresponding time-point on the aEEG is indicated with a red line, demonstrating elevation in the lower margin indicative of a seizure. (Sensitivity: 70 µV/cm; high-frequency filter: 70 Hz; low-frequency filter: 0.5 Hz; time base: 15 mm/sec.)

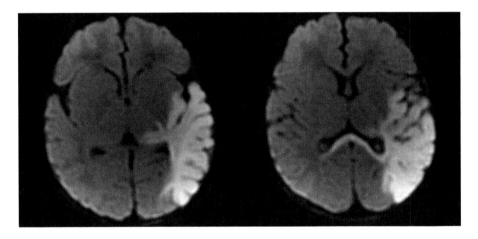

Figure C3.3 Axial diffusion weighted brain MRI images showing an extensive acute infarction in the posterior left middle cerebral artery territory.

Neonatal Intracranial Hemorrhage

Erin Fedak Romanowski and Renée A. Shellhaas

Clinical Presentation

A 2535 g infant girl was born at 36 weeks gestational age via repeat cesarean section due to oligohydramnios, discovered at 35 weeks' gestation. Her Apgar scores were 8 and 9 at 1 and 5 minutes, respectively. She required continuous positive airway pressure (CPAP) at 8 minutes of life for grunting and retractions. She required intubation within 2 hours of life, received surfactant due to increasing oxygen demands, and was later transitioned to high-frequency oscillatory ventilation. Due to further decompensation, she required transfer to a Level IV NICU for extracorporeal membrane oxygenation (ECMO). A cranial ultrasound on day of life 2 revealed increased periventricular white matter echotexture with associated poor cortical and subcortical differentiation. A repeat head ultrasound on day of life 8 revealed a new large left frontal and parietal extra-axial hemorrhage and left parietal intraparenchymal hemorrhage with resultant mass effect and collapse of the left lateral ventricle, confirmed on MRI (Figure C4.1). Continuous video EEG monitoring was performed on day of life 9 due to the known risk of seizures associated with intracranial hemorrhage; EEG revealed subclinical status epilepticus, which resolved after treatment with phenobarbital (Figure C4.2). Her interictal EEG was moderately abnormal due to excessive background discontinuity, excessive multifocal negative sharp waves, occasional brief rhythmic discharges, and positive sharp waves over the right temporal region (Figure C4.3). She ultimately developed chronic, large, left greater than right, subdural fluid collections requiring left subdural-peritoneal shunt placement. She

remained on phenobarbital upon hospital discharge with no clinically apparent seizures.

Discussion

The American Clinical Neurophysiology Society guideline recommends consideration of continuous video EEG monitoring for neonates who have known or suspected acute brain injury *accompanied by encephalopathy*, since they are at high risk for seizures and most such seizures are subclinical (e.g., can only be detected with EEG monitoring). Clinical settings in which acute brain injury and associated symptomatic seizures are likely include intracranial, subarachnoid, subdural, or intraventricular hemorrhage. Other high-risk scenarios that should trigger consideration of EEG monitoring include hypoxic-ischemic encephalopathy, inborn errors of metabolism, CNS infection, trauma, arterial ischemic or venous strokes, premature infants with additional risk factors, clinically suspected seizures, or clinically suspected neonatal epilepsy syndromes [1].

Key Neuromonitoring Findings

Intracranial hemorrhage is one of the most common etiologies of neonatal seizures after hypoxic-ischemic encephalopathy and ischemic stroke [2]. As with seizures of any etiology, newborns with intracranial hemorrhage are at risk for both clinical and subclinical seizures. The interictal EEG in neonates with intracranial hemorrhage may reveal focal slowing or attenuation over the area of bleed, as well as focal or multifocal negative sharp waves. Positive sharp waves, indicating underlying white matter injury, may also be seen.

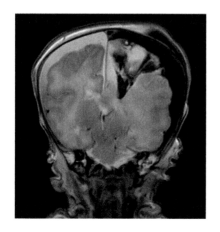

A. Coronal plane: T2 TSE

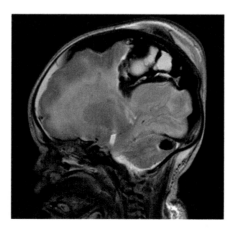

B. Sagittal plane: T2 TSE

Figure C4.1 MRI brain acquired on day of life 8 for a 36-weeks gestational age infant in coronal (panel A), and sagittal (panel B) planes revealed a large intraparenchymal hemorrhage in the left parietal lobe, and a large subdural hematoma over the left cerebral convexity causing mass effect on the left frontal, parietal, and occipital lobes. There is a smaller right subdural hematoma overlying the right cerebral convexity. There is 6 mm of rightward sub-falcine herniation and left uncal herniation. The left lateral ventricle temporal horn is dilated suggestive of entrapment.

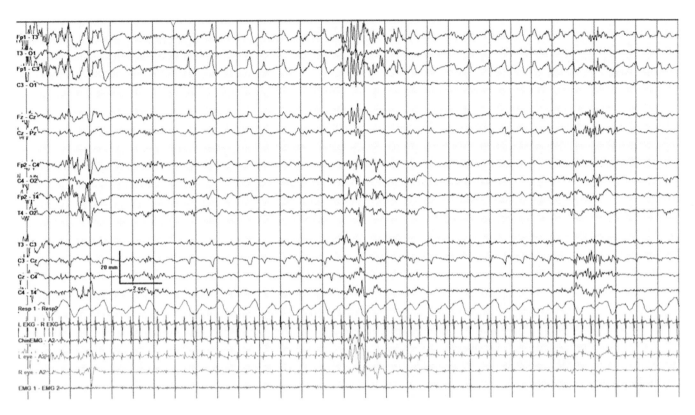

Figure C4.2 Continuous EEG on day of life 9 with a subclinical seizure recorded at Fp1 with a field to Fz and Cz.

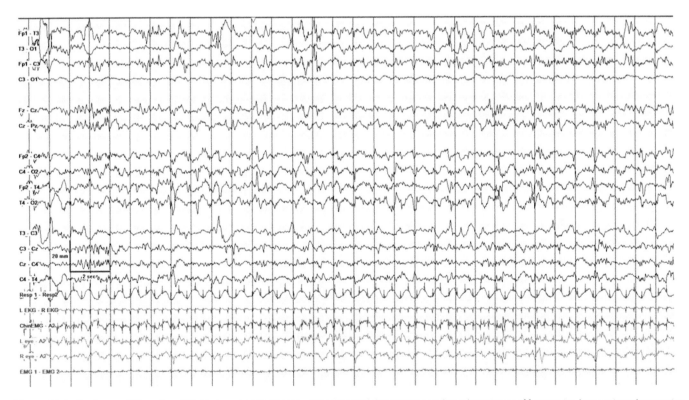

Figure C4.3 Continuous EEG on day of life 11 demonstrating improved background discontinuity, with a richer mixture of frequencies, but persistently excessive negative sharp waves.

References

1. Shellhaas RA, Chang T, Tsuchida T, et al. The American Clinical Neurophysiology Society's Guideline on Continuous Electroencephalography Monitoring in Neonates. *J Clin Neurophysiol.* 2011;**28**:611–17.

2. Glass HC, Shellhaas RA, Wusthoff CJ, et al. Contemporary profile of seizures in neonates: a prospective cohort study. *J Pediatr.* 2016;**174**:98–103.

Neonatal Birth Trauma

Diane Wilson and Cecil D. Hahn

Clinical Presentation

An infant was born by emergency caesarean section following prolapse of the umbilical cord. The mother was a healthy primigravid woman who had an uneventful pregnancy. She presented to hospital at 37 weeks' gestation with ruptured membranes. A cord prolapse was noted 9 hours after membranes ruptured and emergency cesarean section was commenced. There was difficulty extracting the baby as the head was well engaged; significant force was used. The baby was unresponsive at delivery with no respiratory effort or heart rate. The heart rate improved following 15 seconds of positive pressure ventilation and no cardiopulmonary resuscitation was needed. Apgar scores were 2 at one, 3 at five, and 4 at ten minutes. The baby required intubation and the first gasp was noted at 18 minutes of age. At 30 minutes of age the baby continued to have a decreased level of consciousness, was hypotonic, and had depressed primitive reflexes. There was a compound fracture of the left femur. Therapeutic hypothermia was administered for a total of 72 hours post-admission to NICU. At 9 hours of age there was onset of rhythmic leg jerking correlating with a rhythmic pattern on amplitude-integrated EEG (aEEG). Continuous EEG monitoring was started, and the baby was treated with lorazepam followed by phenobarbital for then ongoing subclinical seizures until approximately 20 hours of age. The initial head ultrasound revealed cerebral edema and a parenchymal hematoma with subarachnoid hemorrhage and occipital extracranial collection. A skull radiograph showed a right parietal skull fracture. There was evidence of multi-organ dysfunction. Dobutamine was required for 24 hours. MRI performed following rewarming on day of life 5 demonstrated a right epidural frontoparietal epidural hematoma with mass effect on the adjacent right parietal lobe and overlying extracranial scalp hematoma (Figure C5.1). In addition, there was subarachnoid hemorrhage bilaterally in the frontal and occipital regions and diffusion restriction in the right peritrigonal region and the right temporal lobe (not shown). The patient recovered well and was discharged home on day of life 9. At 14 months of age the patient was making steady developmental progress. On the Alberta Infant Motor Scale, his skills were age appropriate. Socio-adaptive behavior and language were also screened with no concerns noted. There was significant plagiocephaly; a referral was made to the helmet clinic.

Discussion

Emergent delivery following a perinatal sentinel event, such as umbilical cord prolapse, can precede significant hypoxic-ischemic encephalopathy. In this case, there was a confounding factor of birth trauma. Patients with Sarnat stages II–III encephalopathy from an acute perinatal event often develop seizures within 12 hours following delivery. Seizures may be difficult to control. Furthermore, electroclinical uncoupling may occur following treatment with anti-seizure medications, as in this case. Therapeutic hypothermia is standard treatment in these cases to reduce metabolic demands and suppress excitatory neuronal activity. Seizures are usually controlled within 36 hours, but in some cases, rewarming has been associated with recurrence of seizures. To screen for these so-called "rebound seizures," some guidelines recommend continuation of cEEG monitoring until 12 hours after rewarming has been completed.

Key Neuromonitoring Findings

Neuroimaging findings of the skull fracture and significant intra- and extra-axial hematoma confirmed significant birth trauma; areas of diffusion restriction likely represented hypoxic-ischemic injury. Initial focal clonic seizures correlated with a pattern suspicious for seizures on aEEG (not shown), but by the time cEEG monitoring was commenced the neonate had received lorazepam and his subsequent seizures were all subclinical. The cEEG tracing initially showed excessive background discontinuity with an inter-burst interval of up to 22 seconds. Subclinical seizures arose from the vertex (Figure C5.2) and independently from the right temporal head region (Figure C5.3).

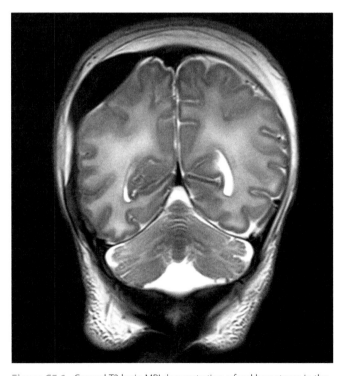

Figure C5.1 Coronal T2 brain MRI demonstrating a focal hematoma in the right parietal region with an intracranial extra-axial, likely epidural, component with overlying extracranial component. The intracranial extra-axial component has some mass effect on the adjacent right parietal lobe.

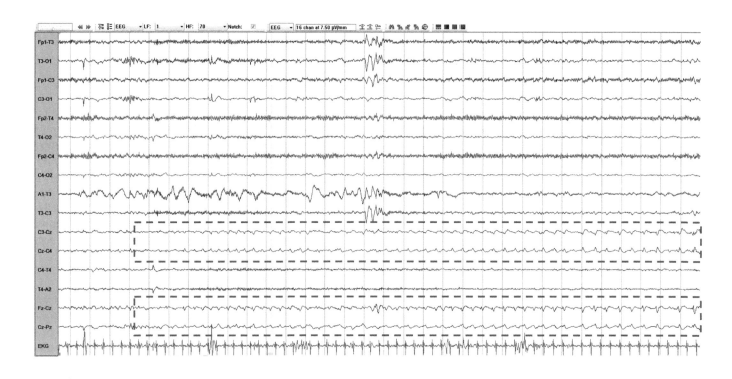

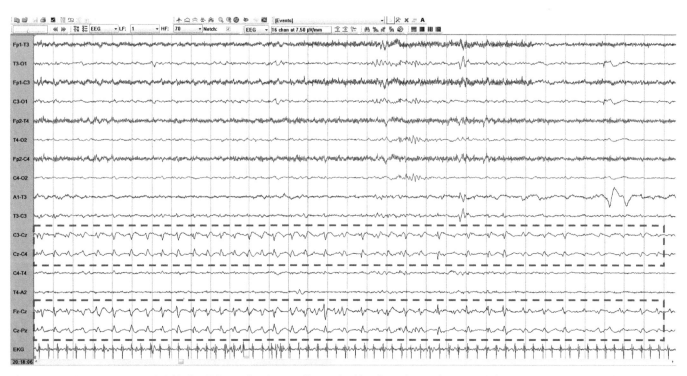

Figure C5.2 Consecutive pages (a & b) of a cEEG recording (neonatal longitudinal bipolar and coronal montages) demonstrating a 1-minute subclinical seizure highlighted in red arising from the vertex at Cz characterized by rhythmic sharp waves at 2 Hertz that evolved in frequency, amplitude, and morphology.

By 24 hours of age the pattern had evolved to discontinuous background with centrotemporal sharp waves suggestive of global cerebral dysfunction with epileptogenic potentials arising from the midline. By 36 hours of age the spikes noted at Cz did not evolve in frequency or amplitude and remained localized.

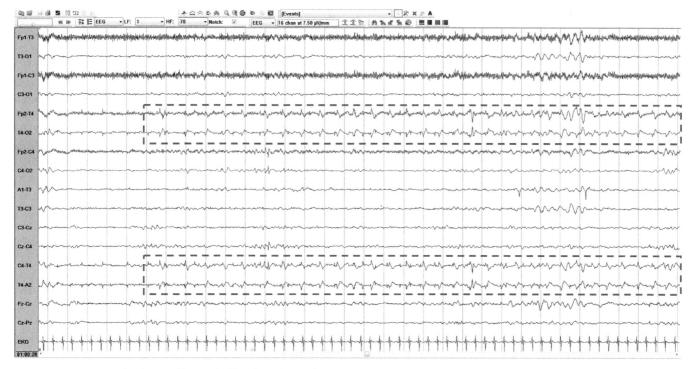

Figure C5.3 cEEG recording (neonatal longitudinal bipolar and coronal montages) demonstrating a subsequent subclinical seizure highlighted in red arising from the right temporal head region at T4 characterized by rhythmic sharp waves at 1 Hertz that evolved in frequency, amplitude, and morphology. Note the positive phase reversal of the sharp waves, which is characteristic of some neonatal seizures.

References

1. Tsuchida TN, Wusthoff CJ, Shellhaas RA, et al. American Clinical Neurophysiology Society standardized EEG terminology and categorization for the description of continuous EEG monitoring in neonates: report of the American Clinical Neurophysiology Society critical care monitoring committee. *J Clin Neurophysiol*. 2013;**30** (2):161–73.

2. Scheibl A, Calderon EM, Borau MJ, et al. Epidural hematoma. *J Pediatr Surg*. 2012;**47**(2):e19–21.

3. Hong HS, Lee JY. Intracranial hemorrhage in term neonates. *Childs Nerv Sys*. 2018;**34**(6): 1135–43.

4. Heyman R, Heckly A, Magagi J, Pladys P, Hamlat A. Intracranial epidural hematoma in newborn infants: clinical study of 15 cases. *Neurosurgery*. 2005;**57**(5):924–9; discussion 9.

Neonatal Intraventricular Hemorrhage

Courtney J. Wusthoff

Clinical Presentation

A neonate was born at 26 weeks and 5 days gestation via emergency caesarian section due to placental abruption. Resuscitation at delivery included 10 minutes of chest compressions. After transfer to a tertiary NICU, admission head ultrasound was normal. On day 3, the patient developed a worsening acidosis; head ultrasound showed bilateral grade 4 intraventricular hemorrhages (IVH), left worse than right. Discovery of grade 4 IVH prompted amplitude-integrated EEG (aEEG) application by the NICU team; at bedside this identified recurrent episodes of abrupt elevation in the activity band with patterns suspicious for seizure on the corresponding EEG. Continuous EEG (cEEG) monitoring was initiated, which confirmed the diagnosis of seizures, all of which were subclinical. Phenobarbital administration resulted in seizure cessation, with cEEG confirming seizure freedom for >48 hours before the recording was stopped. Ventricle size was monitored by serial head ultrasounds; no surgical intervention was required.

One month later, while still in the NICU, the patient suffered necrotizing enterocolitis. The bedside nurse noticed episodes of "increased jitteriness" with mouth opening and closing,

prompting repeat cEEG monitoring. This demonstrated a return of both electroclinical and electrographic-only seizures. Seizures continued despite increased phenobarbital, and also fosphenytoin and levetiracetam. Midazolam infusion was initiated, which controlled seizures. Concurrently, necrotizing enterocolitis was first managed medically, but ultimately surgical bowel resection was required. After returning from surgery, the patient had no further seizures, and midazolam was decreased. Phenytoin was discontinued shortly thereafter. The baby was ultimately discharged to home 4 months later, still on levetiracetam and phenobarbital. Her follow-up plan included ongoing monitoring of ventricle size by neurosurgery, care with neurology for further reduction of seizure medications and management of emerging axial hypotonia with appendicular spasticity, and with high-risk infant developmental follow-up (see Figures C6.1–C6.6).

Discussion

Lloyd and colleagues (2017)[1] conducted a prospective study using cEEG to monitor preterm neonates born <32 weeks; they found seizures in approximately 5% of babies. Intraventricular hemorrhage has long been recognized to increase the risk for seizures in preterm

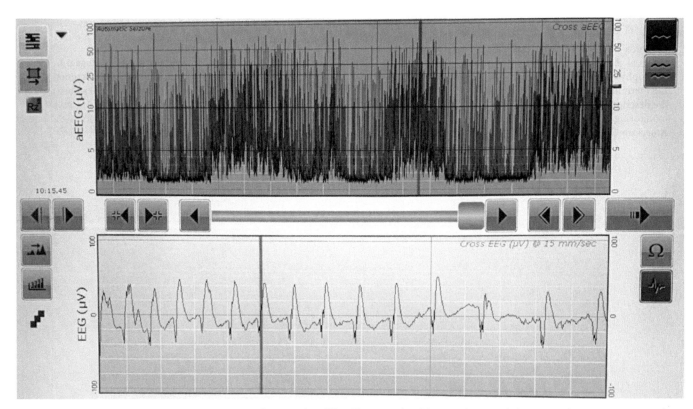

Figure C6.1   aEEG display during screening prior to start of cEEG on day of life 4. The activity band (top panel) is typical of an extremely preterm neonate, with very low amplitudes (lower margin <5 μV) alternating with frequent bursts of much higher amplitude activity (upper margin >50 μV). There are at least two areas in the activity band where the lower margin abruptly increased, suspicious for seizure. The vertical cursor indicates the segment selected for source EEG review in the bottom panel. On EEG, a rhythmic, repetitive pattern of discharges is seen, suspicious for seizure.

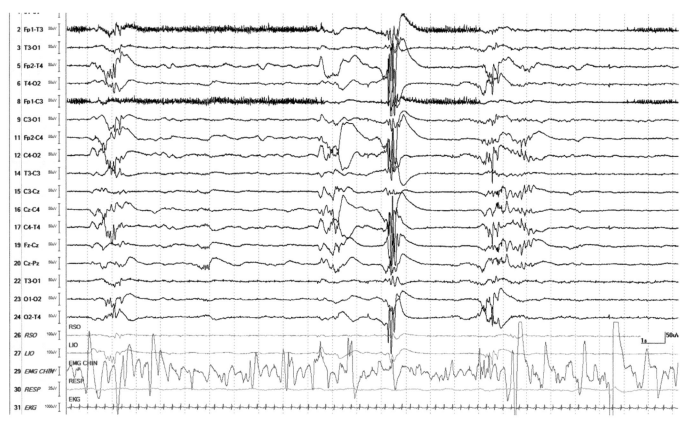

Figure C6.2 Initial EEG background demonstrates the marked discontinuity that is typical of neonates <28 weeks conceptional age. Activity is suppressed with amplitudes <25 μV for several seconds in the inter-burst interval, with activity brief and of much higher amplitude during active bursts lasting only a few seconds. (Sens 7 μV, Tc 0.1, HF 70 Hz, 30 s/page.)

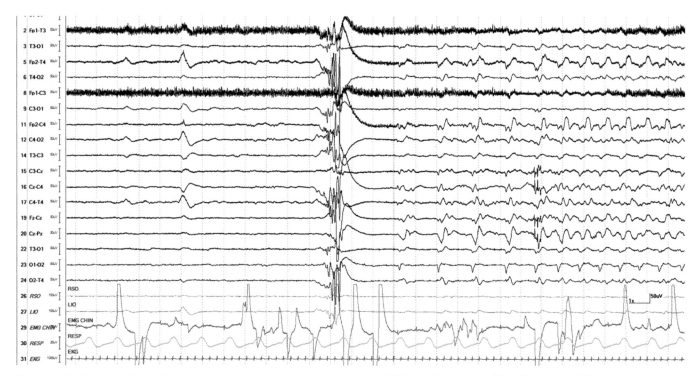

Figure C6.3 Electrographic, subclinical seizures were captured within the first hours of cEEG recording on day of life 4. Here, there is diffuse onset of seizure in the second half of the screen, with slowly repetitive discharges initially of approximately 0.5/second evolving in frequency. (Sens 7 μV, Tc 0.1, HF 70 Hz, 30 s/page.)

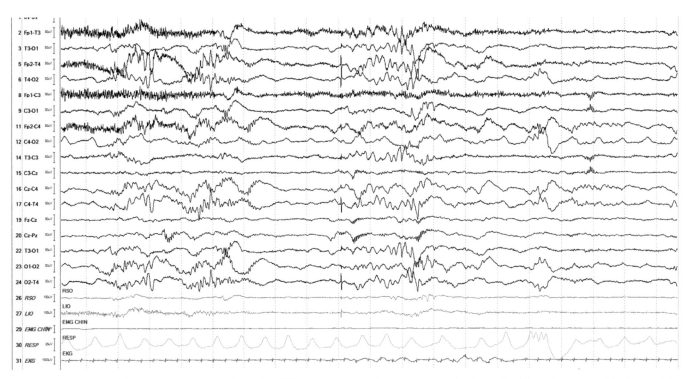

Figure C6.4 One month later, at conceptional age 31 weeks, cEEG shows a more continuous background with sustained faster frequency activity. Note subtle respiratory artifact at O2, corresponding to the respiratory channel (RESP). (Sens 7 μV, Tc 0.1, HF 70 Hz, 20 s/page.)

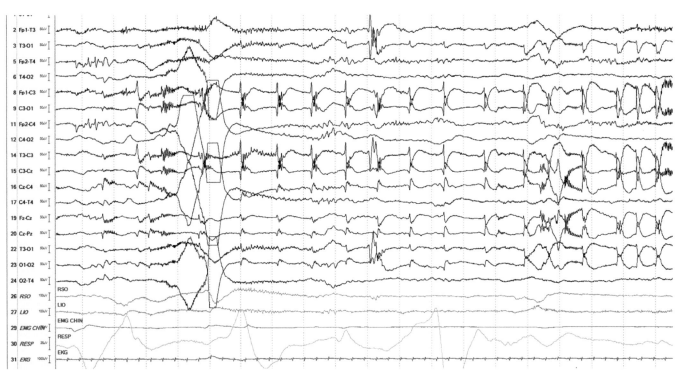

Figure C6.5 During the period of worsened illness with necrotizing enterocolitis, EEG captured recurrent focal seizures at C3/Cz, as shown here. (Sens 10 μV, Tc 0.1, HF 70 Hz, 20 s/page.)

neonates, though there is no consensus whether all preterm neonates with high-grade IVH should undergo EEG screening for seizures. While aEEG may be used as a screening tool, cEEG confirmation of suspected seizures is preferred. Preterm neonates commonly have rhythmic patterns on EEG that are not clearly ictal, making seizure diagnosis with a limited channel recording particularly challenging.

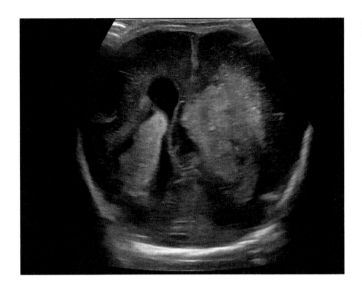

Figure C6.6 Head ultrasound from day 4 (coronal view) showing bilateral intraventricular hemorrhage.

Key Neuromonitoring Findings

Among preterm newborns, IVH is the most common risk factor for seizure. Because IVH most commonly occurs in the first 7 days after birth, the window of greatest risk for seizure extends across this period. For this patient, while there were no clinical events suspicious for seizure, the new, large, bilateral IVH prompted the use of aEEG to screen for seizures. cEEG monitoring confirmed seizures. Similarly, later in the patient's course, she suffered overall decompensation due to necrotizing enterocolitis. At that time, there was a return of seizures, now manifesting with clinical signs.

References

1. Lloyd RO, O'Toole JM, Pavlidis E, Filan PM, Boylan GB. Electrographic seizures during the early postnatal period in preterm infants. *J Pediatr.* 2017 Aug;**187**:18–25.e2. PMID: 28366355.

2. Scher MS, Aso K, Beggarly ME, et al. Electrographic seizures in preterm and full-term neonates: clinical correlates, associated brain lesions, and risk for neurologic sequelae. *Pediatrics.* 1993 Jan;**91**(1):128–34. PMID: 8416475.

3. Weeke LC, van Ooijen IM, Groenendaal F, et al. Rhythmic EEG patterns in extremely preterm infants: classification and association with brain injury and outcome. *Clin Neurophysiol.* 2017 Dec;**128**(12):2428–35. PMID: 29096216; PMCID: PMC5700118.

Neonatal Hypoglycemia

Elana F. Pinchefsky and Emily W. Y. Tam

Clinical Presentation

A full-term baby girl was noted at 60 hours of life to have lethargy, poor feeding, and shaking movements of her arms. The pregnancy and delivery were unremarkable. Birth weight was 2665 grams (below the 10th percentile). Her parents brought her to the emergency department where she was found to be mottled, hypotonic, and hypothermic (temperature 32.1°C). Blood glucose was 0.7 mmol/L (12.6 mg/dL). Blood glucose slowly normalized after two intravenous boluses of normal saline and two intravenous boluses of dextrose. A full septic workup including lumbar puncture was completed. She was started on ampicillin, cefotaxime, and acyclovir. On admission to the neonatal intensive care unit, significant findings on examination were a sunken anterior fontanelle and lethargy. Shortly after admission, the nurse noted a one-minute episode of jerking of the left arm and leg. A glucometer check immediately afterward showed a glucose of 6.5 mmol/L (117 mg/dL). A loading dose of phenobarbital was given and cEEG monitoring was started. Within an hour of commencing the cEEG, there was a short subclinical seizure from the right occipital region. An additional loading dose of phenobarbital was given. She continued to have multiple electrographic seizures, and subsequently a midazolam infusion was required in order to achieve seizure control. Brain MRI on the fifth day of

life revealed cortical and subcortical diffusion restriction in the bilateral parieto-occipital regions (more prominent on the right), and associated axonal swelling in the posterior corpus callosum. Blood and cerebrospinal fluid (CSF) bacterial cultures and herpes simplex virus (HSV) polymerase chain reaction (PCR) test were negative. The endocrine workup (including cortisol level) and newborn screen were normal. She was discharged home on a maintenance dose of phenobarbital. A follow-up EEG performed at 4 months of age was normal and phenobarbital was discontinued. There were no developmental concerns at her clinical follow-up at 12 months of age (Figures C7.1–C7.4).

Discussion

Neonatal hypoglycemia leads to a highly specific pattern of posterior white matter and pulvinar edema on early brain MRI. Consequently, neonatal hypoglycemia can result in cortical blindness, epilepsy, cerebral palsy, and cognitive impairment. Seizures are a common presenting symptom in neonates with profound hypoglycemia; however, the acute effects of blood glucose disturbances on the EEG remain poorly understood. In preterm and term newborns at risk for hypoglycemia, mild neonatal hypoglycemia has been shown to have no effect on amplitude-integrated EEG

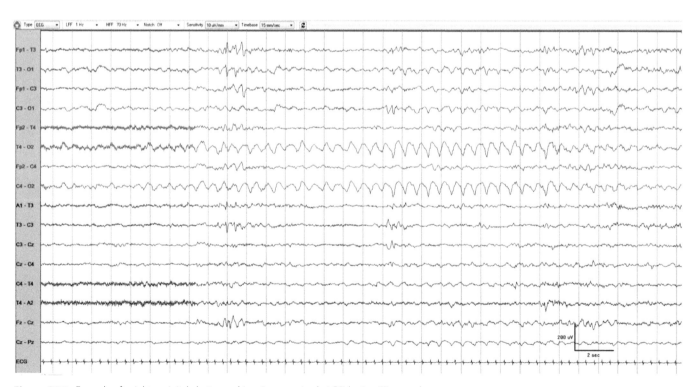

Figure C7.1 Example of a right occipital electrographic seizure maximal at O2, lasting 25 seconds.

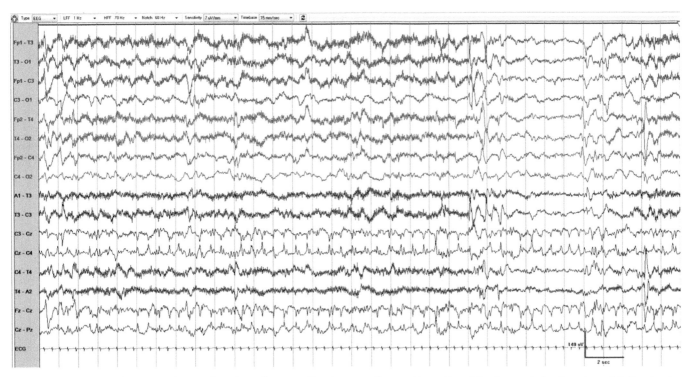

Figure C7.2 Electrographic seizures also arose from the midline central head region as illustrated here, although less frequently than from the occipital head region.

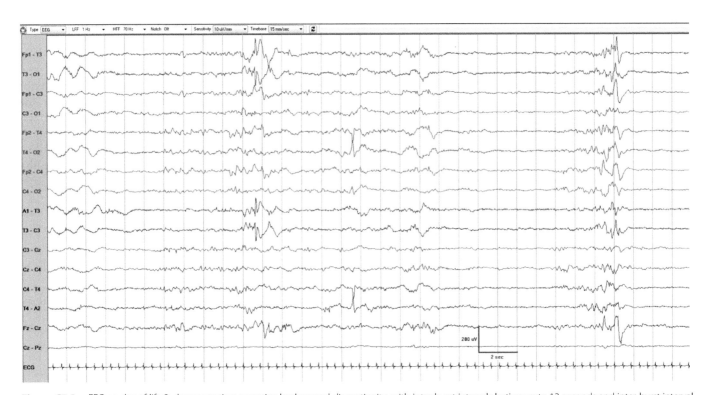

Figure C7.3 cEEG on day of life 3, demonstrating excessive background discontinuity, with inter-burst intervals lasting up to 13 seconds and inter-burst interval amplitude <25 μV. The bursts were occasionally asynchronous. Sharp waves were seen independently at T3 and T4, and also in the central head regions (not demonstrated in this epoch).

background. Epilepsy in children secondary to neonatal hypoglycemia is often focal, most frequently occipital lobe epilepsy associated with parieto-occipital gliosis, and usually has a good prognosis. However, it can occasionally lead to refractory seizures and epileptic encephalopathy, with epileptic spasms, and atonic and tonic seizures

(a) (b)

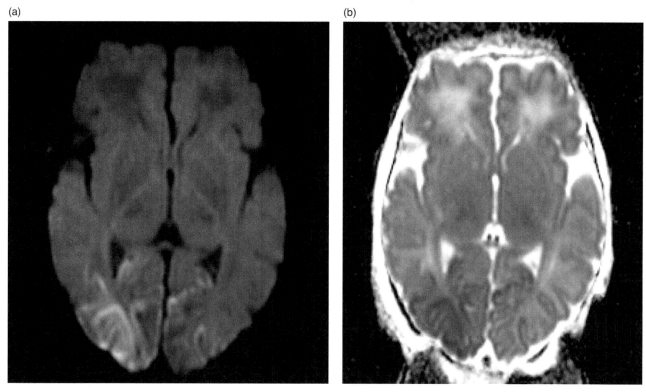

Figure C7.4 Brain MRI on the fifth day of life demonstrating bilateral cortical and subcortical diffusion restriction in the parieto-occipital regions including the (a) axial diffusion weighted image (DWI), and the corresponding (b) apparent diffusion coefficient (ADC) map.

reported. There has not been a clear relationship identified between seizure outcome and the severity, duration, or cause of neonatal hypoglycemia.

Key Neuromonitoring Findings

The EEG background showed excessive discontinuity with inter-burst intervals lasting up to 13 seconds and an inter-burst interval amplitude <25 µV. Frequent sharp waves were seen independently over the bilateral central and temporal head regions. There was frequent semi-rhythmic, non-evolving irregular delta activity noted over the right occipital head region. Multiple electrographic seizures were recorded, mainly arising from the right occipital head region, as well as several over the midline central head region. The background discontinuity improved over the 4 days of recording.

References

1. Wong DS, Poskitt KJ, Chau V, et al. Brain injury patterns in hypoglycemia in neonatal encephalopathy. *Am J Neuroradiol.* 2013;34(7):1456–61.

2. Tam EWY, Widjaja E, Blaser SI, et al. Occipital lobe injury and cortical visual outcomes after neonatal hypoglycemia. *Pediatrics.* 2008;122:507–12.

3. Udani V, Munot P, Ursekar M, Gupta S. Neonatal hypoglycemic brain injury – a common cause of infantile-onset remote symptomatic epilepsy. *Indian J Pediatr.* 2009;46:127–32.

4. Duvanel CB, Fawer CL, Cotting J, Hohlfeld P, Matthieu JM. Long-term effects of neonatal hypoglycemia on brain growth and psychomotor development in small-for-gestational-age preterm infants. *J Pediatr.* 1999;134:492–8.

5. Harris DL, Weston PJ, Williams CE, et al. Cot-side electroencephalography monitoring is not clinically useful in the detection of mild neonatal hypoglycemia. *J Pediatr.* 2011;159(5):755–60.

6. Caraballo RH, Sakr D, Mozzi M, et al. Symptomatic occipital lobe epilepsy following neonatal hypoglycemia. *Pediatr Neurol.* 2004;31(1):24–9.

7. Fong CY, Harvey AS. Variable outcome for epilepsy after neonatal hypoglycaemia. *Dev Med Child Neurol.* 2014;56(11):1093–9.

8. Montassir H, Maegaki Y, Ohno K, Ogura K. Long term prognosis of symptomatic occipital lobe epilepsy secondary to neonatal hypoglycemia. *Epilepsy Res.* 2010;88(2–3):93–9.

Acute Bilirubin Encephalopathy

Shavonne L. Massey and Courtney J. Wusthoff

Clinical Presentation

A 2700 g boy was born to a 26-year-old primigravid mother. An uneventful labor was followed by normal spontaneous vaginal delivery, with Apgar scores of 8 and 9. The baby was discharged home with his family on the day after birth with a plan for routine follow-up. On day 5, the patient was sent to the emergency room by his pediatrician for lethargy and poor feeding. He had presented for his well-baby check-up that morning, with parents reporting that despite attempts to breastfeed, the baby seemed too sleepy to feed over the prior day. The baby was visibly jaundiced and sent immediately for admission. A serum total bilirubin level in the emergency room was 34 mg/dL. The patient was admitted to the NICU for phototherapy and exchange transfusion.

Upon arrival in the NICU, the patient was noted to be lethargic, with a high-pitched cry only with stimulation. He was hypertonic with stiff, arched posturing. Exchange transfusion was initiated. Peripheral blood smear showed hemolytic anemia with a negative direct antiglobulin test. Subsequent quantitative testing showed abnormal glucose-6-phosphtate dehydrogenase activity, confirming G6PD deficiency. Given ongoing encephalopathy, cEEG monitoring was initiated. EEG showed frequent multifocal spikes with excessive background discontinuity. Posturing and arching episodes had no ictal correlate on EEG. Approximately 12 hours into the recording, subclinical seizures were captured. These responded to a phenobarbital loading dose of 20 mg/kg. Maintenance dosing was continued for an additional week, then discontinued. MRI demonstrated characteristic abnormal signal in the basal ganglia (Figure C8.1). Over the following week, the patient became less lethargic and by the time of hospital discharge was bottle feeding well. A hearing screen was abnormal; audiology follow-up for further evaluation was arranged. At hospital discharge, there remained a jerky quality to the baby's general movements; follow-up with neurology was scheduled for age 4 weeks.

Discussion

Acute bilirubin encephalopathy reflects abnormal brain function in a newborn with severe hyperbilirubinemia. The long-term sequelae of acute bilirubin encephalopathy are often termed kernicterus, and can include epilepsy, hearing impairment, visual impairment, and athetoid cerebral palsy. Acute bilirubin encephalopathy is rare in high-resource settings, but does occur. Among term and near-term infants, the underlying cause is often hemolysis, sepsis, and/or dehydration. G6PD deficiency is a common cause of severe hyperbilirubinemia which develops 3–5 days after birth. In moderate acute bilirubin encephalopathy, lethargy and

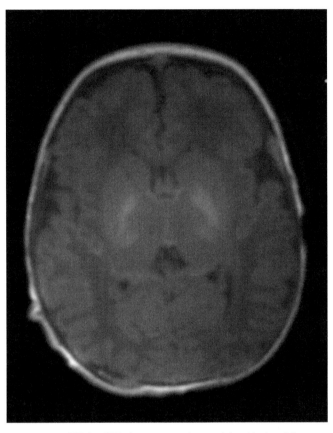

Figure C8.1 MRI (axial T1) demonstrates abnormal signal in the globus pallidus bilaterally.

opisthotonos with retrocollis may be observed. Distinguishing these abnormal movements from seizures is necessary to select appropriate treatment. Similarly, twitching, jerky movements are common but do not always represent seizures. cEEG is useful for acute management to distinguish these seizure mimics while also identifying subtle or subclinical seizures.

Key Neuromonitoring Findings

In this case, the initial EEG background confirmed acute encephalopathy, manifesting as an excessively discontinuous background activity (Figure C8.2). An increased risk of seizures was indicated by the presence of frequent sharp waves occurring in runs (Figure C8.3). While for this neonate abnormal posturing was not associated with seizures on EEG, there were separate subclinical seizures, arising in the left temporal region (Figure C8.4).

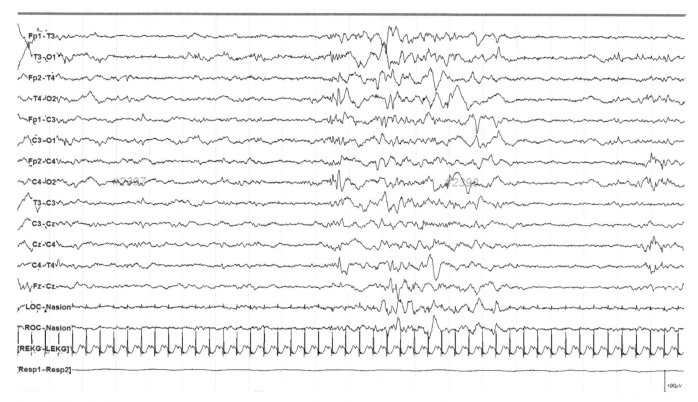

Figure C8.2 Initial EEG background was excessively discontinuous, with inter-burst intervals greater than 8 seconds separating active segments lasting a few seconds each.

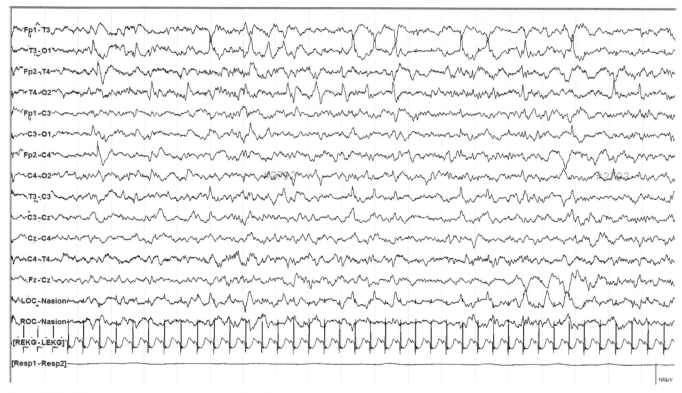

Figure C8.3 EEG background in the first hours of recording showed frequent negative sharp waves, clustered in runs independently in the left and right temporal regions, indicating an increased risk for seizures.

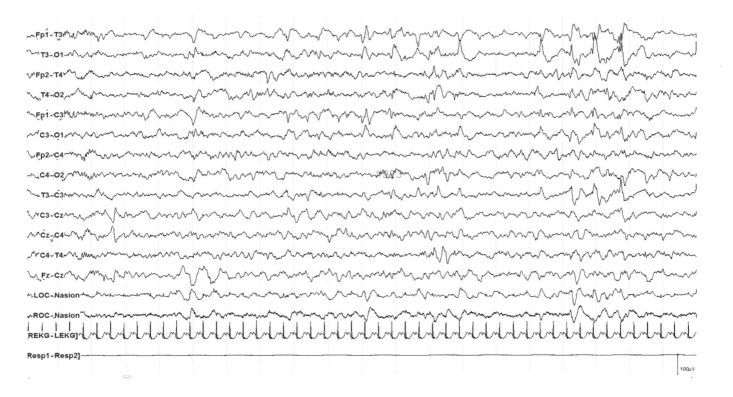

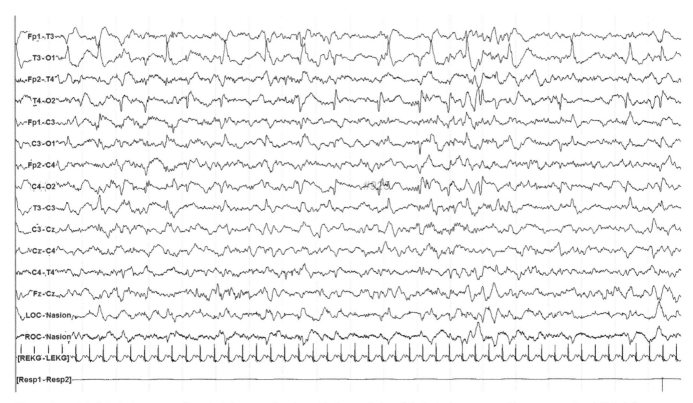

Figure C8.4 Subclinical seizures arose from the left temporal region, with slow evolution of rhythmic sharp waves without any associated clinical change.

References

1. AlOtaibi SF, Blaser S, MacGregor DL. Neurological complications of kernicterus. Can J *Neurol Sci.* 2005 Aug;32(3): 311–15.

2. Gourley GR. Bilirubin metabolism and kernicterus. *Adv Pediatr.* 1997; 44:173–229.

KCNQ2-Related Seizures

Courtney J. Wusthoff

Clinical Presentation

A term-born infant with normal spontaneous delivery following uncomplicated pregnancy presents to the local ER on day of life 4. He had been home for two days. After an initial period of good feeding and alertness, on the day of admission he had two episodes of jerking and trembling movements lasting about one minute each, followed by "sleepiness." In the ER, three additional episodes were observed, prompting administration of phenobarbital 20 mg/kg and admission to the NICU. On arrival in the NICU, the patient was drowsy but arousable. There were no focal abnormalities on neuro exam. Glucose and electrolytes were normal. Continuous EEG monitoring was initiated. Initial EEG background showed only mild discontinuity, which improved over time. While there were no further clinical episodes in the night of admission, after approximately 20 hours of monitoring the patient had a confirmed electroclinical seizure, characterized by tonic stiffening of both arms followed by clonic jerks. Four such seizures were confirmed on EEG over the course of the day, prompting administration of additional phenobarbital, levetiracetam, and phenytoin. This resulted in a decrease in seizure duration and frequency, but not complete seizure resolution. Head ultrasound and brain MRI were normal.

On hospital day 5, at age 9 days, the patient's father provided additional history that he had seizures as an infant himself – he only learned of this from his family when discussing the patient's admission. Genetic testing for neonatal onset epilepsy was sent. The patient was transitioned to oral oxcarbazepine. Additional events of various clinical movements were identified by parents as possible seizures – these were shown on EEG to be non-epileptic. Review of video with parents helped in distinguishing features of electroclinical seizures from other movements. After an additional 5 days, the patient had seizures controlled for at least 3 days, and showed improved alertness with ability to take oral feeds. He was discharged to outpatient care. Three weeks after hospital discharge, genetic results returned showing a pathogenic mutation in *KCNQ2*. He continued on oral oxcarbazepine for 12 months, during which time he had occasional breakthrough seizures, but ultimately remission of epilepsy, and normal development at last follow-up at age 4 years.

Discussion

KCNQ2 mutations are the most common genetic cause of neonatal seizures. The gene *KCNQ2* encodes a voltage-gated potassium channel expressed in neurons. This gene is highly expressed in fetal and newborn brain, then less so later in life. A spectrum of phenotypes has been described in association with *KCNQ2* mutations. Some patients have a clinical syndrome characterized as benign familial neonatal epilepsy, further characterized by a relatively normal interictal EEG but frequent

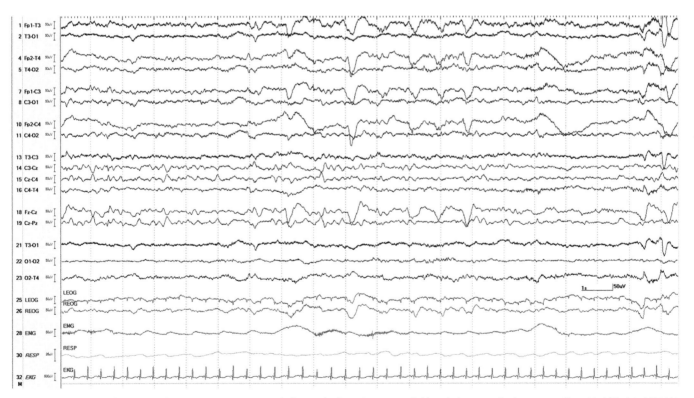

Figure C9.1   Initial awake EEG on admission was continuous and of normal voltage. It was remarkable only for excess Cz sharp waves. (Sens 10 μV, Tc 0.1s, HF 70 Hz, 20s per page.)

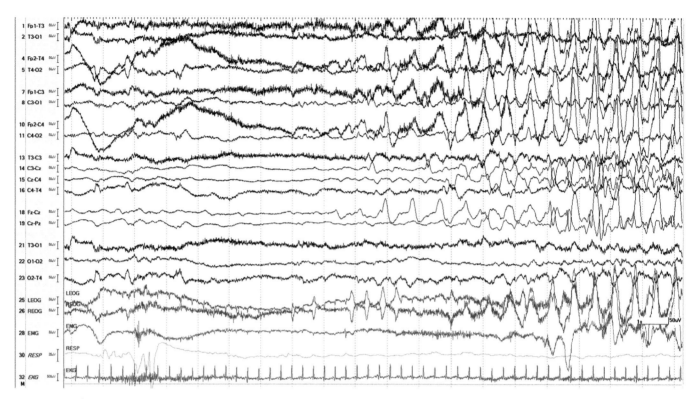

Figure C9.2 The patient's electroclinical seizures were highly stereotyped. These began with EEG attenuation corresponding to tonic stiffening, followed by evolution of high-amplitude central sharp waves and rapid spread across both hemispheres, accompanied by clinical clonic jerks of the extremities. (Sens 10 μV, Tc 0.1s, HF 70 Hz, 20s per page.)

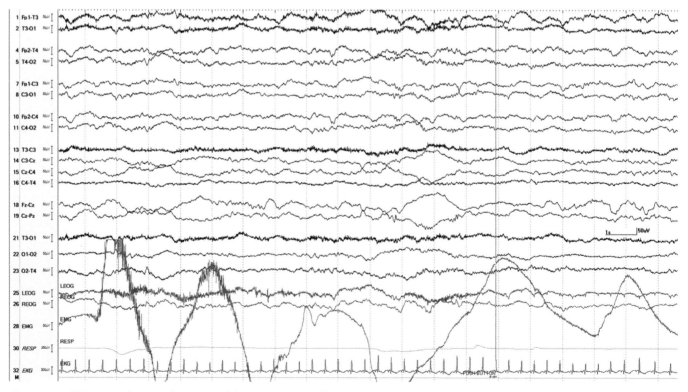

Figure C9.3 EEG segment during a subsequent push button patient event for lip smacking and body movement. There is no corresponding change in the EEG; this event was not seizure. (Sens 10 μV, Tc 0.1s, HF 70 Hz, 20s per page.)

electroclinical seizures beginning in the first few days of birth. Other patients are more severely affected, with neonatal onset epileptic encephalopathy and frequent refractory seizures. EEG monitoring is helpful to distinguish epileptic encephalopathy from isolated seizures, and to guide seizure treatment.

Key Neuromonitoring Findings

Patients with benign familial neonatal epilepsy due to *KCNQ2* mutations characteristically have frequent seizures with normal EEG background in the interictal period. In this patient, initial mild discontinuity likely reflected effects of phenobarbital administration. Early EEG was continuous, though with excess focal sharp waves (Figure C9.1). Clinical seizures were highly stereotyped, with corresponding EEG signature (Figure C9.2). Video EEG was additionally helpful in this case for clarifying which events were *not* seizures (Figure C9.3). After the initial diagnosis of seizures, raising caregiver concern, a number of push button events for various movements followed. These were proven not to be seizure on EEG; review of the corresponding video with parents was helpful in reassuring them of features they could use to identify their baby's electroclinical seizures.

References

1. Allen NM, Mannion M, Conroy J, et al. The variable phenotypes of KCNQ-related epilepsy. *Epilepsia*. 2014 Sep;**55**(9):e99–105. PMID: 25052858.

2. Pisano T, Numis AL, Heavin SB, et al. Early and effective treatment of KCNQ2 encephalopathy. *Epilepsia*. 2015 May;**56** (5):685–91. PMID: 25880994.

3. Shellhaas RA, Wusthoff CJ, Tsuchida TN, et al.; Neonatal Seizure Registry. Profile of neonatal epilepsies: Characteristics of a prospective US cohort. *Neurology*. 2017 Aug 29;**89**(9):893–9. PMID: 28733343; PMCID: PMC5577964.

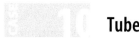

Tuberous Sclerosis

Jonathan D. Santoro and Courtney J. Wusthoff

Clinical Presentation

A term born infant with cardiac rhabdomyoma and asymmetric intrauterine growth restriction (IUGR) diagnosed on 35 week prenatal ultrasound was admitted to the NICU to evaluate signs concerning for tuberous sclerosis (TS). The patient had normal admission neurological and dermatological examinations. There were no clinical events concerning for seizures. A continuous EEG was performed on day of life five as a baseline to assess for epileptiform activity. EEG demonstrated several subclinical seizures arising from the right central region; none had visible correlate on accompanying video. The patient was treated with phenobarbital, which resulted in seizure cessation. MRI of the brain demonstrated numerous bilateral cortical, subcortical, and subependymal foci of abnormal signal, consistent with tubers. The infant was discharged home following cardiac and genetic evaluations in the NICU, with plans in place for outpatient follow-up. The patient was found to have a mosaic deletion in the *TSC2* gene (Figures C10.1–C10.4).

Discussion

Cardiac rhabdomyoma is a common first presenting sign of tuberous sclerosis (TS); it is the most common feature prompting diagnosis in newborns. The majority of children with TS have some degree of cortical dysplasia; most will develop epilepsy at some point in their lives. However, clinical seizures occur in only a small percentage of newborns. It is unknown if this reflects that seizures are truly rare in neonates with TS, or that seizures are difficult to diagnose clinically in the newborn period. Most children with TS will have obvious seizures within the first year. Close neurological follow-up is critical for newborns with TS, as up to a third will develop infantile spasms later in infancy. There is growing interest in the use of regular screening EEG in neonates and infants with TS in order to identify infants and risk of developing seizures and infantile spasms, and create opportunities for possible preemptive therapy.

Key Neuromonitoring Findings

In this case, continuous EEG monitoring was used to assess baseline seizure risk, and identified multiple brief seizures. The seizures were focal in the right central region, though imaging revealed many individual lesions in other areas as well. The background was otherwise continuous and symmetric. Although a brief routine EEG may not have captured the subclinical neonatal seizures, the focal repetitive sharp waves would

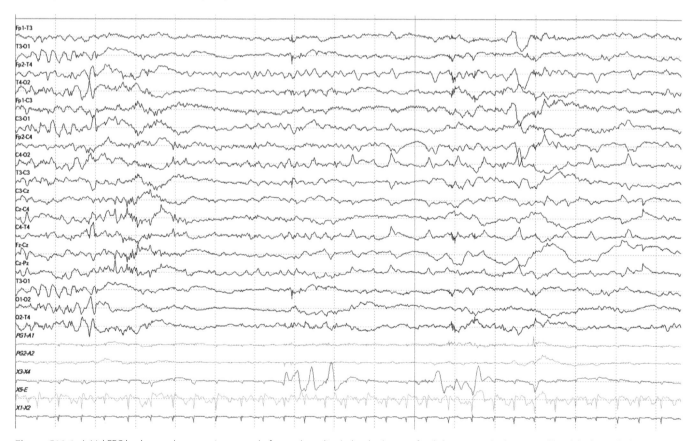

Figure C10.1 Initial EEG background was continuous and of normal amplitude, but had excess focal sharp wave discharges and brief rhythmic discharges in the right central region at C4. (All EEGs displayed with Sens 7μV Tc 0.1s, HF 70 Hz, 20 sec per page.)

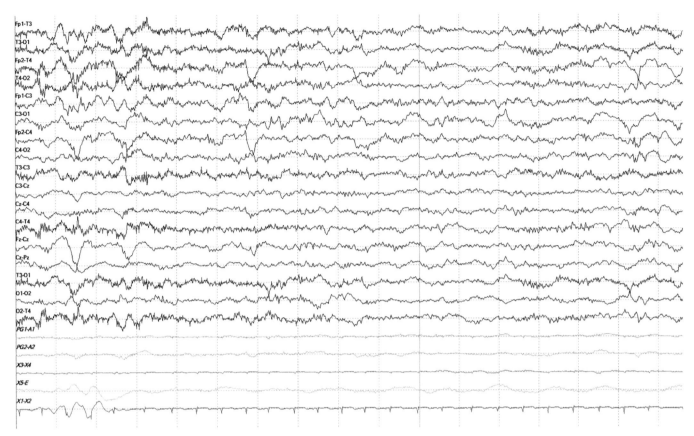

Figure C10.2 Periods of the initial EEG were normal; seizures were not apparent in the first 20 minutes of recording.

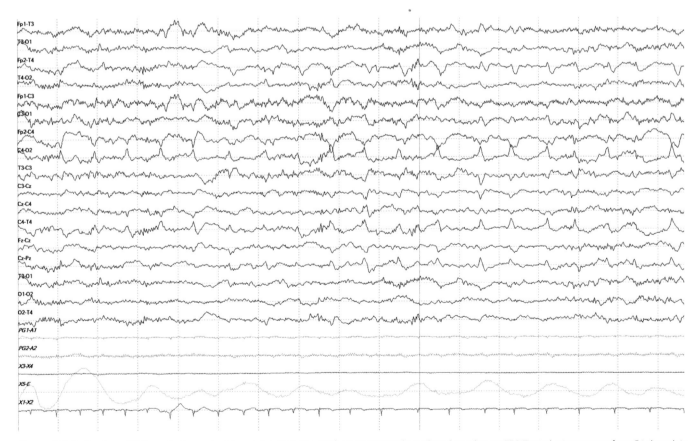

Figure C10.3 Continued EEG monitoring captured many brief (<1 minute) focal seizures without clinical correlate on EEG. Typical seizures arose from C4, though in some instances also involved Cz or T4.

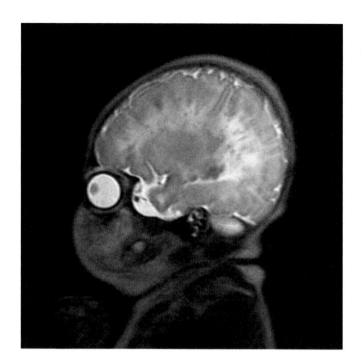

Figure C10.4 MRI on day 2 showed multiple cortical and subcortical tubers, evident on this sagittal view as multiple areas of decreased signal intensity on a T2-weighted sequence.

have been seen, indicating a propensity for seizures and likely prompting close clinical and EEG surveillance during infancy.

References

1. Davis PE, Filip-Dhima R, Sideridis G, et al.; Tuberous Sclerosis Complex Autism Center of Excellence Research Network. Presentation and diagnosis of tuberous sclerosis complex in infants. *Pediatrics*. 2017 Dec;**140**(6):e20164040. PMID: 29101226; PMCID: PMC5703775.

2. Miller SP, Tasch T, Sylvain M, et al. Tuberous sclerosis complex and neonatal seizures. *J Child Neurol*. 1998 Dec;**13**(12):619–23. PMID: 9881532.

3. Datta AN, Hahn CD, Sahin M. Clinical presentation and diagnosis of tuberous sclerosis complex in infancy. *J Child Neurol*. 2008 Mar;**23**(3):268–73. PMID: 18230839.

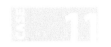

Hemimegalencephaly

Jonathan D. Santoro and Courtney J. Wusthoff

Clinical Presentation

A term born infant presented at two weeks of age for paroxysmal "spells" of repetitive movements. The events lasted up to 20 seconds in duration, consisting of left upper extremity jerks. The parents had initially been advised that these were normal baby movements, but when the events increased in frequency, they brought the baby to the ER for further evaluation. An initial EEG showed background asymmetry, prompting admission for continuous EEG monitoring to capture a typical event. While no clinical events occurred the first evening of monitoring, the EEG background was abnormal, with asymmetry and excess focal sharp waves occurring in runs. Monitoring was therefore continued into a second day. On the second day, brief electroclinical seizures were captured, each lasting up to 30 seconds on EEG, but with accompanying left upper extremity clonic jerks only for the last few seconds. The patient received phenobarbital, resulting in good seizure control. MRI demonstrated asymmetric enlargement of the right cerebrum, particularly in the posterior hemisphere, with cortical thickening of the occipital and temporal lobes, consistent with pachygyria and polymicrogyria.

In the months following presentation, the patient received close follow-up, with EEGs consistently showing nearly continuous sharp waves in the right posterior quadrant. There was no return of clinical seizures, with the patient receiving a combination of levetiracetam and topiramate. The patient had slow developmental progress over the subsequent two years; it was uncertain to what degree this was the result of epileptic encephalopathy. Eventually he underwent a right hemispherotomy at age two years. Following this procedure, the patient experienced a rapid improvement in language, cognition, and milestone acquisition, despite a left hemiparesis (Figures C11.1–C11.3).

Discussion

Hemimegalencephaly is an uncommon malformation of cortical development. It is characterized by an enlarged, dysplastic hemisphere. The condition may be complete, involving the entire hemisphere, or partial, involving only certain lobes. It has been suggested that partial hemimegalencephaly may fall on a spectrum with multilobar cortical dysplasia. Hemimegalencephaly has been reported in a number of syndromes of abnormal cell proliferation, including neurocutaneous syndromes. Hemimegalencephaly can also be an isolated finding. Most patients present with refractory seizures in infancy; epileptic encephalopathy has also been reported. Case series have suggested that early hemispherotomy may be associated with better developmental outcomes and higher rates of seizure freedom.

Key Neuromonitoring Findings

Hemimegalencephaly typically presents early in infancy with frequent seizures. In this case, the clinical events

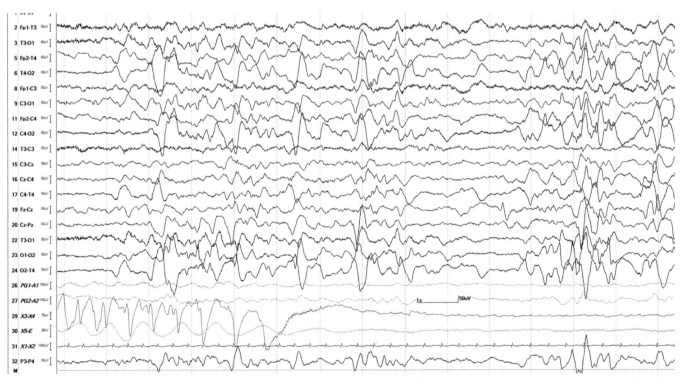

Figure C11.1 The first evening of EEG did not capture typical clinical events, but demonstrated frequent, high-amplitude right posterior quadrant epileptiform discharges. (Sens 10 µV, Tc 0.1 s, HF 70 Hz, 15 s per page.)

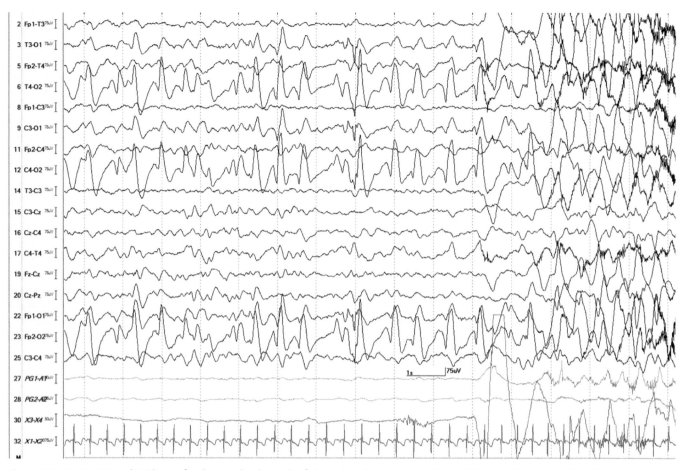

Figure C11.2 Approximately 12 hours after the recording began, brief electroclinical seizures were observed. These each lasted less than 30 seconds, and were characterized by gradually increasing frequency of right posterior quadrant discharges, culminating in left upper extremity clonic jerks. (Sens 10 µV, Tc 0.1 s, HF 70 Hz, 15 s per page.)

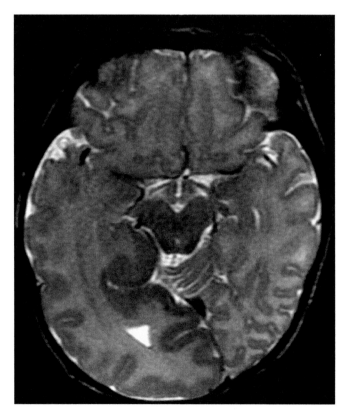

Figure C11.3 Axial view of T2 MRI demonstrating right hemimegalencephaly, most prominent in the posterior quadrant.

were not witnessed in the emergency room, but the very abnormal EEG prompted further monitoring. An asymmetric EEG background is characteristic of hemimegalencephaly. Some neonates will have frequent epileptiform discharges in the affected hemisphere; others will have a suppression burst background pattern. In this case, there were both runs of sharp waves in the right central region and frequent right occipital epileptiform discharges. While these only rarely evolved into seizures, an early hemispherotomy was pursued given the persistence of near-continuous epileptiform discharges in the setting of developmental impairment.

References

1. Flores-Sarnat L. Hemimegalencephaly: part 1. Genetic, clinical, and imaging aspects. *J Child Neurol*. 2002 May;**17**(5):373–84. PMID: 12150586.

2. D'Agostino MD, Bastos A, Piras C, et al. Posterior quadrantic dysplasia or hemi-hemimegalencephaly: a characteristic brain malformation. *Neurology*. 2004 Jun 22;**62**(12):2214–20. PMID: 15210885.

3. Di Rocco C, Battaglia D, Pietrini D, Piastra M, Massimi L. Hemimegalencephaly: clinical implications and surgical treatment. *Childs Nerv Syst*. 2006 Aug;**22**(8):852–66. PMID: 16821075.

4. Honda R, Kaido T, Sugai K, et al. Long-term developmental outcome after early hemispherotomy for hemimegalencephaly in infants with epileptic encephalopathy. *Epilepsy Behav*. 2013 Oct;**29**(1):30–5. PMID: 23933627.

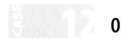

Ohtahara Syndrome

Carlos I. Salazar and Cecil D. Hahn

Clinical Presentation

A term newborn female presented on day 5 of life with unusual movements. Family history was negative for epilepsy. The pregnancy and delivery were uncomplicated. The episodes of concern were first observed by the parents on day 2 of life, described as sudden head and eye deviation to the left, mouthing, generalized body stiffening, and either flexion or extension of the arms, lasting less than 1 minute. The baby was also lethargic, needed to be woken up for feeding, and lost 13% of her birth weight in 5 days. She was admitted to the NICU for neurological assessment and management of suspected seizures. She received a loading dose of phenobarbital and then maintenance therapy. Conventional video-EEG monitoring showed a burst suppression background pattern and captured the clinical events, which were confirmed to represent seizures. Infectious and metabolic workups and brain MRI were unremarkable. Despite therapy, the seizures persisted with tonic head deviation, right hemifacial spasms, and tonic extension of the limbs. Pyridoxine was started by day of life 7, associated with a partial improvement in seizures. She had further clusters of seizures at age 4 weeks of life in the context of necrotizing enterocolitis, and levetiracetam was added. She continued to have daily brief self-resolving seizures so topiramate was added by age 6 weeks. At age 8 weeks, she remained hypotonic, required feeding by nasogastric tube, and was also started on vigabatrin in the context of hypsarrhythmia seen in a follow-up EEG. An epilepsy gene panel subsequently revealed a *KCNQ2* gene mutation. Treatment was adjusted and sodium-channel blocking medications were added, with a loading dose of IV fosphenytoin followed by oral carbamazepine therapy, with significant improvement in seizure control (Figures C12.1–C12.2).

Discussion

Ohtahara syndrome, also known as early infantile epileptic encephalopathy (EIEE), is characterized by severe recurrent seizures and encephalopathy beginning in the first weeks of life (from the neonatal period to up to age 3 months). The classic seizure semiology is tonic spasms, occurring either in isolation or in clusters, with either symmetric or asymmetric tonic posturing. Focal motor seizures may also be present. Ohtahara syndrome is caused primarily by structural brain lesions (dysgenetic or encephaloclastic), but may also be caused by mutations in genes such as *STXBP1*, *KCNQ2*, and *ARX*. *KCNQ2* encephalopathy has a broad phenotypic spectrum, from benign familial neonatal epilepsy (BFNE), which responds well to treatment and is associated with normal outcomes, to a neonatal epileptic encephalopathy with recurrent seizures, neurological impairment, and overall poor prognosis with profound developmental delay. Patients with *KCNQ2* encephalopathy may present with an electroclinical phenotype

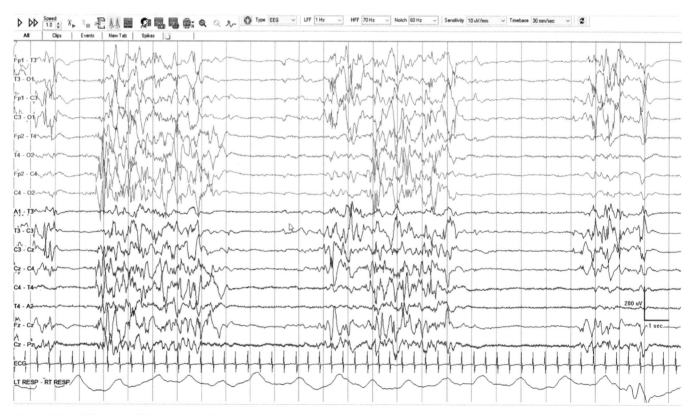

Figure C12.1 EEG on day of life 7 demonstrating a burst suppression background pattern with the bursts containing multifocal high-amplitude sharp waves. Neonatal montage. LFF = 1 Hz, HFF = 70 Hz, Sensitivity 10 μV/mm, Time base 10 mm/second.

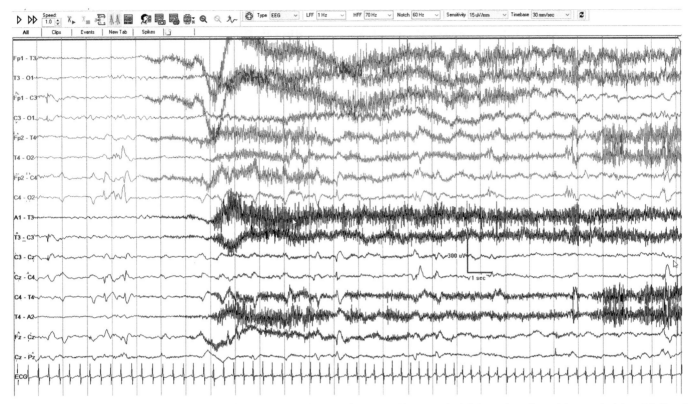

Figure C12.2 EEG on day of life 7 demonstrating a focal electroclinical seizure characterized by onset of subtle low-voltage fast activity over the left occipital head region, followed by diffuse muscle artifact associated with asymmetric tonic posturing. Neonatal montage. LFF = 1 Hz, HFF = 70 Hz, Sensitivity 15 μV/mm, Time base 10 mm/second.

resembling either Ohtahara syndrome or early myoclonic encephalopathy (EME). Sodium channel blockers, particularly carbamazepine, have been shown to be particularly effective in patients with *KCNQ2* encephalopathy, resulting in a successful reduction of seizures and even seizure freedom.

Key Neuromonitoring Findings

The classic EEG feature of Ohtahara syndrome is a burst suppression background pattern that persists during the awake and sleep states, characterized by high-voltage bursts. Over the first weeks to months of life, this pattern commonly evolves into hypsarrhythmia, and infantile spasms may ensue. In *KCNQ2* encephalopathies, background EEG patterns described include burst suppression and multifocal epileptiform activity, and seizures are characterized by unilateral hemispheric onset with low-voltage fast activity followed by either voltage attenuation or focal spike and wave complexes.

References

1. Abend N, Jensen F, Inder T, Volpe J. Neonatal seizures. In Volpe J, Inder T, Darras B, et al., editors. *Volpe's Neurology of the Newborn*, 6th ed. Philadelphia: Elsevier; 2018, pp. 275–321.

2. Cilio MR Neonatal epilepsies and epileptic encephalopathies. In Nagarajan L, editor. *Neonatal Seizures: Current Management, Future Challenges*. London: Mac Keith Press; 2016, pp. 100–13.

3. Beal JC, Cherian K, Moshe SL. Early-onset epileptic encephalopathies: Ohtahara syndrome and early myoclonic encephalopathy. *Pediatr Neurol*. 2012 Nov;47(5):317–23.

4. Kim HJ, Yang D, Kim SH, et al. Clinical characteristics of KCNQ2 encephalopathy. *Brain Dev*. 2021 Feb;43(2): 244–50.

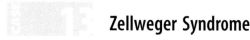

Zellweger Syndrome

Elena Pavlidis, Andreea M. Pavel, and Geraldine B. Boylan

Clinical Presentation

A baby boy was born at term (39+3 weeks) by vaginal delivery, birth weight 2.95 kg (9th centile) and head circumference 34 cm (25th centile). The baby had poor respiratory effort, HR 80–90 bpm, and poor tone and required positive pressure ventilation. Apgar scores were 1, 6, and 7 at the first, fifth, and tenth minutes, respectively. He was born to a 32-year-old, G2P1, with well-controlled gestational diabetes. The pregnancy was notable for polyhydramnios. The parents were first cousins.

On the basis of a poor initial blood gas (pH 6.97, BE –10.4, lactate 7.2), low Apgar scores, hypotonia, lethargy, weak suck, and suspected clinical seizures, he was commenced on therapeutic hypothermia at 3 hours of age for a duration of 72 hours. He received a loading dose of phenobarbital (20 mg/kg). Dysmorphic features were noted: up-slanting palpebral fissures, hypertelorism, a broad nasal bridge, bilateral single palmar creases, and a sandal gap. Due to difficulties with oxygenation, he was intubated and ventilated.

EEG started at 4 hours of age revealed a severely abnormal background pattern, with no sleep–wake cycling (Figure C13.1). Brief electrographic seizures started at 46 hours of age, subsequently increasing in frequency and duration (Figure C13.2). Two additional loading doses of phenobarbitone (10 mg/kg

each) were administered and seizures stopped a few hours later. However, seizures reappeared with a similar pattern on day of life 8, and phenobarbital treatment was recommenced.

Cerebral ultrasound scan showed lenticulostriate vascular hyperechogenicity, a mild increase of white matter hyperechogenicity, and cava septum pellucidum and vergae. Brain MRI showed bilateral perisylvian polymicrogyria, further possible areas of polymicrogyria in the frontal regions (Figure C13.3), and normal spectroscopy.

Karyotype and microarray were normal. A full metabolic screen showed increased levels of alanine, proline, glutamine, and very long chain fatty acids (VLCFA).

Despite intensive care, he remained unstable and on day of life 11 care was redirected and the infant died. Zellweger syndrome, suspected because of clinical, neuroimaging, and laboratory findings, was confirmed postmortem by the presence of a pathogenic variant of *PEX12* gene on chromosome 17.

Discussion

Zellweger syndrome is the most severe condition in the group of peroxisomal biogenesis disorders [1, 2]. It is an autosomal recessive disorder caused by defects in one of several *PEX* genes [1, 2]. It usually manifests in the neonatal period with characteristic craniofacial dysmorphic features, hypotonia, hepatic

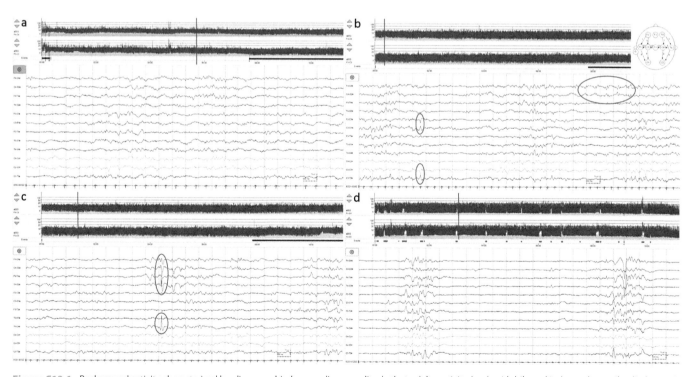

Figure C13.1 Background activity characterized by oligomorphic, low-medium amplitude theta-delta activity (a–c), with bilateral independent spike discharges in the centro-temporal regions [red circles] (b–c). Periods of burst suppression were also evident (d). The time-point of the corresponding aEEG is indicated with a red line; red bars below the aEEG in (d) indicate the seizures. (Sensitivity: 70 µV; high-frequency filter: 70 Hz; low-frequency filter: 0.5 Hz; time base: 15 mm/sec; montage depicted at top right.)

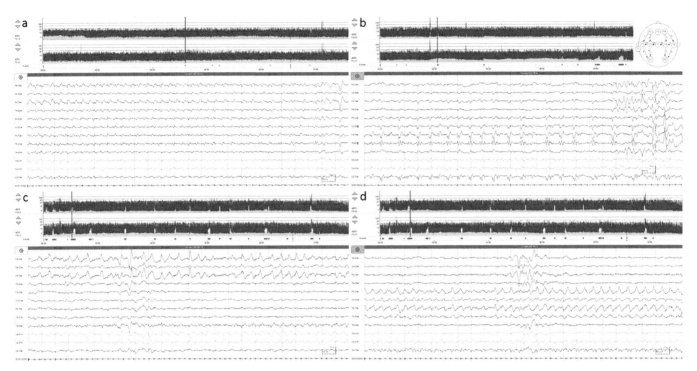

Figure C13.2 Seizures always had a focal onset in frontal or centro-temporal regions, sometimes starting in one hemisphere (c) and then moving to the contralateral hemisphere (d). The time-point of the corresponding aEEG is indicated with a red line (a, b, d); red bars below the aEEG represent the seizures) (Sensitivity: 70 μV; high-frequency filter: 70 Hz; low-frequency filter: 0.5 Hz; time base: 15 mm/sec; montage depicted at top right.)

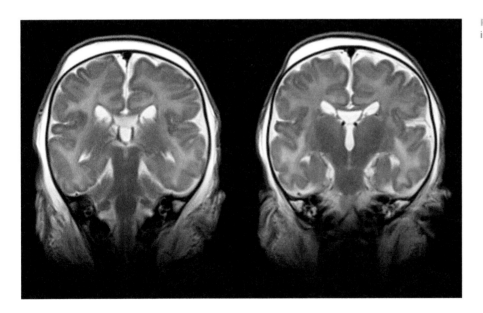

Figure C13.3 T2-weighted coronal brain MR images showing bilateral perisylvian polymicrogyria.

dysfunction (with subsequent prolonged jaundice and poor feeding), and often seizures [2, 3]. An accumulation of VLCFA is typically found in blood plasma [1–3].

Key Neuromonitoring Findings
Neuronal migration defects are common in Zellweger spectrum disorders. Neuroimaging typically detects cortical gyral abnormalities (such as perisylvian polymicrogyria and pachygyria), or generalized or focal leukoencephalopathy [1–3]. The functional correlate of this is evident on EEG. Seizures starting in the neonatal period are common [1–3]. Negative sharp waves and spikes over the Rolandic regions, with phase reversal at the vertex, have been reported [4,5].

Elena Pavlidis, Andreea M. Pavel, and Geraldine B. Boylan

References

1. Klouwer FC, Berendse K, Ferdinandusse S, et al. Zellweger spectrum disorders: clinical overview and management approach. *Orphanet J Rare Dis.* 2015;**10**:151.

2. Braverman NE, Raymond GV, Rizzo WB, et al. Peroxisome biogenesis disorders in the Zellweger spectrum: an overview of current diagnosis, clinical manifestations, and treatment guidelines. *Mol Genet Metab.* 2016 Mar;**117**(3):313–21.

3. Lee PR, Raymond GV. Child neurology: Zellweger syndrome. *Neurology.* 2013;**80**(20):e207–10.

4. Govaerts L, Colon E, Rotteveel J, Monnens L. A neurophysiological study of children with the cerebro-hepato-renal syndrome of Zellweger. *Neuropediatrics.* 1985;**16**(4):185–90.

5. Panjan DP, Meglic NP, Neubauer D. A case of Zellweger syndrome with extensive MRI abnormalities and unusual EEG findings. *Clin Electroencephalogr.* 2001;**32**(1):28–31.

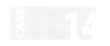

Pyridoxine-Dependent Epilepsy

Saadet Mercimek-Andrews and Cecil D. Hahn

Clinical Presentation

A newborn boy with a history of progressive bilateral asymmetrical severe ventriculomegaly on serial prenatal head ultrasounds was admitted to the neonatal intensive care unit for evaluation and monitoring following delivery. A postnatal head ultrasound and brain MRI showed bilateral asymmetric dilation of the lateral ventricles with bilateral large subependymal cysts at 4 days of age. He had poor feeding, vomiting, and hyponatremia (Na 127; reference range 133–142 mmol/L) at age 4 days.

Clusters of multifocal clonic seizures started at age 7 days, which were successfully treated with lorazepam and phenobarbital. He remained seizure free on phenobarbital monotherapy until 17 days of age, when he had four generalized tonic-clonic seizures lasting 5 to 10 seconds responding to lorazepam. At age 18 days, he had lip smacking and eye rolling. At age 19 days, he had multiple generalized tonic-clonic seizures lasting 15 to 30 seconds, consistent with status epilepticus, for which he was treated with phenytoin, lorazepam, and midazolam (5 mcg/kg/min). Levetiracetam and pyridoxine (14 mg/kg/

day) were added at age 21 days. Midazolam was weaned off at age 24 days. He had no further seizures. Investigations for infectious and acute metabolic causes were normal. He was discharged home at age 30 days on phenobarbital, levetiracetam, and pyridoxine therapy.

Because of his treatment-refractory neonatal seizures, he underwent extensive metabolic investigations. He was found to have elevated urine α-aminoadipic acid semialdehyde (α-AASA), suggesting a diagnosis of pyridoxine-dependent epilepsy. Subsequent genetic evaluation at age 3 months revealed compound heterozygous likely pathogenic variants in *ALDH7A1*, confirming the diagnosis of pyridoxine-dependent epilepsy (Figures C14.1–C14.2).

Discussion

Pyridoxine-dependent epilepsy due to mutations in *ALDH7A1* is an autosomal recessively inherited disease of lysine catabolism. The majority of patients present with neonatal onset seizures, usually not responsive to anti-seizure medications. The treatment consists of pyridoxine, a lysine-restricted diet,

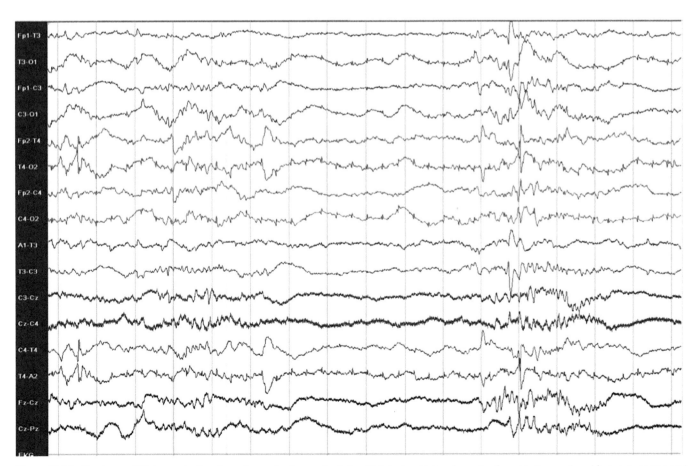

Figure C14.1   Continuous EEG demonstrating discontinuous background activity with inter-burst intervals ranging from 4 to 6 seconds and frequent negative and positive sharp waves over the bilateral centrotemporal head regions.

245

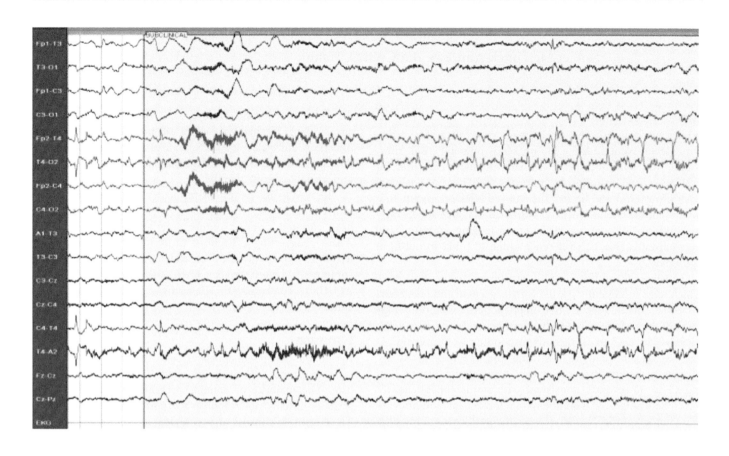

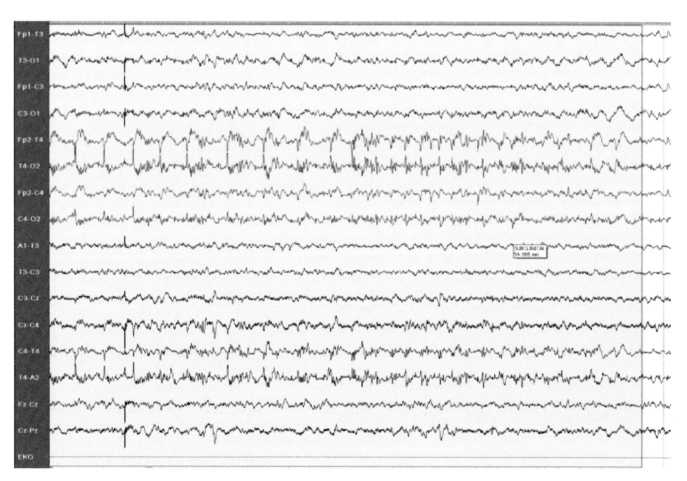

Figure C14.2   (a, continued in b) Continuous EEG demonstrating a typical subclinical seizure lasting 54 seconds consisting of rhythmic spike wave discharges arising from the right temporal head region (T4) evolving in frequency, amplitude, and morphology.

and arginine. More than 90% of patients are seizure free on pyridoxine monotherapy. Initiation of a lysine-restricted diet and arginine in the early infantile period improves neurodevelopmental outcome and cognitive function.

White matter abnormalities, corpus callosum dysgenesis, mega cisterna magna, cortical dysplasia, heterotopias, hemorrhage, hydrocephalus, and subependymal cysts on brain MRI have been reported in various patients.

Due to specific therapy, pyridoxine-dependent epilepsy should be included in the differential diagnosis of neonatal or infantile onset medically refractory seizures, even in the presence of structural brain malformations or a transient response to phenobarbital. Pyridoxine should be initiated and continued until disease-specific investigations exclude the diagnosis.

Key Neuromonitoring Findings

Continuous EEG for 15 hours revealed discontinuous background activity with inter-burst interval ranging from 4 to 6 seconds with several subclinical electrographic seizures and frequent negative and positive sharp wave transients over the bilateral temporal and central head region.

References

1. Gospe SM, Jr. (2014) Pyridoxine-dependent epilepsy. In Pagon RA, Adam MP, Ardinger HH, et al., editors. *GeneReviews* ® [Internet]. Seattle: University of Washington; 1993–2015. 2001 Dec 07 [updated 2014 Jun 19]

2. Coughlin CR 2nd, van Karnebeek CD, Al-Hertani W, et al. Triple therapy with pyridoxine, arginine supplementation and dietary lysine restriction in pyridoxine-dependent epilepsy: neurodevelopmental outcome. *Mol Genet Metab*. 2015;**116**:35–43.

3. Jain-Ghai S, Mishra N, Hahn C, Blaser S, Mercimek-Mahmutoglu S. Fetal onset ventriculomegaly and subependymal cysts in a pyridoxine dependent epilepsy patient. *Pediatrics*. 2014;**133**(4):E1092–E96.

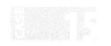

Metabolic Encephalopathy

Jonathan D. Santoro and Courtney J. Wusthoff

Clinical Presentation

A term infant born following uncomplicated pregnancy presented on day of life four to a local hospital with lethargy and decreased feeding. The newborn had an initial ammonia level of 215 μmol/L that, despite initiation of IV fluids with nothing by mouth, by day six had risen 900 μmol/L. At the same time, there was clinical deterioration to obtundation requiring intubation. The patient was transferred to a tertiary NICU. Neurological examination demonstrated profound encephalopathy, symmetric hyperreflexia and clonus, and symmetric withdrawal in the horizontal plane to noxious stimulation. With progression of liver failure of unclear etiology, IV carnitine and IV sodium benzoate with sodium phenylacetate were initiated. Due to continued hyperammonemia, continuous renal replacement therapy (CRRT) was initiated. Upon admission to NICU on day six, screening aEEG was initiated. Within the first evening, aEEG revealed rhythmic patterns without clinical correlate (Figure C15.1); continuous video EEG was initiated to clarify the findings. No seizure activity was captured on EEG (Figure C15.2). With use of CRRT and the above interventions, the patient's ammonia decreased to less than 150 μmol/L, with corresponding transient improvement of EEG background (Figures C15.3 & C15.4). The patient's newborn screen results returned indicating a propionyl CoA carboxylase deficiency as the cause of propionic acidemia. Unfortunately, while receiving maximal therapy for liver failure the patient developed bacteremia and sepsis that was ultimately fatal.

Discussion

Neonatal onset propionic acidemia an inborn error of metabolism that presents as lethargy in the first few days after birth. Hyperammonemia is typical, with disease progressing to hepatic failure without early treatment. In many countries, newborn screening can detect neonates with this condition, though clinical symptoms may arise before newborn screen results are reported. EEG monitoring is recommended for all patients with propionic aciduria at the time of initial presentation and during periods of metabolic decompensation, both to detect seizures and to assess brain function while the clinical exam is limited. Similarly, EEG monitoring can be useful for neonates with hyperammonemia due to other inborn errors of metabolism.

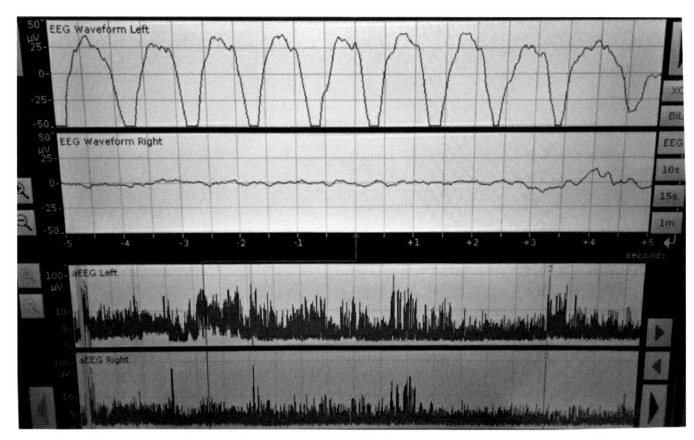

Figure C15.1 aEEG recording from the first 4 hours after admission to the tertiary NICU. The top two panels show a 10-second segment of EEG; a rhythmic pattern across the left hemispheric channel is evident in the uppermost panel, suspicious for possible seizure. The bottom two panels display 3 hours of aEEG trend from the left and right hemispheric channels. Overall, amplitudes are abnormally low, with the lower margin of the activity band less than 5 μV and the upper margin often less than 10 μV. This is a severely abnormal background pattern.

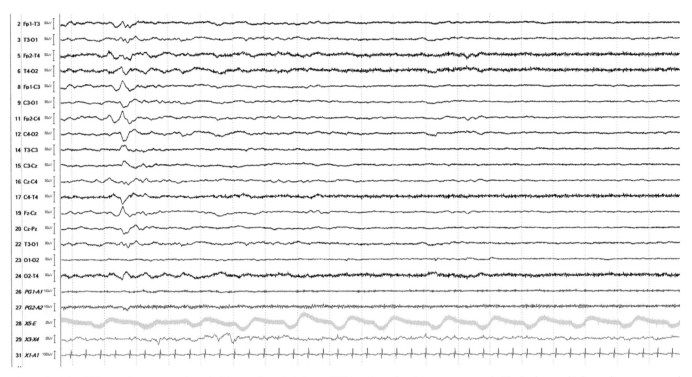

Figure C15.2 cEEG recording at approximately 8 hours after admission to NICU, at time of peak hyperammonemia. The background is low-voltage suppressed; activity is almost entirely below 10 µV in amplitude. (Sens 7, Tc 0.1s, HF 70 Hz, 20s/screen.)

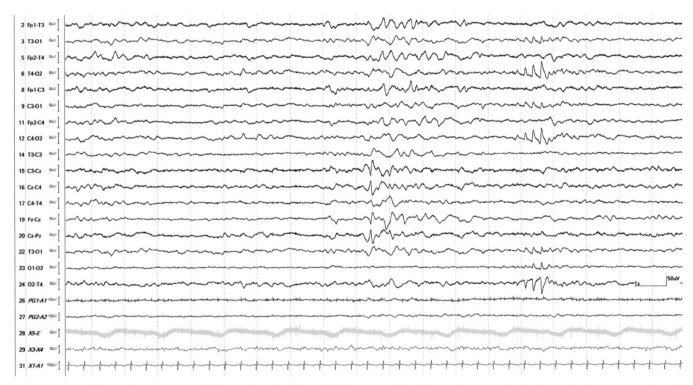

Figure C15.3 cEEG recording approximately 24 hours after admission to NICU, as ammonia levels began to improve. The background voltages are now above 25 µV in amplitude and activity is increasingly continuous. There are excess sharp waves, including in a run at O2, but no seizures.

Key Neuromonitoring Findings

Neonates with inborn errors of metabolism and those with hyperammonemia are at high risk for seizures. These patients are often obtunded or comatose; EEG monitoring is essential for accurate diagnosis of seizures. In this case, while limited array aEEG showed rhythmic patterns, full array continuous EEG monitoring did not identify electrographic seizures. Even as the patient's examination was limited by sedation, the evolution

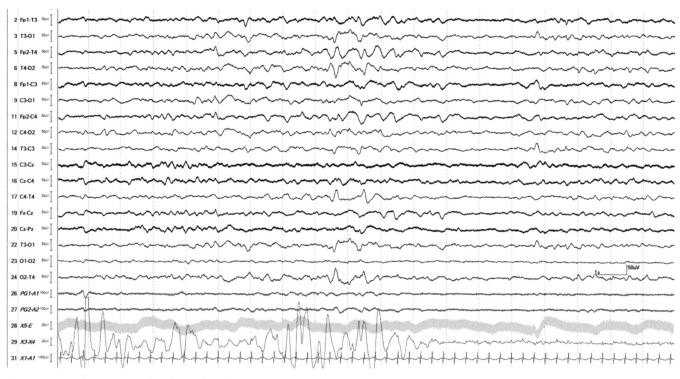

Figure C15.4 cEEG approximately 36 hours after admission, when ammonia levels were at a nadir. The background is continuous and of normal amplitude. Some sharp waves are present, but no longer occur in runs.

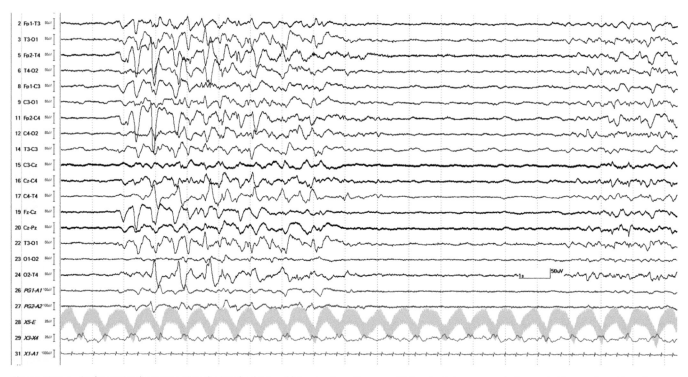

Figure C15.5 As the patient became septic, the EEG background became discontinuous, with bursts of sharp waves lasting up to 7 seconds and inter-burst intervals with amplitude less than 25 μV.

of the EEG background provided real-time information regarding brain function. Initially, this reflected severe encephalopathy, with transient improvement as ammonia levels improved. As the patient became septic, brain function again worsened (Figure C15.5), providing an early indication to the clinical team that the patient was deteriorating.

References

1. Olischar M, Shany E, Aygün C, et al. Amplitude-integrated electroencephalography in newborns with inborn errors of metabolism. *Neonatology*. 2012;**102**(3):203–11. PMID: 22797054.

2. Schreiber J, Chapman KA, Summar ML, et al. Neurologic considerations in propionic acidemia. *Mol Genet Metab*. 2012 Jan;**105**(1):10–15. doi: PMID: 22078457.

3. Wiwattanadittakul N, Prust M, Gaillard WD, et al. The utility of EEG monitoring in neonates with hyperammonemia due to inborn errors of metabolism. *Mol Genet Metab*. 2018 Nov;**125**(3):235–40. PMID: 30197275.

Glycine Encephalopathy

Puneet Jain and Cecil D. Hahn

Clinical Presentation

The patient was born to a non-consanguineous couple at 40 weeks' gestation following unremarkable pregnancy with uncomplicated delivery. He showed persisting lethargy and poor feeding since day 1 of life. Examination showed normal head circumference, poor state-to-state variability, global hypotonia, and depressed muscle stretch reflexes. On day 6, he was noted to have very frequent, brief, fragmentary body jerks involving the distal extremities both during awake and sleep states. There were associated frequent hiccups and occasional brief episodes of tonic posturing of the left arm. Continuous EEG monitoring was initiated to characterize these events.

Basic investigations showed normal blood sugar, calcium, pH, lactate, ammonia, and urine organic acids. Glycine was markedly elevated in CSF (321 μmol/L [normal range, 6–19]) and plasma (1571 μmol/L [normal range, 178–248]) with a high CSF/plasma glycine ratio of 0.2:1. A ratio of >0.08 is highly suggestive of non-ketotic hyperglycinemia. Urinary glycine was also elevated (13,242 mmol/mol Cr [normal range, 563–2563]). MRI brain showed increased T2 hyperintensity throughout the bilateral cerebral white matter, posterior limbs of the internal capsule, subthalamic region, midbrain and within the dorsal tegmental tracts. EEG suggested early myoclonic encephalopathy (EME) (Figures C16.1–C16.4). Clinical phenotype and investigations suggested a diagnosis of non-ketotic hyperglycinemia, or glycine encephalopathy. The baby was treated with multiple anti-seizure medications, sodium benzoate, carnitine, dextromethorphan, and supportive care.

Discussion

EME is a rare epileptic encephalopathy. Seizures usually start within 1 month of age. Erratic, fragmentary myoclonia is the defining seizure type. Mycolonus often involves the face and limbs and is usually very frequent. Myoclonus has been reported even antenatally, often described as fetal "hiccups" during the pregnancy. Other seizure semiologies may include focal seizures (eye deviation, apnea, clonic, asymmetric tonic movement) and rarely epileptic spasms. Seizures remain refractory to treatment, with severe subsequent neurodevelopmental impairment. EME may evolve into infantile spasms syndrome or epilepsy with multiple independent spike foci

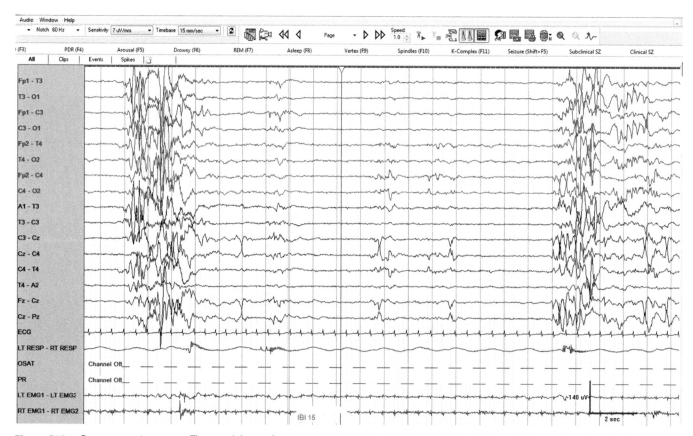

Figure C16.1 Burst suppression pattern: The record shows a burst suppression pattern with inter-burst interval of around 15 seconds and amplitude <10 μV. Also note sharp waves at Cz (negative) and C4 (positive) during the suppression phase. (Neonatal bipolar montage with a time base of 15 mm/sec, sensitivity 7 μV/mm, high-frequency filter at 70 Hz, low-frequency filter at 1 Hz.)

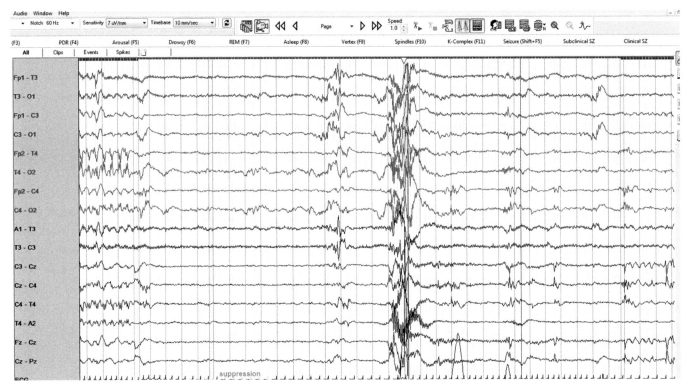

Figure C16.2 Epileptic spasm: The record shows generalized high-amplitude slow waves with superimposed faster frequencies [arrow head at top] on a background of suppression with the clinical correlate of a flexor spasm. (Neonatal bipolar montage with a time base 10 mm/sec, sensitivity 7 μV/mm, high-frequency filter at 70 Hz, low-frequency filter at 1 Hz.)

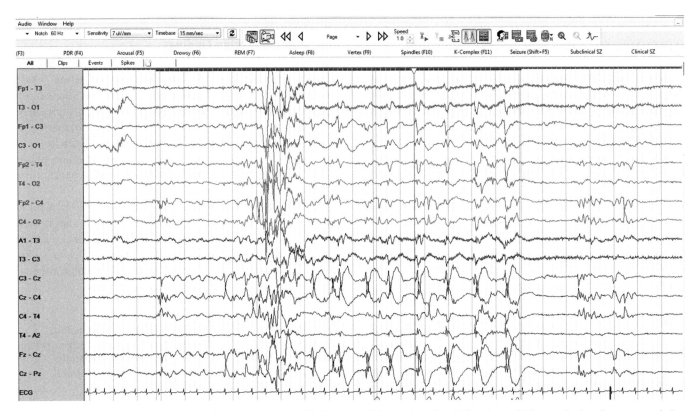

Figure C16.3 Subclinical seizure: The record shows sudden onset of rhythmic 2 Hz delta activity at Cz, which evolves to higher amplitude spike wave morphology with fields at C3 and C4. It lasts for 15 seconds with abrupt termination. There was no clinical correlate. (Neonatal bipolar montage with a time base 15 mm/sec, sensitivity 7 μV/mm, high-frequency filter at 70 Hz, low-frequency filter at 1 Hz.)

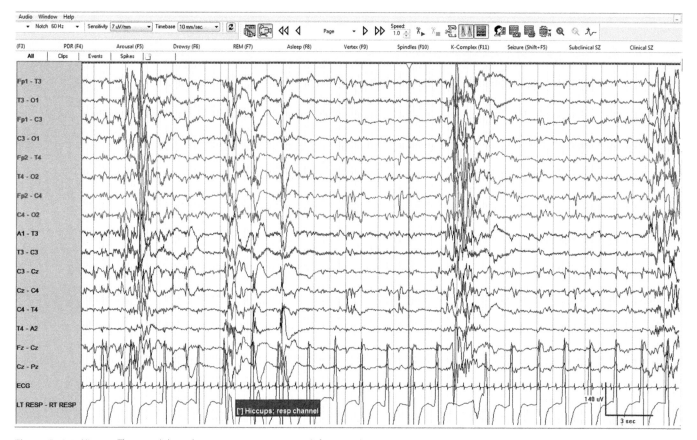

Figure C16.4 Hiccups: The record shows burst suppression pattern with frequent sharp waves at Cz, C4 and T3. The baby was having around 1 per second hiccups during this epoch as evident on the respiratory channel but with no EEG change. (Neonatal bipolar montage with a time base 10 mm/sec, sensitivity 7 μV/mm, high-frequency filter at 70 Hz, low-frequency filter at 1 Hz.)

(MISF). More than half of patients with EME die before 2 years of age.

Many cases are familial. Metabolic causes predominate, though the etiology remains unknown in majority of the cases. Reported causes include non-ketotic hyperglycinemia, organic acidemias, sulfite and xanthine oxidase deficiency, molybdenum cofactor deficiency, Menkes disease, and Zellweger syndrome.

Glycine encephalopathy is an autosomal-recessive disorder caused by deficient activity of the multimeric glycine cleavage enzyme with resultant accumulation of excessive of glycine in all body tissues, including the brain. The majority of patients present in the neonatal period (usually within in the first hours to days of life) with progressive lethargy, hypotonia, and myoclonic jerks leading to apnea and often death. The diagnosis is made by elevated CSF-to-plasma glycine ratio, enzymatic analysis in biopsied liver tissue, or genetic testing. Treatment is symptomatic.

Key Neuromonitoring Findings

The interictal EEG in EME characteristically shows a burst suppression pattern, which consists of bursts lasting 1 to 5 seconds alternating with periods of background suppression lasting 3 to 10 seconds. This pattern may be more prominent or only seen during sleep state. As compared to Ohtahara syndrome, EME shows longer inter-burst intervals, asynchronous bursts, and more multifocal spikes in the suppression phase. The EEG during wakefulness usually shows slow background activity with frequent multifocal spike waves.

Myoclonia are not associated with ictal EEG change but may coincidentally occur with bursts of burst suppression pattern. Focal seizures may have variable ictal EEG patterns including alphoid rhythm, theta activity, or irregular spike-waves. Tonic spasms may be associated with voltage attenuation, also known as a desynchronization pattern.

References

1. Ohtahara S, Yamatogi Y. Epileptic encephalopathies in early infancy with suppression-burst. *J Clin Neurophysiol.* 2003;**20**:398–407.

2. Beal JC, Cherian K, Moshe SL. Early-onset epileptic encephalopathies: Ohtahara syndrome and early myoclonic encephalopathy. *Pediatr Neurol.* 2012;**47**:317–23.

3. Rossi S, Daniele I, Bastrenta P, Mastrangelo M, Lista G. Early myoclonic encephalopathy and nonketotic hyperglycinemia. *Pediatr Neurol.* 2009;**41**:371–4.

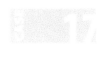

Newborn Heart Surgery
Hypoplastic Left Heart Syndrome

Shavonne L. Massey and Robert Clancy

Clinical Presentation

A term newborn with prenatally-diagnosed hypoplastic left heart syndrome (HLHS) was born via spontaneous vaginal delivery. The Apgar scores were 9 at both 1 and 5 minutes. Weight was 3480 grams (25th percentile), length 48 centimeters (25th percentile), but head circumference was only 32 centimeters (5th percentile). The baby was stabilized with a normal neurological examination and transferred to the cardiac intensive care unit. Echocardiogram confirmed HLHS with mitral and aortic valve atresia, a diminutive ascending aorta, patent foramen ovale, and a large patent ductus arteriosus. Baseline pre-operative magnetic resonance imaging (MRI) of the brain on day of life 3 showed immature, underdeveloped opercula. MR spectroscopy revealed elevated lactate peaks in the posterior periventricular white matter in both hemispheres, though no actual leukomalacia was visible on imaging. The patient underwent stage 1 HLHS palliation with a Sano shunt. Newborn heart surgery was conducted after the patient was placed on cardiopulmonary bypass, cooled, and transitioned to deep hypothermic circulatory arrest (DHCA) for a total of 50 minutes.

Continuous video EEG monitoring was initiated immediately after return from the operating room, as recommended by the American Clinical Neurophysiology Society (ACNS) [1]. Initially, the EEG background was invariant with excessive discontinuity for age. The inter-burst intervals were 7 to 10 seconds in duration with amplitudes less than 10 μV. There was minimal improvement of the background over the first 24 hours of monitoring. Multiple, brief subclinical seizures arising from the right posterior region (temporal-occipital) started around 30 hours post-operatively. The patient was initially loaded with 40 mg/kg of levetiracetam with no reduction in seizure frequency, followed by a loading dose of 20 mg/kg of phenobarbital, given as four 5 mg/kg aliquots to avoid hypotension. There was no improvement, and the subclinical electrographic seizures eventually escalated to status epilepticus and finally ceased after a single dose of 20 mg/kg of fosphenytoin, administered slowly at a rate of 1 mg/kg/minute to avoid cardiotoxicity and bradycardia. The infant remained seizure free for an additional 24 hours of EEG monitoring, which was then discontinued. The background remained excessively discontinuous with prolonged and attenuated inter-burst intervals and excessive sharp waves in the T4-O2 channel. A repeat brain MRI 8 days post-operatively showed ischemic injury in the right thalamus and bilateral occipital lobes (right greater than left), evidenced by restricted diffusion and hemorrhage within the right occipital lobe, the right occipital horn, and the choroid plexus of the left lateral ventricle. The patient was

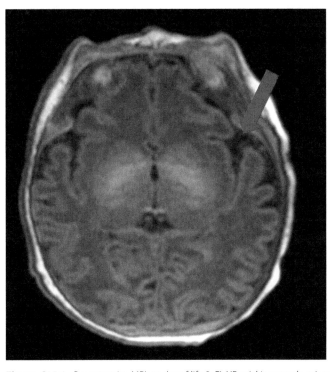

Figure C17.1 Pre-operative MRI on day of life 3. FLAIR axial images showing some brain immaturity with incompletely closed cerebral opercula [arrow].

maintained on 6 mg/kg/day of phenobarbital with no further seizures (Figures C17.1–C17.5).

Discussion

Infants born with serious forms of congenital heart disease (CHD) are considered at high risk of neurological injury even before newborn heart surgery. This infant had a relatively small head circumference at birth, in contrast with age-appropriate percentiles for weight and length. Small head circumferences correlate significantly with the diameter of the ascending aorta which is decreased in HLHS and results in obstructed cerebral blood flow during a period of normally rapid head growth. Similarly, the brain appeared immature on imaging with operculae that had not fully closed. Lactate peaks shown by MR spectroscopy indicated relative ischemia within those white matter areas, present even before the stress of newborn heart surgery. The duration of DHCA depends on the complexity of the cardiac defect and the skill of the surgeon. A duration of 50 minutes is common, but times above 40 minutes increase the chance of post-operative seizures. The need for full anticoagulation during and after DHCA increases the risk for secondary hemorrhagic transformation after ischemic injury. Modern CHD cohorts have demonstrated post-operative

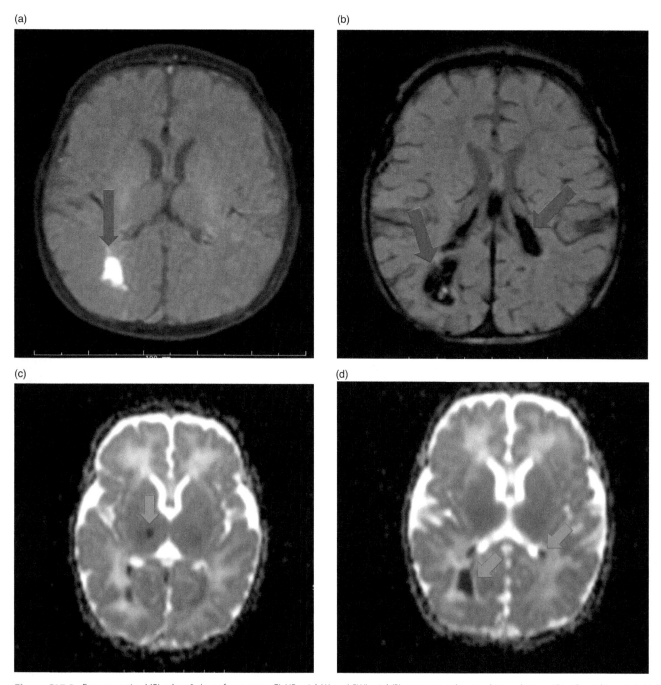

(a)

(b)

(c)

(d)

Figure C17.2 Post-operative MRI, taken 8 days after surgery. FLAIR axial (A) and SWI axial (B) sequences showing hemorrhage within the right occipital lobe and bilateral occipital horns of the lateral ventricles [red arrows]. ADC axial (C) and (D) show areas of ischemia involving the right thalamus [blue arrow, C], right occipital lobe and bilateral occipital lobes [blue arrows, D].

seizure incidences up to 23%, with over 80% of those seizures being subclinical. Seizures in the CHD population are treated with the same medications used in other neonatal populations: phenobarbital, levetiracetam, fosphenytoin (or phenytoin), and benzodiazepines. The practitioner must remember the potential side effects of hypotension from myocardial depression from phenobarbital. Fosphenytoin and phenytoin can induce cardiac arrhythmias such as bradycardia, heart block, ventricular tachycardia, and ventricular fibrillation, which can lead to asystole and death. Rapid intravenous administration of phenytoin or fosphenytoin can also cause a sharp drop in blood

pressure from peripheral vasodilation and a negative inotropic myocardial effect and these iatrogenic consequences need to be fastidiously avoided in this cardiovascularly delicate group.

Key EEG Findings

Excessively discontinuous EEG background activity is common soon after newborn heart surgery (Figure C17.3). In addition to the stress of the surgery itself, the infants are still recovering from the effects of prolonged general anesthesia and hypothermia. Medications which act on the central nervous system administered in the immediate post-operative

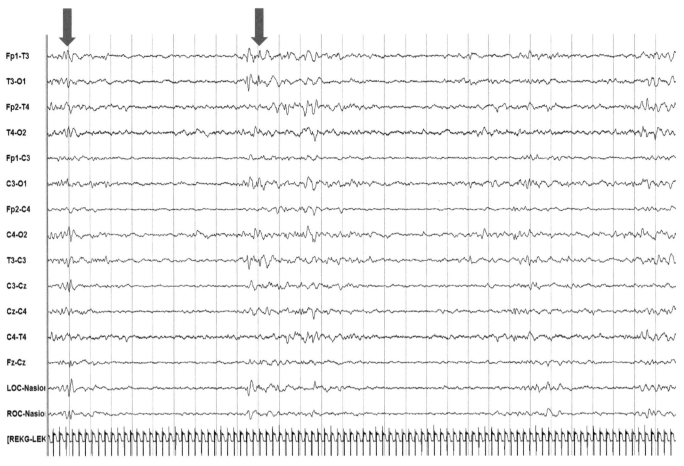

Figure C17.3 The EEG background activity is excessively discontinuous, consisting of bursts with normal patterns and graphoelements separated by inter-burst intervals [between red arrows] longer than 6 seconds and less than 25 microvolts in amplitude.

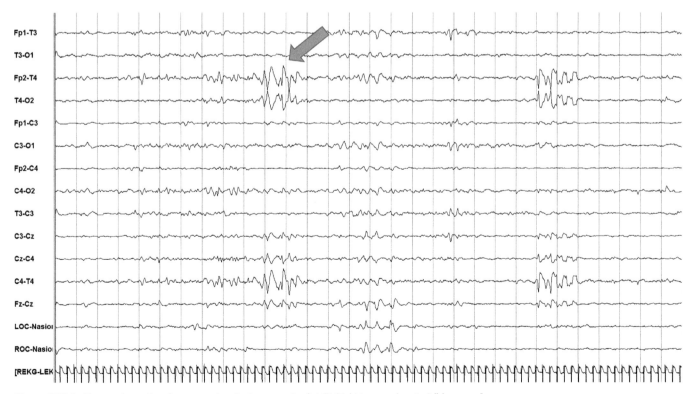

Figure C17.4 Abnormal negative sharp wave transients are maximal at T4 (right temporal region) [blue arrow].

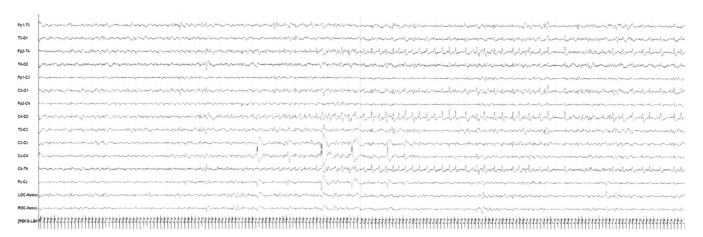

Figure C17.5 An electrographic neonatal seizure has abrupt onset of rhythmic 1–2 Hz delta activity in T4 and C4 channels, which evolves in amplitude and frequency into 1.5 Hz spike and wave discharges, maximal in the right temporal (T4) and occipital (O2) regions. (15 mm/sec.). Separately, there is a non-evolving run of sharp-wave discharges at Cz (central vertex) in the center of the image.

period typically include narcotics for pain control and benzodiazepines for anxiolysis. Post-operatively, infants may also experience a prolonged period of hypotension since the myocardium is still "stunned" from the effects of cardiac surgery. In this case, the EEG was notable for the persistence of a moderate degree of discontinuity at a time when patients typically begin to recover a continuous EEG background (24–48 hours post-operatively). Furthermore, all of the EEG seizures were originating from a single focal location. Follow-up MRI showed diffuse signs of injury but also a focal hemorrhagic infarct in the right posterior region concordant with EEG seizure focus.

References

1. Shellhaas RA, Chang T, Tsuchida T, et al. The American Clinical Neurophysiology Society's Guideline on Continuous Electroencephalography Monitoring in Neonates. *J Clin Neurophysiol.* 2011;**28**(6): 611–17.

2. Tsuchida TN, Wusthoff CJ, Shellhaas RA, et al. American Clinical Neurophysiology Society standardized EEG terminology and categorization for the description of continuous EEG monitoring in neonates: report of the American Clinical Neurophysiology Society Critical Care Monitoring Committee. *J Clin Neurophysiol.* 2013;**30**(2):161–73.

Extracorporeal Membrane Oxygenation

Nicholas S. Abend

Clinical Presentation

A 7-month-old unvaccinated male infant was previously healthy and developmentally normal until he presented with persistent cough and fever. Other family members were also experiencing similar symptoms. His initial workup demonstrated leukocytosis, a right upper lobe pneumonia, and positive pertussis polymerase chain reaction. His respiratory status worsened on day 5 of hospital admission, and he was transferred to the pediatric intensive care unit. On day 7 of admission, he was intubated for respiratory failure with bi-lobar pneumonia. On day 8 of admission, he developed a life-threatening pulmonary hypertensive crisis requiring emergent cannulation for veno-arterial extracorporeal membrane oxygenation (ECMO). Given the acute clinical change and known risk of seizures during ECMO, continuous EEG monitoring was initiated. EEG demonstrated continuous 1–3 Hz delta activity with symmetric sleep spindles but without variability or reactivity. During the ECMO course, the EEG pattern changed to show new left posterior quadrant attenuation (Figures C18.1 & C18.2). A portable CT scan demonstrated a 33 mm intraparenchymal hemorrhage in the left occipital lobe surrounded by vasogenic edema producing local mass effect with sulcal effacement in the left posterior parietal and occipital region (Figure C18.3). Anticoagulation was adjusted through the ECMO circuit to minimize the risk of hemorrhage expansion, and the patient's target platelet goal was increased. Sedation was transiently decreased to permit clinical neurological assessment, and the patient moved his extremities purposefully. He was maintained under sedation, and a repeat head CT two days later did not show hemorrhage expansion. The patient underwent

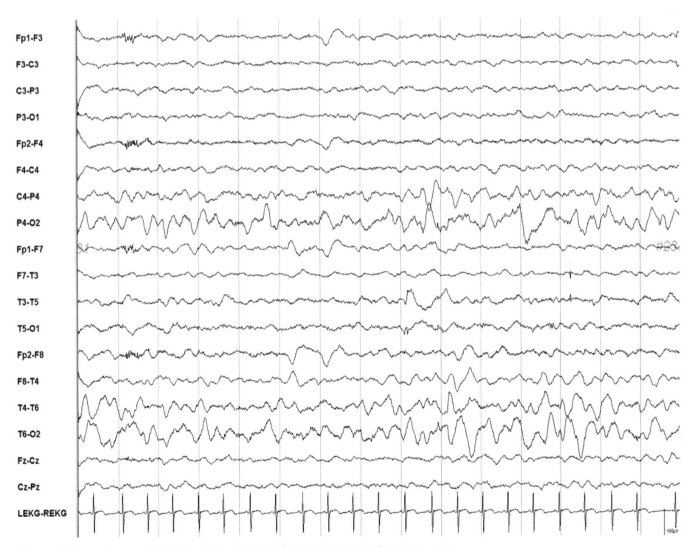

Figure C18.1 Bipolar longitudinal montage demonstrating left posterior quadrant voltage attenuation.

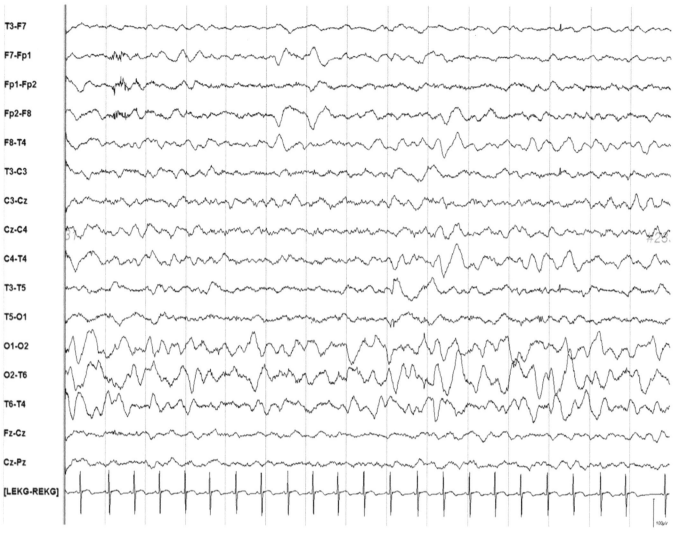

Figure C18.2 Circumferential montage demonstrating left posterior quadrant voltage attenuation.

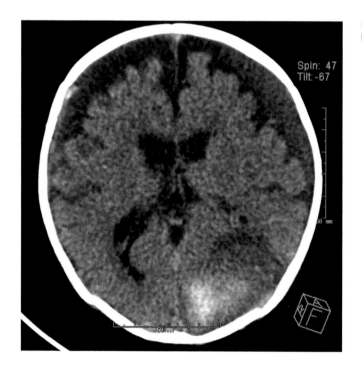

Figure C18.3 Non-contrast CT head demonstrating acute left occipital hemorrhage with surrounding edema.

a 24-day ECMO course, after which he was successfully decannulated.

Discussion

Electrographic seizures occur in up to 30% of neonates and children undergoing ECMO. Critical illness precipitating the need for ECMO, the cannulation procedure, and complications of ECMO itself each creates a risk for brain injury in children. Consensus statements recommend use of cEEG monitoring during ECMO in neonates[1] and children[2, 3]. While cEEG monitoring is mainly directed at seizure detection, it can also provide useful information regarding evolution of brain function over time.

Key Neuromonitoring Findings

While this patient did not have seizures during ECMO, EEG data were important in guiding management. EEG monitoring elucidated focal findings – left posterior attenuation – that would not have been apparent clinically in a patient requiring high levels of sedation and paralytic infusion. This EEG finding directly prompted earlier imaging and adjustment of anticoagulation parameters, potentially preventing expansion of the hemorrhage.

References

1. Shellhaas RA, Chang T, Tsuchida T, et al. The American Clinical Neurophysiology Society's Guideline on Continuous Electroence-phalography Monitoring in Neonates. *J Clin Neurophysiol.* 2011;**28** (6):611–17.

2. Herman ST, Abend NS, Bleck TP, et al; Critical Care Continuous EEG Task Force of the American Clinical Neurophysiology Society. Consensus statement on continuous EEG in critically ill adults and children, part I: indications. *J Clin Neurophysiol.* 2015a;**32**(2):87–95.

3. Herman ST, Abend NS, Bleck TP, et al Consensus statement on continuous EEG in critically ill adults and children, part II: personnel, technical specifications, and clinical practice. *J Clin Neurophysiol.* 2015b;**32**(2):96–108.

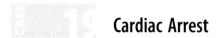

Cardiac Arrest

Courtney J. Wusthoff

Clinical Presentation

A 7-month-old female had been put in her crib for a nap; her father returned to the room 40 minutes later to wake her and found her limp and cyanotic. Parents began chest compressions and rescue breaths; on arrival by emergency medical services there was no palpable pulse, but return of spontaneous circulation occurred after 3 additional minutes of CPR. On arrival to ER, the patient was found to be RSV positive with patchy opacities on chest X-ray. Head CT was normal. The parents recalled preceding rhinorrhea but no fever or notable cough. In the ER, the patient had episodes of right hemibody extension and stiffening without associated vital sign changes. The patient was intubated and sedated; EEG monitoring was initiated in the pediatric ICU.

Upon initiation of EEG, generalized occipitally predominant periodic discharges (PDs) were present. These were treated empirically with benzodiazepines, with improvement of the EEG although no corresponding clinical change. The background activity became slow and disorganized. There were no further episodes of body stiffening/extension captured. Approximately 30 hours after admission, subclinical seizures began. These had a subtle evolution on EEG, and required treatment with benzodiazepines, IV fosphenytoin 20 mg PE/

kg, and levetiracetam 60 mg/kg before remitting. They never reached the threshold for status epilepticus. EEG after resolution of seizures showed diffuse slowing with intermittent multifocal sharp waves.

Repeat head CT at 48 hours after admission showed bilateral areas of ischemia in a watershed distribution as well as mild diffuse cerebral edema. The patient remained on EEG until, at 72 hours after admission, she had been seizure free for over 24 hours on maintenance dosing of levetiracetam. Sedation was weaned over the following four days with extubation to high flow nasal cannula.

Discussion

Seizures are common following cardiac arrest, occurring in up to 50% of children. They are most often subclinical. Seizures typically begin within the first 24 hours after cardiac arrest; in this case, the first electrographic seizures were recorded approximately 30 hours after admission. However, the patient had also had clinically suspicious stiffening episodes in the ER prior to EEG initiation, and had received benzodiazepine to treat PDs within the first 12 hours after return of circulation. Although seizures and generalized periodic discharges are associated with worse prognosis, in this case there were some

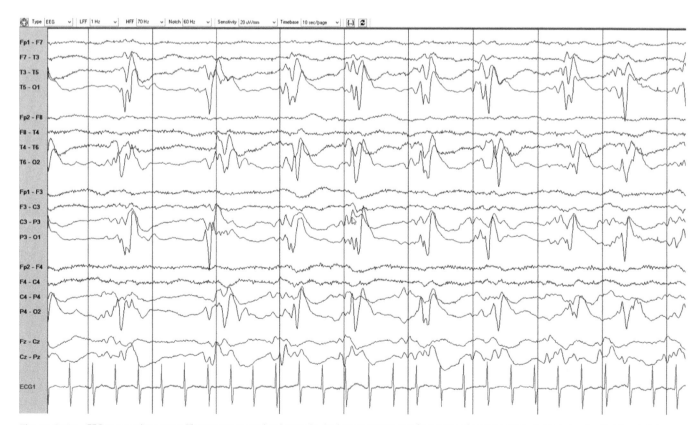

Figure C19.1 EEG at recording onset. There were generalized periodic discharges (GPDs) at a frequency of approximately 1 per second, with bi-occipital predominance. These diminished with benzodiazepine administration. (LFF 1 Hz, HFF 70 Hz, Sens 20 μV/mm, 10 sec/page.)

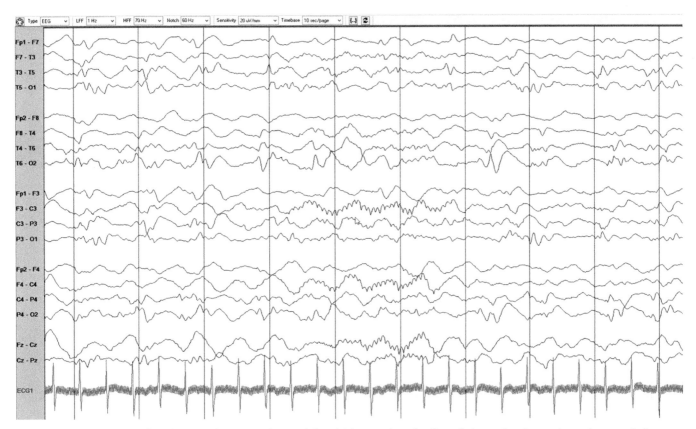

Figure C19.2 EEG 20 hours after admission. There remain frequent left and right posterior epileptiform discharges, but these no longer have a periodic pattern. There has emerged a mixture of background frequencies and symmetric sleep spindles are present.

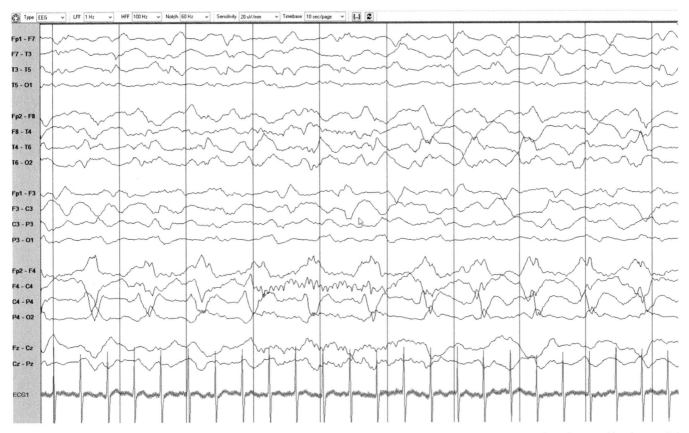

Figure C19.3 EEG 30 hours after admission reveals a subclinical seizure characterized by rhythmic sharp-and-wave activity in the right parietal head region (P4). Over several hours, seizures were seen arising independently from both the left and right parietal head regions.

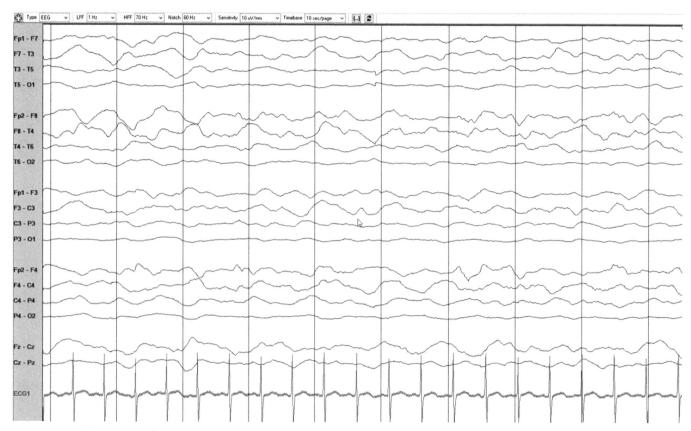

Figure C19.4 EEG at 42 hours after admission, following treatment with multiple anti-seizure medications shows a diffusely slow background, likely at least in part due to medication effect.

encouraging prognostic EEG features in the first 24 hours, including the slow-disorganized background (without suppression or discontinuity), variability, and the presence of sleep transients.

Key Neuromonitoring Findings

EEG was initiated after this patient was intubated and transferred to the ICU; at that time there was no clinical evidence of seizures, and the clinical examination was limited due to sedation. The initial EEG recording showed generalized occipitally predominant periodic discharges (Figure C19.1). This pattern falls on the ictal-interictal continuum:

it indicates a high risk of concurrent seizures, and there is some evidence that this pattern can itself contribute to clinical encephalopathy. While the empiric trial of benzodiazepines did not result in clinical improvement, it led to resolution of the PDs and was followed by significant improvement of the EEG background (Figure C19.2). Continued EEG monitoring allowed the detection of late seizures (Figure C19.3). In this case the early appearance of PDs was a harbinger of later seizures. After multiple medications, the EEG showed diffuse slowing (Figure C19.4), likely reflecting a combination of medication effect and brain dysfunction due to the cardiac arrest.

References

Topjian AA, de Caen A, Wainwright MS, et al. Pediatric post-cardiac arrest care: a scientific statement from the American Heart Association. *Circulation.* 2019 Aug 6;**140**(6):e194–e233. PMID: 31242751.

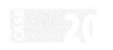

Cerebral Sinovenous Thrombosis

Robyn Whitney and Cristina Go

Clinical Presentation

A 17-month-old boy with gross motor delay, speech delay, and iron deficiency anemia presented acutely with a decreased level of consciousness and seizures. He had three days of gastrointestinal illness and decreased oral intake. His seizures were characterized by rhythmic twitching of the left shoulder and arm. He was seen at a local hospital and treated with multiple doses of midazolam, fosphenytoin, and phenobarbital. He was subsequently transferred to a tertiary pediatric intensive care unit for stabilization. On admission, he was started on maintenance phenobarbital and levetiracetam. A head CT scan revealed thrombosis within the superior sagittal sinus, sulcal subarachnoid hemorrhage within the right posterior frontal lobe, and venous infarction in the right frontal and parietal lobes. These findings were subsequently confirmed on brain MRI and MRV. He was started on enoxaparin with aggressive hydration. His blood gas, glucose, liver enzymes, and urinalysis were all normal. However, his complete blood count showed microcytic anemia, and his sodium and chloride levels were elevated. Continuous EEG monitoring for 72 hours was commenced after return from the CT scan. Ongoing clinical and subclinical seizures were recorded, ultimately controlled after the addition of increased midazolam, levetiracetam, and fosphenytoin.

Upon stabilization, he was transferred out of the intensive care unit. He continued to have intermittent episodes of brief rhythmic twitching of the left upper extremity of uncertain type; continuous EEG clarified that these were seizures. His anti-seizure medications again were adjusted, and his seizures were ultimately controlled on a combination of levetiracetam and carbamazepine. Upon discharge, his neurological exam was normal.

Discussion

Cerebral sinovenous thrombosis (CSVT) is a cause of stroke in children and neonates. Children with CSVT often present with diffuse clinical signs such as lethargy, seizures, and headache. Diagnosis may be delayed due to the lack of focal clinical symptoms. Brain injury from CSVT ranges from venous congestion to parenchymal ischemic injury, which is often hemorrhagic and can occur in the cortical or subcortical areas. Subarachnoid hemorrhage has also been reported, as occurred in this case. Risk factors for CSVT are numerous and include infection, fever, dehydration, anemia, head trauma, and underlying medical conditions such as malignancy and congenital heart disease. In this case, the presence of dehydration, recent illness, and anemia likely contributed to the development of venous thrombosis. Continuous EEG in encephalopathic patients with CSVT monitors for clinical and subclinical seizures. EEG findings in CSVT are variable. The EEG may be normal, may show generalized background slowing, or, in the case of unilateral infarction, may show focal slowing or focal epileptiform discharges. Treatment of CSVT is supportive and aimed at managing underlying contributing factors and complications (e.g., infection, seizures, electrolyte imbalance). Antithrombotic agents are generally recommended in children with CSVT.

Key Neuromonitoring Findings

Continuous EEG monitoring revealed rhythmic delta activity over the right central-temporal-parietal regions. There was persistent delta/theta slowing over the right central-temporal-parietal regions (Figure C20.1) and sleep features were poorly formed over the right hemisphere (Figure C20.2). Two subclinical seizures lasting 3–4 minutes each with onset from the right central-temporal-parietal head regions were recorded on the first day of monitoring (Figure C20.3). Two clinical seizures with left-sided extremity twitching were also recorded on the second and third day of recording, one of which was prolonged, lasting 25 minutes.

References

1. Cardenas J, Rho J, Kirton A. Pediatric stroke. *Childs Nerv Syst.* 2011;**27**:1375–90.

2. Dlamini N, Billinghurst L, Kirkham F. Cerebral venous sinus (sinovenous) thrombosis in children. *Neurosurg Clin N Am.* 2010; **21**:511–27.

3. Ichord R, Benedict SL, Chan AK, Kirkham FJ, Nowak-Göttl U; International Paediatric Stroke Study Group. Pediatric cerebral sinovenous thrombosis: findings of the international pediatric stroke study. *Arch Dis Child.* 2015;**100**(2):174–9.

4. Moharir M, Shroff M, Stephens D, et al. Anticoagulants in pediatric cerebral sinovenous thrombosis a safety and outcome study. *Ann Neurol.* 2010;**67**:590–9.

5. Niedermeyer E. Cerebrovascular disorders and EEG. In *Electroencephalography Basic Principles, Clinical Applications and Related Fields.* Philadelphia: Lippincott Williams & Wilkins; 2005, pp. 339–62.

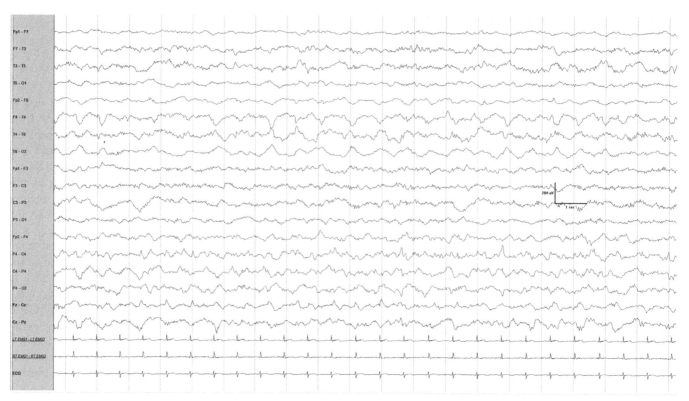

Figure C20.1 cEEG upon admission to the intensive care unit, demonstrating sharply contoured rhythmic delta activity over the right central-temporal-parietal head regions.

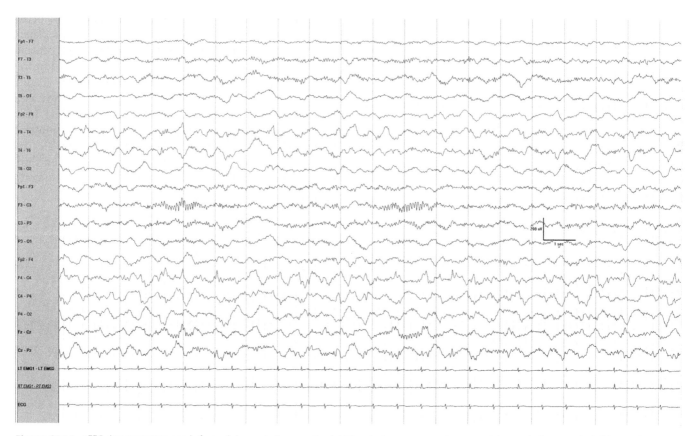

Figure C20.2 cEEG demonstrating poorly formed sleep spindles over the right hemisphere, compared to normal sleep spindles over the left hemisphere.

A

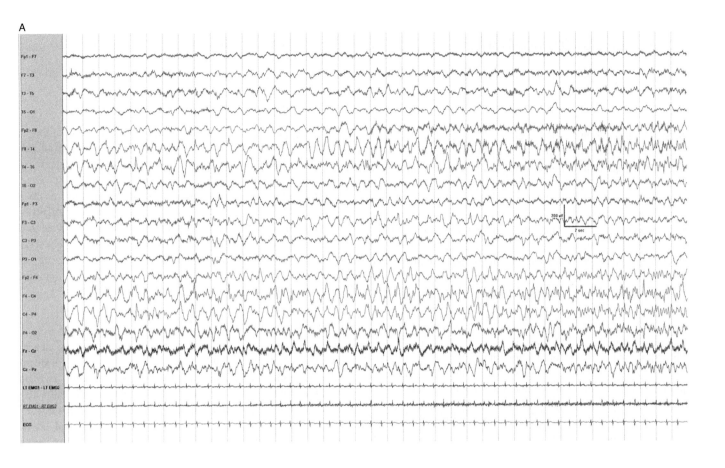

B

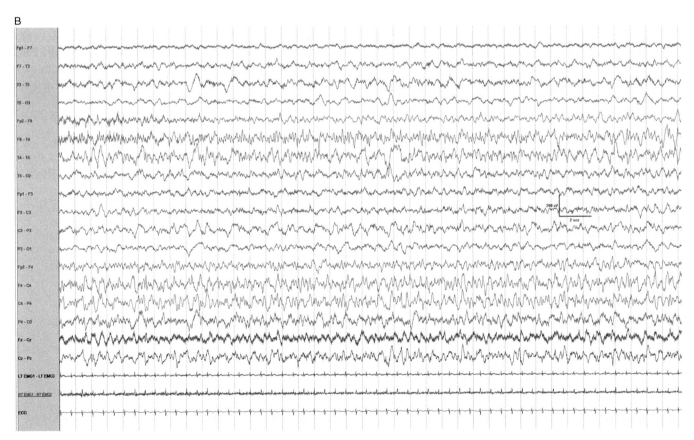

Figure C20.3 Example of a subclinical seizure captured on the first day of monitoring with onset from the right central-temporal-parietal head regions (A), and subsequent evolution in frequency and morphology (B).

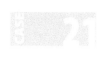

Mitochondrial Encephalomyopathy, Lactic Acidosis, and Stroke-Like Episodes (MELAS)

Shatha Shafi and Blathnaid McCoy

Clinical Presentation

A 16-year-old male with mitochondrial encephalomyopathy, lactic acidosis, and stroke-like episodes (MELAS) (*A3243G* mutation) and end-stage renal disease on hemodialysis presented with headache, vomiting, and recurrent seizures. His seizures were characterized by left eye deviation, secondary generalization, and post-ictal left extremity weakness. He was admitted to the intensive care unit. On initial examination he was awake and oriented with a left upper motor neuron facial palsy, left homonymous hemianopia, and left hemiparesis with exaggerated deep tendon reflexes. Blood gases, serum glucose, electrolytes, liver enzymes, complete blood count, toxicology screen, urine and serum amino acids, urine organic acids, and serum lactate and pyruvate were all normal. His deficits markedly improved two hours after high-dose L-arginine was given. However, he continued to have intermittent confusion and blurred vision. Brain MRI, MRA, and MRV showed a new stroke within the left basal ganglia and abnormal FLAIR/T2 signal involving the posteromedial aspect of the right temporal lobe and the right mesial occipital lobe. Continuous EEG monitoring was commenced after return from MRI. This revealed nonconvulsive states epilepticus as the etiology of ongoing intermittent confusion. Upon further increase of the midazolam infusion seizures stopped, and after several hours of seizure control, midazolam reduced with return to normal mentation.

Discussion

Both convulsive status epilepticus (CSE) and nonconvulsive status epilepticus (NCSE) have been reported in MELAS [1, 2].

When individuals with MELAS present with acute changes in behavior or confusion, continuous EEG monitoring should be considered if there is a clinical suspicion of NCSE. There are no pathognomonic EEG features described in MELAS; however, occipital status epilepticus has previously been reported in a patient with this particular mutation [3, 4]. The mechanism of status epilepticus in MELAS is postulated to involve a cycle that develops after an inciting event, such as fever, glucose alterations, or headache, or cause a stroke-like episode, which may in turn trigger a seizure, thereby increasing metabolic demand and as consequence increased neuronal injury [3].

Key Neuromonitoring Findings

At the onset of continuous video EEG monitoring, nearly continuous electrographic seizures were observed, around 80% of which were associated with clinical confusion and the remaining without any clinical signs. Electrographically, the seizures were characterized by spiky alpha activity arising from the right occipital region (Figure C21.1), which evolved to spike-wave discharges involving bilateral posterior head regions. Seizures were 40–60 seconds in duration and occurred every 2–5 minutes. Following initiation of a midazolam infusion, the morphology of the seizures changed to rhythmic spiky 6–7 Hz theta activity at the right occipital region without any clinical signs (Figure C21.2). Upon further increase of the midazolam infusion rate, his seizures stopped, and the EEG showed normal background activity with a posterior dominant rhythm of 9–10 Hz, which was reactive to eye opening and eye closure and no interictal epileptiform discharges.

References

1. Kaufman KR, Zuber N, Rueda-Lara MA, Tobia A. MELAS with recurrent complex partial seizures, nonconvulsive status epilepticus, psychosis, and behavioral disturbances: case analysis with literature review. *Epilepsy Behav.* 2010 Aug; 18(4):494–7.

2. Ribacoba R, Salas-Puig J, González C, Astudillo A. Characteristics of status epilepticus in MELAS. Analysis of four cases. *Neurologia.* 2006 Jan-Feb;21(1): 1–11.

3. Demarest ST, Whitehead MT, Turnacioglu S, Pearl PL, Gropman AL. Phenotypic analysis of epilepsy in the mitochondrial encephalomyopathy, lactic acidosis, and strokelike episodes-associated mitochondrial DNA A3243G mutation. *J Child Neurol.* 2014 Sep;29 (9):1249–56.

4. Karkare S, Merchant S, Solomon G, Engel M, Kosofsky B. MELAS with A3243G mutation presenting with occipital status epilepticus. *J Child Neurol.* 2009 Dec;24(12):1564–7.

A

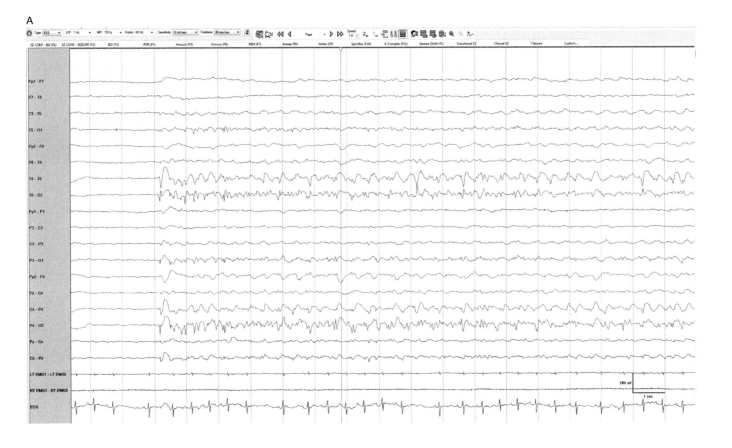

B

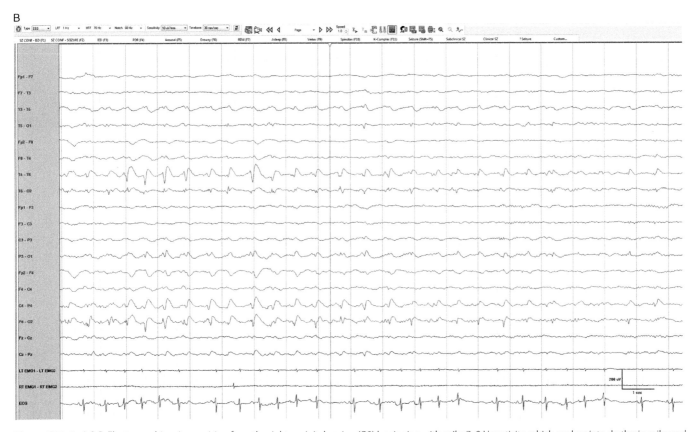

Figure C21.1 A & B: Electrographic seizure arising from the right occipital region (O2) beginning with spiky 7–8 Hz activity, which evolves into rhythmic spike and waves which spread to the left occipital head region.

A

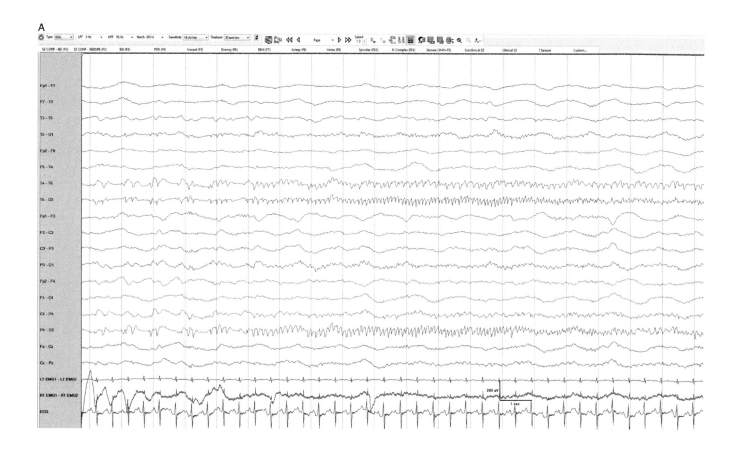

B

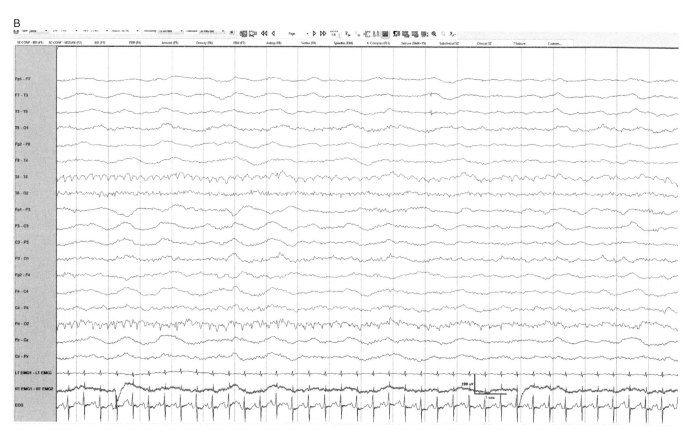

Figure C21.2 A & B: Altered seizure morphology at the right occipital head region following initiation of midazolam: spiky 6–7 Hz theta activity, which initially increases in frequency to 8 Hz and then gradually decreases in frequency and amplitude.

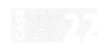

Parenchymal Hemorrhage with Subarachnoid Hemorrhage

Jonathan D. Santoro and Courtney J. Wusthoff

Clinical Presentation

A previously healthy 12-year-old girl developed sudden onset headache with dizziness, nausea, and emesis while at the park with her family. Approximately one hour later, she collapsed. On arrival of emergency medical services, she had a Glasgow Coma Scale score of 7 and was responsive only to sternal rub. By arrival in the ER, she had sluggishly reactive pupils bilaterally, was hemiparetic on the right side, but could provide thumbs up/down for responses to some questions. CT head scan revealed a large left fronto-parietal parenchymal hemorrhage with subarachnoid hemorrhage and midline shift (Figure C22.1). A repeat CT scan at six hours was unchanged. Approximately 12 hours after initial symptoms, the patient had a generalized convulsion for which she received 4 mg of lorazepam. She received a 1 g loading dose of levetiracetam and was continued on 70 mg/kg/day. Angiography identified an arterio-venous malformation (AVM) at the nidus of hemorrhage. The patient underwent a left hemicraniectomy for decompression with external ventricular drain placement the night of admission to the ICU, after which EEG electrodes were placed. EEG monitoring continued for the next several days while the patient remained sedated; no further seizures occurred. On day 10, after clinical stabilization, the patient underwent resection of her AVM. She underwent heavy sedation with pentobarbital for 48 hours after her procedure to reduce cerebral metabolic demand and swelling. Subsequently, sedation was weaned over three days. Follow-up neuroimaging demonstrated no neurovascular residua of the resected AVM except for the initial hemorrhage. The patient remained hemiparetic on the right side but had intact receptive language, although she remained expressively aphasic. She was transferred to neurorehabilitation on post-hemorrhage day 24.

Discussion

Cerebral arteriovenous malformations typically have clinical presentation in childhood as intraparenchymal hemorrhage, often with concurrent subarachnoid hemorrhage. This may manifest as headache, collapse, and/or as seizure. Seizures are more common when AVMs have cortical involvement. While there is no evidence to support prophylactic anti-seizure medication for all children with ruptured AVM, given the risk of seizures after hemorrhage, EEG monitoring is warranted for early seizure detection and to facilitate prompt treatment. During and immediately after cerebrovascular neurosurgery, heavy sedation including barbiturate-induced coma may be applied to reduce cerebral metabolic demand and potential edema. Continuous EEG monitoring can be useful for titrating these agents to achieve burst suppression without excessive doses that may increase the risk of adverse effects such as hypotension.

Key Neuromonitoring Findings

In this case, the evolution of EEG findings mirrored the patient's clinical progression. The first night of EEG recording followed a clinical convulsive seizure and emergency hemicraniectomy. EEG confirmed there were no ongoing electrographic seizures after the patient returned

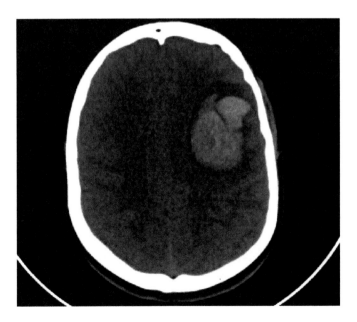

Figure C22.1 Initial CT scan on arrival demonstrating left-sided parenchymal hemorrhage (3.0 × 5.8 × 2.7 cm) and 6 mm of midline shift.

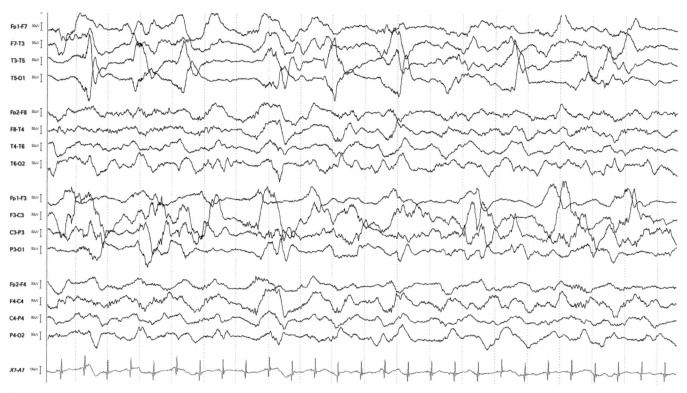

Figure C22.2 EEG recording on the first night of admission, shortly after left hemicraniectomy. Breach rhythm is evident in the left-sided channels, characterized by higher amplitude fast frequencies. There are superimposed left lateral periodic discharges, occurring approximately one every 2 seconds. Note electrodes Fz, Cz, and Pz are omitted due to the external ventricular drain. (Sensitivity 10 μV, Tc 0.1s, HF 70 Hz, 20 seconds per page.)

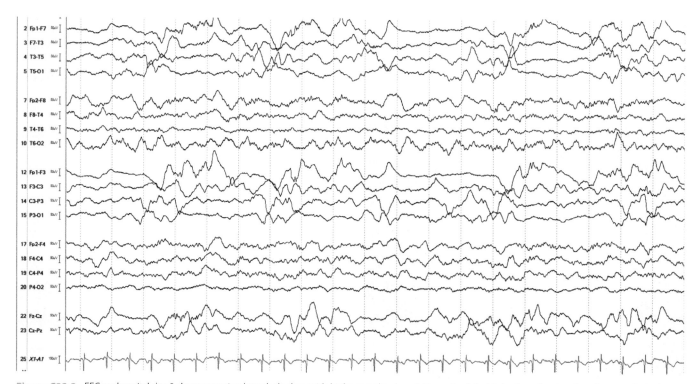

Figure C22.3 EEG on hospital day 8 shows ongoing breach rhythm, with higher amplitude activity on the left side ipsilateral to hemicraniectomy. Periodic discharges have improved; left slowing remains.

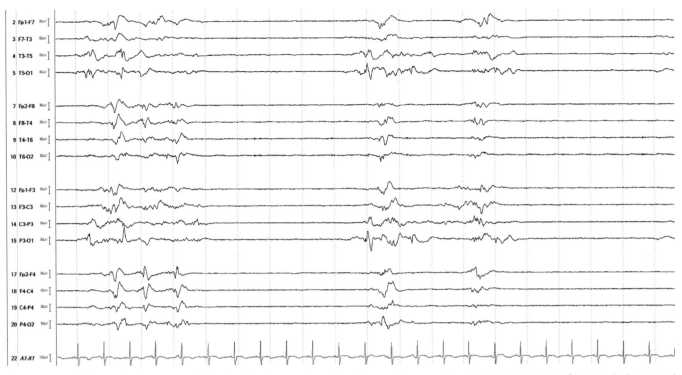

Figure C22.4 EEG immediately post-operatively reflects burst suppression achieved by use of heavy sedation. Suppressed segments of ~5 seconds alternate with bursts of activity lasting 1–4 seconds.

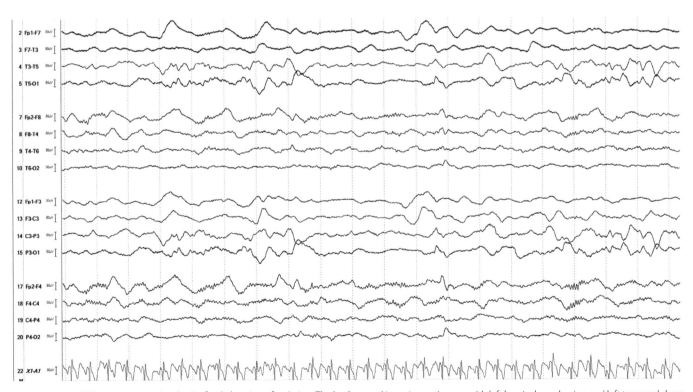

Figure C22.5 EEG on post-operative day 3, after lightening of sedation. The background is again continuous, with left hemisphere slowing and left temporal sharp waves. Fast frequencies are more evident in the right channels.

from the operating room, though it did display findings reflective of focal injury, ongoing risk for seizures, as well as expected breach rhythm (Figure C22.2). EEG subsequently improved as the patient became clinically stable, with reduction of periodic discharges though ongoing asymmetry (Figure C22.3). Immediately post-operatively, EEG was used to titrate sedation with the goal of maintaining burst suppression (Figure C22.4). As sedation was reduced, the EEG became more continuous, though with ongoing asymmetry reflective of the resected lesion (Figure C22.5).

References

1. Fullerton HJ, Achrol AS, Johnston SC, et al.; UCSF BAVM Study Project. Long-term hemorrhage risk in children versus adults with brain arteriovenous malformations. *Stroke.* 2005 Oct;36(10):2099–104. PMID: 16141419.

2. Garcin B, Houdart E, Porcher R, et al. Epileptic seizures at initial presentation in patients with brain arteriovenous malformation. *Neurology.* 2012 Feb 28;78(9):626–31. PMID: 22345217.

3. Hemphill JC 3rd, Greenberg SM, Anderson CS, et al.; American Heart Association Stroke Council; Council on Cardiovascular and Stroke Nursing; Council on Clinical Cardiology. Guidelines for the management of spontaneous intracerebral hemorrhage: a guideline for healthcare professionals from the American Heart Association/ American Stroke Association. *Stroke.* 2015 Jul;46(7):2032–60. PMID: 26022637.

Non-Accidental Injury

Cecil D. Hahn

Clinical Presentation

A previously healthy 9-week-old boy was being breastfed by his mother when he became unresponsive and apneic. The mother called emergency medical services; upon arrival they could not find a pulse. Cardiopulmonary resuscitation was started. The pulse returned, but the baby remained apneic and received bag and mask ventilation while transported to a community hospital. Upon arrival, the baby was awake and moving but lethargic. Twitching movements of the limbs were noted, and he was given a loading dose of fosphenytoin. The baby was sedated, paralyzed, and intubated, then transferred to a specialty pediatric hospital for further care. Upon arrival, he was sedated on midazolam and morphine infusions. Upon exam, the fontanel was bulging. There was no spontaneous eye opening or limb movement, only slight withdrawal to noxious stimuli in all four extremities. There was diffuse hypotonia of the trunk and limbs. Deep tendon reflexes were very brisk throughout, with 2–3 beats of ankle clonus bilaterally. A complete blood count, venous blood gas, serum lactate, liver enzymes, and tests of clotting function were all normal. A CT head (Figure C23.1) demonstrated loss of gray-white differentiation within both cerebral hemispheres with some effacement of the sulci at the vertex. A subdural hematoma was noted adjacent to the superior sagittal sinus, along the posterior falx, tentorium, and posterior fossa. Because of persistent altered mental status, high risk for seizures in the context of acute brain injury, and compromised clinical assessment due to ongoing sedation, continuous EEG monitoring was commenced. Continuous EEG demonstrated recurrent seizures of multifocal onset (Figure C23.3). An MRI the following day (Figure C23.2) demonstrated extensive cortical and subcortical diffusion restriction with sparing of the thalami and basal ganglia, and an extensive subdural hematoma as initially demonstrated on CT.

Discussion

Children with traumatic brain injury are at risk for early post-traumatic seizures (occurring within 7 days of injury). Those with non-accidental mechanisms of injury, younger age, and intra-axial hemorrhage appear to be at particularly high risk [1, 2, 3]. Electrographic seizures have been reported in 42% of children with mild-severe acute traumatic brain injury requiring intensive care who were monitored prospectively with continuous EEG, with electrographic-only (subclinical) seizures in 16% [1]. The occurrence of seizures has been associated with increased duration of hospital stay and worse functional outcome. Consequently, continuous EEG monitoring has been recommended for all children with traumatic brain injury requiring intensive care, particularly those who present with altered mental status (e.g., a Glasgow Coma Scale score of ≤8). Continuous EEG monitoring can also assist with prognostication. Absence of EEG background reactivity has been associated with poor outcome, particularly if the EEG background does not improve over the course of the EEG recording [4]. Preservation of sleep architecture (e.g., sleep spindles, vertex waves) is a favorable prognostic sign [3].

Key Neuromonitoring Findings

Recurrent, bilateral independent electroclinical seizures consisting of subtle right and left hand twitching were apparent

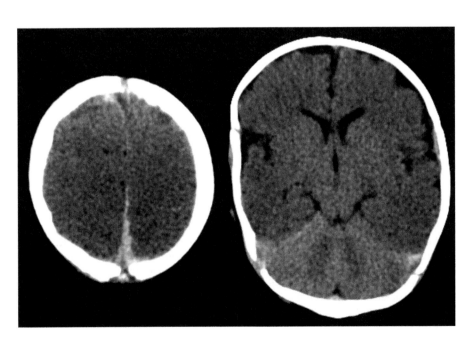

Figure C23.1 Unenhanced CT head obtained on the day of presentation demonstrating loss of gray-white matter differentiation within both cerebral hemispheres diffusely, with effacement of the sulci at the vertex. There is hyperdense subdural hematoma to the left of the superior sagittal sinus, along the posterior falx, along the tentorium, and in the posterior fossa. There was no evidence of venous sinus thrombosis.

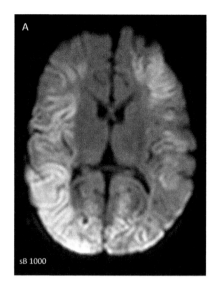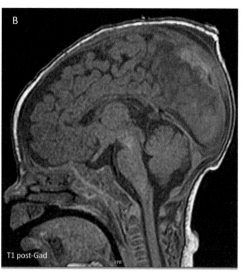

Figure C23.2 MRI brain obtained the following day. Panel A (sB 1000) demonstrates extensive cortical and subcortical diffusion restriction involving all lobes of the cerebral hemispheres. The basal ganglia, thalami, and posterior limbs of the internal capsule appeared normal. Panel B (T1-weighted, post-gadolinium) again demonstrates the extensive subdural hematoma initially visualized on CT.

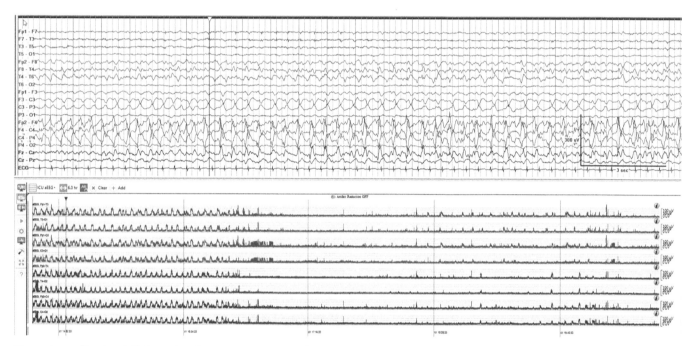

Figure C23.3 First day of cEEG recording demonstrating recurrent left and right electroclinical seizures lasting on average 2 minutes, which persisted for about 2 hours. (Top panel: longitudinal AP bipolar montage, Sensitivity 7 μV/mm, Time base 10 mm/sec, LFF 1 Hz, HFF 70 Hz. Bottom panel: 8-channel amplitude-integrated EEG, 6-hours per page, with blue cursor corresponding to the raw EEG displayed in the top panel.)

from the onset of EEG monitoring on both the raw EEG and amplitude-integrated EEG tracings (Figure C23.3). Following administration of phenobarbital 20 mg/kg, the seizures stopped and the background activity become attenuated (Figure C23.4). About one hour later, focal seizures recurred, initially over the left frontal and then right frontal head regions (Figures C23.5 & C23.6). Following an additional two doses of 10 mg/kg of phenobarbital, these seizures stopped.

References

1. Arndt DH, Lerner JT, Matsumoto JH, et al. Subclinical early posttraumatic seizures detected by continuous EEG monitoring in a consecutive pediatric cohort. *Epilepsia*. 2013;**54**(10):1780–8.

2. Liesemer K, Bratton SL, Zebrack CM, Brockmeyer D, Statler KD. Early post-traumatic seizures in moderate to severe pediatric traumatic brain injury: rates, risk factors, and clinical features. *J Neurotrauma*. 2011;**28** (5):755–62.

3. Vaewpanich J, Reuter-Rice K. Continuous electroencephalography in pediatric traumatic brain injury: Seizure characteristics and outcomes. *Epilepsy Behav*. 2016;**62**:225–30.

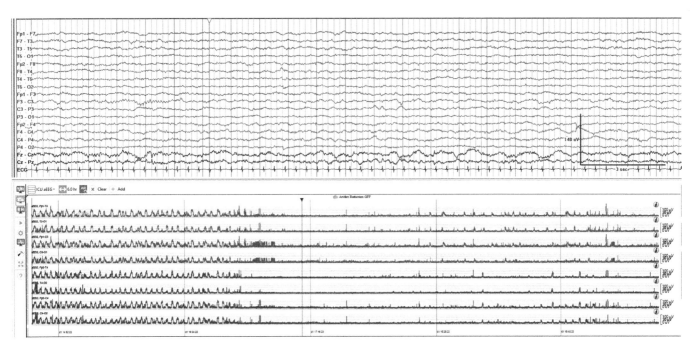

Figure C23.4 Following administration of phenobarbital, seizures cease and the background activity becomes attenuated, with occasional sleep spindles visible over the right central head region.

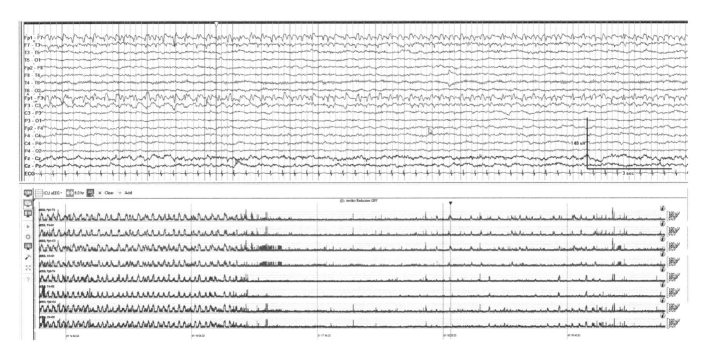

Figure C23.5 One hour later, focal seizures recur, initially over the left frontal head region, lasting 60 seconds.

4. Ramachandrannair R, Sharma R, Weiss SK, Cortez MA. Reactive EEG patterns in pediatric coma. *Pediatr Neurol.* 2005;**33**(5): 345–9.

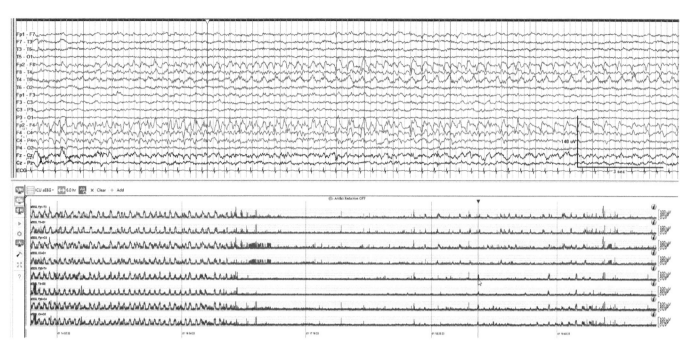

Figure C23.6 Shortly thereafter, focal seizures recurred over the right frontal head region lasting 45–60 seconds.

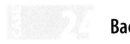

Bacterial Meningitis

Adam Wallace and Eric T. Payne

Clinical Presentation

Following a normal pregnancy and delivery, an 11-day-old term neonate suffered an out-of-hospital acute respiratory arrest and multiple clinical seizures after several days of poor feeding. The patient received cardiopulmonary resuscitation and upon arrival to hospital was intubated and treated for septic shock. Physical exam revealed a Glasgow Coma Scale score of 6, hypothermia to 36°C, and fixed and dilated pupils. His corneal and gag reflexes were present, and his anterior fontanelle was flat. Early head CT demonstrated mild hydrocephalus and large diffuse areas of hypodensity suspicious for ischemia. Cerebral spinal fluid analysis showed 27,000 nucleated cells and grew *E. coli*. Continuous EEG monitoring demonstrated refractory non-convulsive status epilepticus (Figures C24.1–C24.3). Subclinical seizures subsided after treatment with a midazolam infusion. Over the next 12 hours, frequent repetitive clinical paroxysms suspicious for cortically generated myoclonus *vs.* hiccups emerged (Figure C24.4). A brief rocuronium infusion confirmed non-cortical hiccups and diffuse cerebral inactivity. Repeat neuroimaging revealed complete cerebral ischemia, intraventricular debris, and tonsillar herniation. Care was withdrawn 72 hours after hospital admission following demonstration of clinical brain death.

Discussion

Central nervous system infections (meningitis, encephalitis, brain abscess, etc.) can cause direct cell damage and secondary brain injury through seizures, hydrocephalus, increased intracranial pressure, and strokes (ischemic and hemorrhagic). These patients are often obtunded or even comatose, and at high risk for subclinical seizures, thus necessitating the use of continuous EEG monitoring. Post-anoxic brain injury is frequently associated with myoclonus and myoclonic status epilepticus. In a critical care setting it can be challenging to differentiate cortical from non-cortical myoclonus, especially when repositioning the patient is not feasible. The brief use of a paralytic agent (when possible to safely administer) can help eliminate movement artifact and allow for a more reliable assessment of cortical activity [1]. Since paralytic medications (i.e., rocuronium) have no impact on cortical activity, if the paroxysmal movement is cortically generated, then the EEG discharge would persist during pharmacological paralysis. If the EEG activity is due to movement artifact, then it would resolve with pharmacological paralysis.

Key Neuromonitoring Findings

Continuous EEG monitoring was applied within a few hours of hospital admission and identified a highly suppressed, non-reactive background with multifocal subclinical seizures arising independently from both hemispheres (Figure C24.1).

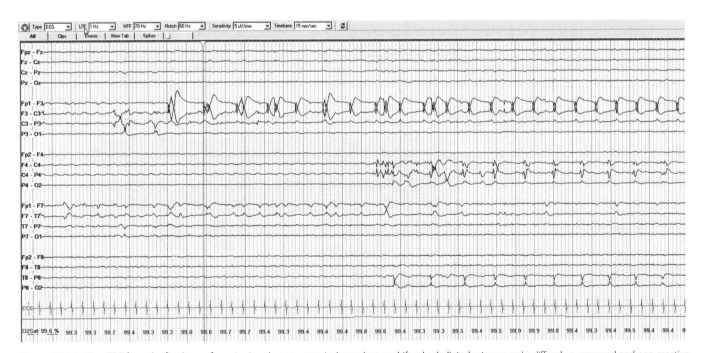

Figure C24.1 Raw EEG from the first hour of monitoring demonstrates independent, multifocal subclinical seizures and a diffusely suppressed and non-reactive background. During this brief epoch, focal seizures arise independently over the left frontal (F3), left anterior temporal (F7), right central (C4), and right parietal (P8) regions.

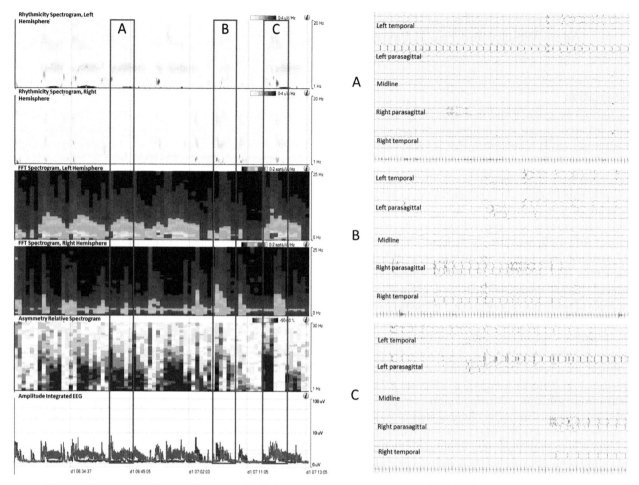

Figure C24.2 A 60-minute quantitative EEG trend panel (left) demonstrates recurrent and prolonged multifocal seizures that are confirmed on raw EEG (right) and consistent with nonconvulsive status epilepticus. (A) Left frontal lobe seizure. (B) Right frontotemporal seizure. (C) Left frontal and independent left temporal seizures are followed by an overlapping but independent right frontotemporal seizure.

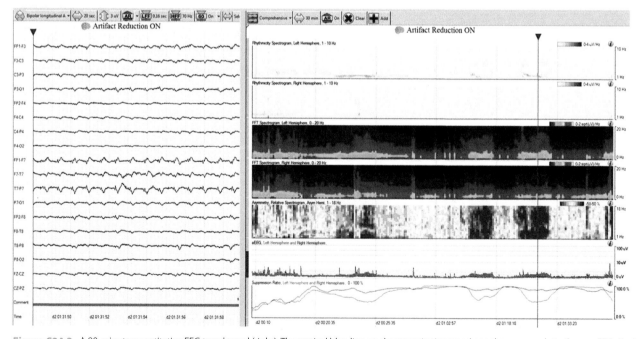

Figure C24.3 A 90-minute quantitative EEG trend panel (right). The vertical blue line on the quantitative trend panel corresponds to the raw EEG displayed on the left during a focal left hemisphere seizure. The suppression ratio on the quantitative trend panel increases to 100% as the anti-seizure medications are titrated and only drops below 100% during left hemisphere seizures.

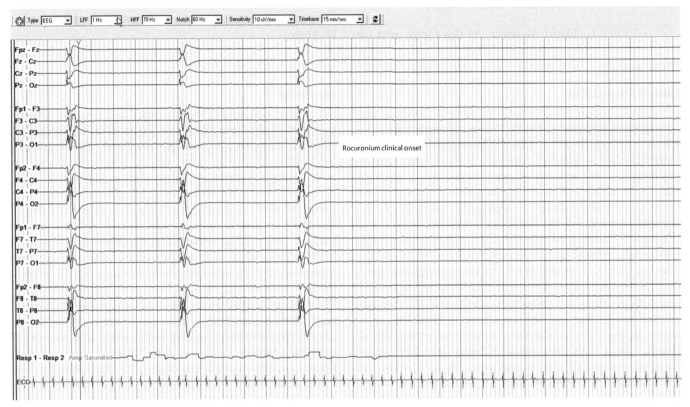

Figure C24.4 Raw EEG during repetitive body jerks. Each jerk correlates electrographically with a posterior predominant generalized "discharge" and is followed by an amplitude elevation on the respiratory belt. After administration of rocuronium, the body jerks and EEG "discharges" cease, confirming their non-cortical origin.

A midazolam infusion was titrated to electrographic seizure cessation. The quantitative EEG trend panels were very accurate and useful at discerning seizure location and duration (Figures C24.2 & C24.3). Repetitive clinical paroxysms consisting of diffuse body jerks emerged, which correlated on EEG with a generalized posterior predominant discharge that resolved after administration with rocuronium (Figure C24.4). Each clinical jerk had caused the posterior head leads to make contact with the bed generating an artifactual EEG "discharge." Since myoclonic seizures often correlate on EEG with frontally predominant spike-wave discharges, the posterior predominance of this patient's discharges was a clue to their non-cortical origin.

References

1. Hirsch L, Brenner R. *Atlas of EEG in Critical Care*. Wiley-Blackwell; 2011.

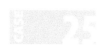

Traumatic Brain Injury

Daad Alsowat, Ayako Ochi, and Cecil D. Hahn

Clinical Presentation

A previously healthy 2-month-old boy was a rear passenger in a high-speed motor vehicle accident. He was restrained in the baby seat and responsive on the scene. When he arrived at a local hospital, he had a Glasgow Coma Scale score of 3 and unequal pupils (left > right) with the left pupil less responsive, left-sided extensor posturing and central apneic episodes. He was transferred to a tertiary pediatric hospital; upon admission to the intensive care unit, his right pupil was 2 mm and reactive and left pupil 3 mm and not reactive. Corneal and oculocephalic reflexes were present, and he demonstrated a weak cough. His tone was flaccid, deep tendon reflexes were exaggerated, there were no spontaneous movements, and there was no response to deep painful stimuli. An initial brain CT showed diffuse subarachnoid hemorrhage and cerebral edema. A second CT performed 9 hours later showed significant interval progression of cerebral edema, likely due to diffuse ischemia with effacement of the ventricles and cisterns. Continuous EEG monitoring was commenced 17 hours after the first CT. Continuous EEG monitoring showed multifocal subclinical status epilepticus. Midazolam infusion was initiated (Figures C25.1–C25.5).

Discussion

Traumatic brain injury (TBI) is a major cause of morbidity and mortality in children. TBI is thought to occur in two phases. The primary injury phase occurs immediately after mechanical forces distort the brain tissue, causing parenchymal and vascular damage. A subsequent, secondary injury phase is associated with failure of cerebral autoregulation and an increase in brain metabolism, leading to cerebral ischemia, release of excitatory neurotransmitters, and cellular energy failure. There is concern that seizures may exacerbate this secondary brain injury; early post-traumatic seizures are associated with increased mortality and worse neurodevelopmental outcomes. Early post-traumatic seizures have been reported in up to 42.5% of children following TBI [1]. Subgroups of children at particularly high risk for seizures include those younger than 2.4 years and victims of abusive head trauma. The majority of early post-traumatic seizures are subclinical, and therefore require continuous EEG monitoring for their identification. The presence of early diffuse slowing on EEG in children with TBI is associated with delayed patient recovery and poor functional outcomes. Continuous EEG monitoring allows for

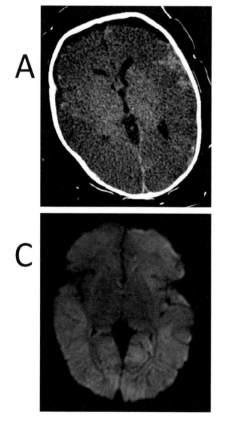

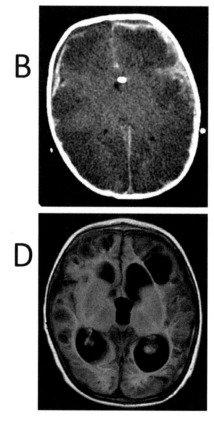

Figure C25.1 (A) Brain CT on day 1 post-injury shows diffuse subarachnoid hemorrhage and cerebral edema. (B) Brain CT 9 hours after the first CT shows significant interval progression of brain swelling, likely related to diffuse ischemia, with effacement of the ventricles and cisterns. Also there is interval increase in size of the subarachnoid hemorrhage and subdural bleed in the posterior fossa. (C) Brain MRI (axial diffusion-weighted imaging) on day 5 post-injury shows diffuse parenchymal edema, and ischemia is again seen in the cerebral hemispheres bilaterally with swelling and diffusion restriction. In addition, there was extensive loss of normal gray-white matter differentiation noted bilaterally involving all lobes (FLAIR sequence, not shown). (D) Five months after the TBI, brain MRI (axial FLAIR) shows interval evolution of supra- and infratentorial extra-axial hemorrhages with small supra- and infratentorial residual collections noted in place. There is extensive supratentorial cystic encephalomalacia with associated laminar necrosis and volume loss.

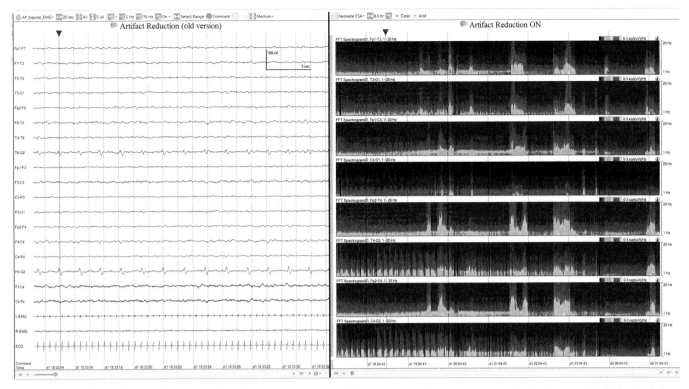

Figure C25.2 cEEG at 17 hours after the first CT. Left panel shows the raw EEG tracing illustrating lateralized periodic discharges at O2. Right panel shows the 8-channel color spectrogram (CSA) at a time scale of 8 hours per page. The corresponding cursors on the EEG and CSA panels indicate the same point in time. The CSA panel illustrates periodic epochs of higher power in the two channels containing O2 electrode corresponding to the lateralized periodic discharges seen on the raw EEG.

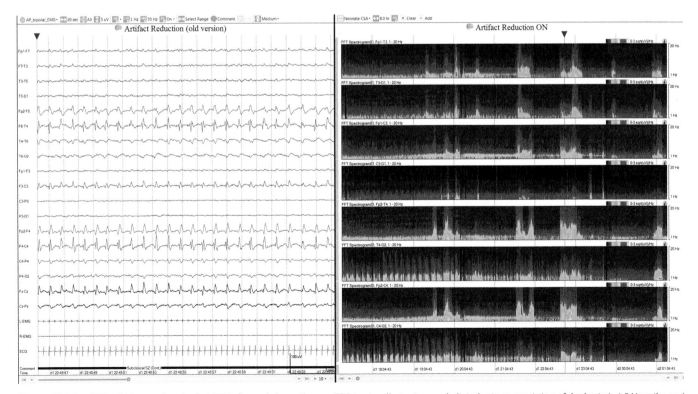

Figure C25.3 cEEG at 21 hours after the first CT. Left panel shows the raw EEG tracing illustrating a subclinical seizure consisting of rhythmic 1–1.5 Hz spike-and-wave activity over the right fronto-central-temporal head region. Right panel shows the 8-channel CSA at a time scale of 8 hours per page, illustrating a sustained epoch of higher power over the right fronto-central head region corresponding to the continuous spike-and-wave discharges seen on the raw EEG.

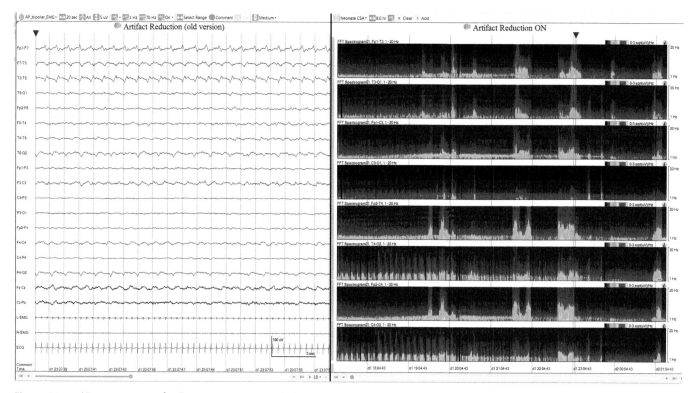

Figure C25.4 Nineteen minutes after Figure 25.3, continuous rhythmic 1–1.5 Hz sharp waves are now seen over the left fronto-temporal head region on the raw EEG in the left panel, and on CSA in the right panel. Note how the higher power activity has shifted from the right to the left hemispheric electrodes on CSA. This seizure lasted a total of 33 minutes.

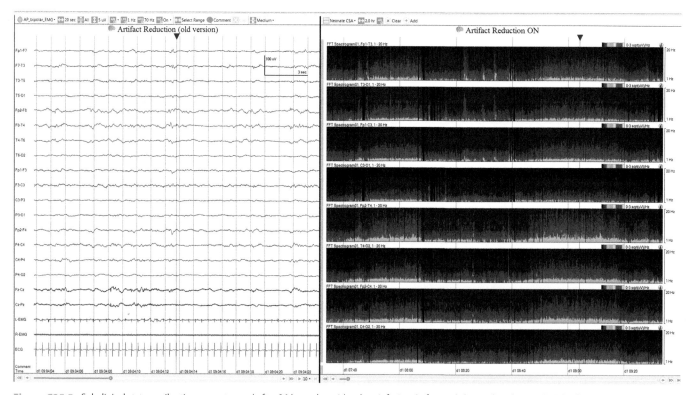

Figure C25.5 Subclinical status epilepticus was stopped after 36 hours by midazolam infusion. Left panel shows that the raw EEG background activity is suppressed, with frequent low amplitude sharp waves at F8-T4, F4, Cz, F7-T3, T5, and F3. There was no reactivity of the EEG to painful stimulation. There was no sleep architecture. The right panel shows the corresponding CSA tracing illustrating diffusely lower power.

accurate diagnosis and timely treatment of post-traumatic seizures, which may mitigate secondary injury [2, 3, 4, 5].

Key Neuromonitoring Findings

EEG findings soon after injury correlate with the location and severity of brain injury and prognosis. For example, a slow monotonous pattern has been associated with a prolonged coma and poor prognosis. Normal sleep architecture and EEG reactivity correlate with favorable outcome. Lack of spontaneous arousal activity correlates with death or a vegetative state. The interictal EEG may be normal or may show focal or multifocal interictal spikes or spike-and-wave discharges over the location(s) of the traumatic brain injury. Risk factors for subclinical seizures include younger age, abusive head trauma, and intra-axial hemorrhage. In this case, continuous EEG monitoring showed multifocal subclinical status epilepticus. The background activity was markedly suppressed. There was no EEG reactivity or spontaneous arousal activity. After midazolam controlled the subclinical status epilepticus, the background activity remained diffusely attenuated and there were multifocal interictal epileptiform discharges.

References

1. Arndt DH, Lerner JT, Matsumoto JH, et al. Subclinical early posttraumatic seizures detected by continuous EEG monitoring in a consecutive pediatric cohort. *Epilepsia*. 2013;**54**(10):1780–8.

2. Nadlonek NA, Acker SN, Bensard DD, Bansal S, Partrick DA. Early diffuse slowing on electroencephalogram in pediatric traumatic brain injury: impact on management and prognosis. *J Pediatr Surg*. 2015;**50**:1338–40.

3. O'Neill BR, Handler MH, Tong S, Chapman KE. Incidence of seizures on continuous EEG monitoring following traumatic brain injury in children. *J Neurosurg Pediatr*. 2015;**16**:167–76.

4. Arndt DH, Goodkin HP, Giza CC. Early posttraumatic seizures in the pediatric population. *J Child Neurol*. 2016;**31**(1):46–56.

5. Vaewpanich J, Reuter-Rice K. Continuous electroencephalography in pediatric traumatic brain injury: seizure characteristics and outcomes. *Epilepsy Behav*. 2016;**62**:225–30.

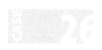

Acute Pediatric Stroke

Saptharishi Lalgudi Ganesan and Cecil D. Hahn

Clinical Presentation

A previously healthy 2-month-old girl presented with a 2-day history of nasal congestion, lethargy, and poor feeding. On the second day of illness, she developed eye deviation and twitching of arms. There was no history of fever or trauma. On presentation to the community hospital, she was found to have right-sided seizures, which were treated with anti-seizure medicines. She developed respiratory failure, requiring endotracheal intubation and ventilation. Her initial CT head showed right cerebral hemispheric hypodensity, loss of gray-white differentiation, and severe edema. In view of her worsening neurological status, with bulging anterior fontanelle and cerebral edema on her scan, she received hypertonic saline, broad-spectrum antibiotics, and antivirals. She was managed with neuroprotective measures and aggressive seizure control. Her MRI scan revealed extensive diffusion restriction with loss of gray-white matter differentiation involving cortex, subcortical, and deep white matter of almost the entire right cerebral hemisphere and left frontal lobe. Diffusion restriction was also seen in the right-sided corpus callosum, posterior limb of internal capsule, and corticospinal tract extending down to the pons. MR angiography showed diffuse vasculopathy with marked attenuation of the supra-clinoid portion of carotid arteries and narrowing of the proximal anterior and middle cerebral arteries bilaterally. Attenuation of proximal basilar

with superimposed beading was also noted. The neuroimaging was suggestive of a diffuse vasculopathic process and large strokes. She received anticoagulation, high-dose steroids (to treat potential inflammatory etiologies), and supportive measures in the intensive care unit. She also had continuous EEG monitoring (Figures C26.1–C26.2) during the two days that she was in the ICU. Despite these interventions, she continued to deteriorate clinically, with her second MRI showing extension of the infarction to her left hemisphere. In view of her severe neurological injury, parents wanted to discontinue aggressive interventions and withdraw life-sustaining therapies. She was extubated in the presence of her family and died peacefully in their arms.

Discussion

Etiology of the large hemispheric infarcts appeared to be unclear and likely related to the vasculopathy evident on MR angiography. Moyamoya disease is a cerebrovascular disorder characterized by the progressive occlusion of the supra-clinoid internal carotid artery and other intracranial vessels. Moyamoya disease in young children could present as rapidly progressing cerebral infarction with neurological deficits or seizures, as in this case [1]. There are descriptions of a similar attack of cerebral infarction on the contralateral side shortly after disease onset [2–4]. The aggressive natural course and

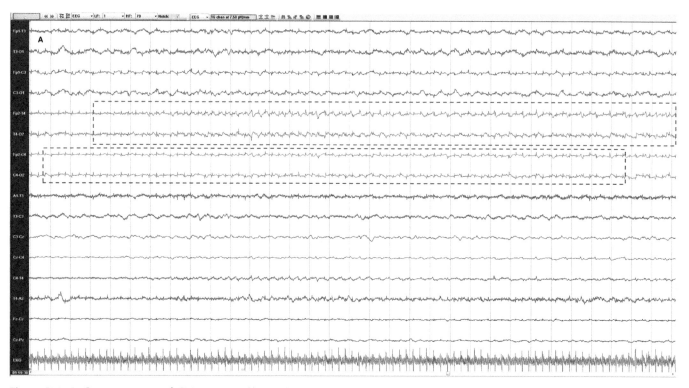

Figure C26.1A Consecutive pages of cEEG in a neonatal longitudinal bipolar montage. A subtle electrographic seizure is noted [highlighted in red] with onset in the right frontal head region (A) and subsequent spread to the right central head region (B). Recognition of this child's seizures was complicated by widespread ECG artifacts [highlighted in blue].

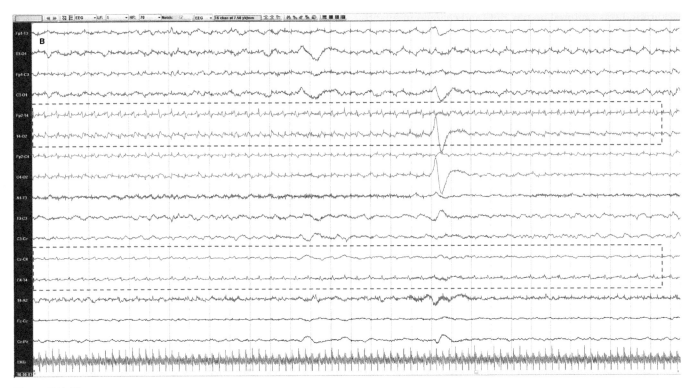

Figure C26.1B

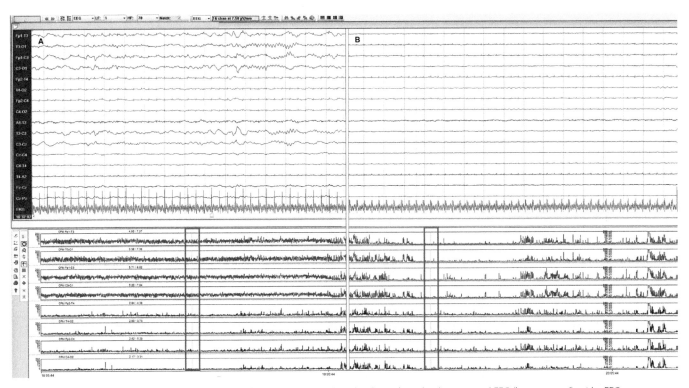

Figure C26.2 Composite figure showing two epochs of raw EEG (top panel) and 8-channel amplitude-integrated EEG (bottom panel), with aEEG segments corresponding to the raw EEG above noted in red. The first segment (A) demonstrates asymmetric background activity with attenuation over the right hemisphere. The second segment (B) approximately 1 hour later demonstrates abrupt onset of diffuse background attenuation due to new left hemispheric ischemia.

poor clinical outcome in this age group are well documented. In this case, the etiology for the vasculopathy could not be identified despite extensive evaluation including genetic

testing. The EEG can be very useful at the bedside in the neurocritical care unit and reflects integrity of the underlying neuronal circuits [5]. In this case, abrupt change in the background was captured on raw EEG and changes in quantitative EEG display trends (amplitude-integrated EEG) suggested acute ischemia in the left hemisphere.

Key Neuromonitoring Findings

EEG background in this case showed continuous, low-amplitude (30–50 μV) delta waves in the right hemisphere and moderate-amplitude (>50 μV) delta and theta waves on the left hemisphere. Sleep spindles were seen only on the left hemisphere. ECG artifacts were most prominent at A1, A2, Fp1, Fp2. Intermittent sharp waves were seen at T3 and C3. Progressively the background became more suppressed with amplitude <25 μV. Three brief focal subclinical seizures were seen originating from the right fronto-temporal region. On day 2 of monitoring, there was an abrupt attenuation of the background over the left hemisphere. Subsequently, over the next hour, it became severely attenuated like the right hemisphere. The MRI done thereafter showed extension of the infarction to the left hemisphere. This case demonstrates the ability of EEG to detect cerebral ischemia in real time.

References

1. Wang KC, Kim SK, Seol HJ, Cho BK. Moyamoya disease in young children. In Cho BK, Tominaga T, editors. *Moyamoya Disease Update*. Springer; 2010.

2. Maki Y, Enomoto T. Moyamoya disease. *Childs Nerv Syst*. 1988;**4**:204–12.

3. Matsushima Y, Aoyagi M, Masaoka H, et al. Mental outcome following encephaloduroarterio-synangiosis in children with Moyamoya disease with the onset earlier than 5 years of age. *Childs Nerv Syst*. 1990;**6**:440–43.

4. Kim SK, Seol HJ, Cho BK, et al. Moyamoya disease among young patients: its aggressive clinical course and the role of active surgical treatment. *Neurosurgery*. 2004;**54**:840–4.

5. Foreman B, Claassen J. Quantitative EEG for the detection of brain ischemia. *Crit Care*. 2012;**16**(2):216.

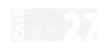

Autoimmune Encephalitis

William B. Gallentine

Clinical Presentation

A 16-year-old female presented with episodic confusion and disorientation. One week prior to symptom onset she had signs of an upper respiratory tract infection. Two days prior to presentation, she began complaining of diffuse headache and seemed to be more forgetful. On the day of presentation, she had episodes of confusion with associated lip smacking and fumbling with both hands. These episodes would last a few minutes, followed by periods of lucidity. She then started having erratic behaviors including paranoia, rapid mood swings with paroxysms of laughter followed by crying, as well as visual and auditory hallucinations. Over the next few days her speech became nonsensical. Head CT and MRI brain scans with contrast were normal. Lumbar puncture revealed 46 WBC (97% lymphocytes), with no organisms seen on gram stain. CSF glucose and protein were normal, and CSF HSV PCR was negative. Twenty-four hours after initial presentation she developed two episodes of generalized stiffening followed by rhythmic jerking, with eye deviation to the right lasting 2 minutes. The previously described behaviors continued, with worsening confusion and shorter periods of lucidity. She also developed oral dyskinesias and severe insomnia. cEEG monitoring revealed frequent focal seizures coming from the left temporal lobe (Figure C27.1) which were refractory to numerous antiepileptic drugs. One week into the illness, CSF tested positive for anti-*N*-methyl-D-aspartate (NMDA) receptor

antibodies. She was found to have an ovarian teratoma that was subsequently resected. She was treated with IV methylprednisolone, IVIG, and rituximab. Six months after initial presentation, she had fully recovered.

Discussion

This case is an excellent example of how bedside QEEG may reduce the time from seizure onset to seizure recognition. In Figure C27.2, the black arrow illustrates when the cEEG was last reviewed by a neurophysiologist at around 1:30 p.m. Because this patient had been on cEEG for 12 hours prior to this review without any evidence of seizures, the next routine review was scheduled for 5:00 p.m. (red arrow). However, at around 2:00 p.m. the patient began having 10–12 seizures per hour, which went undetected until the next scheduled cEEG review. Had QEEG trends been available at this child's bedside, seizure recognition by bedside caregivers may have occurred much sooner, allowing for more rapid intervention.

Key Neuromonitoring Findings

Individuals with anti-NMDA receptor encephalitis commonly have diffuse or focal EEG background slowing. One third of patients have a unique pattern known as extreme delta brush, named for its resemblance to the delta brush pattern commonly seen in preterm neonates. The presence of extreme delta brushes has been associated with worse outcomes.

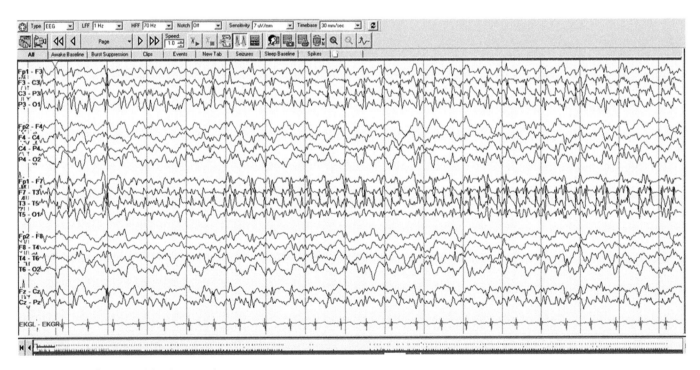

Figure C27.1 Left temporal lobe electrographic seizure.

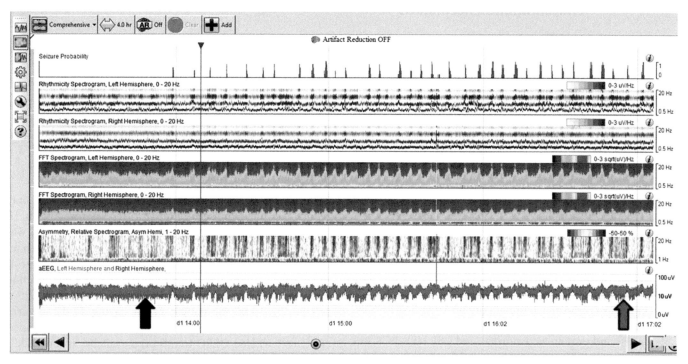

Figure C27.2 QEEG trend panel (from top to bottom: seizure probability index, rhythmicity spectrogram, fast Fourier transform [FFT] spectrogram, relative asymmetry spectrogram, amplitude-integrated EEG) revealing recurrent left temporal lobe electrographic seizures. Black and red arrows indicate the timing of routine cEEG review in this case.

Multifocal interictal spikes are also commonly seen in anti-NMDA receptor encephalitis, as well as in other autoimmune epilepsies. Like many patients with anti-NMDA receptor encephalitis, this patient developed very frequent drug-resistant temporal lobe seizures (Figure C27.1), which were visualized quite well on QEEG trends (Figure C27.2).

References

1. Schmitt SE, Pargeon K, Frechette ES, et al. Extreme delta brush: a unique EEG pattern in adults with anti-NMDA receptor encephalitis. *Neurology*. 2012 Sep 11;**79**(11):1094–100.

2. Quek AM, Britton JW, McKeon A, et al. Autoimmune epilepsy: clinical characteristics and response to immunotherapy. *Arch Neurol*. 2012 May;**69**(5): 582–93.

290

Febrile Infection–Related Epilepsy Syndrome (FIRES)

Eric T. Payne, Adam Wallace, and Cecil D. Hahn

Clinical Presentation

A 12-year-old developmentally and cognitively normal boy presented in clinical status epilepticus (SE) following a week-long febrile (viral) respiratory illness. Treatment with anti-seizure medications led to resolution of clinical SE. However, continuous EEG monitoring (cEEG) quickly confirmed ongoing, refractory, nonconvulsive SE (Figures C28.1 & C28.2). A barbiturate infusion was necessary on day 3 to combat his now super refractory SE. Over the next few weeks, subclinical seizures re-emerged when the barbiturate infusion rate was decreased, despite attempts at control by introducing other anti-seizure medications (levetiracetam, fosphenytoin, topiramate, ketamine, lacosamide, and methylprednisolone), as well as a 4:1 ketogenic diet. During this time, extensive investigations returned normal; the patient was diagnosed with febrile infection–related epilepsy syndrome (FIRES). The barbiturate infusion was weaned off after 6 weeks, although intermittent focal subclinical seizures continued. Sequelae from this prolonged infusion included hypotension requiring multiple pressors, infections (ventilator acquired pneumonia, urinary tract infection), ileus, venous thrombosis, hypersensitivity drug reaction, tracheostomy, and G-tube insertion. Repeat neuroimaging showed only mild diffuse atrophy. One year after discharge, he had refractory epilepsy and remained with severe motor and cognitive deficits requiring ongoing rehabilitation.

Discussion

FIRES is a devastating epileptic encephalopathy of unclear etiology, although evidence for an inflammatory pathophysiology is emerging [1, 2]. FIRES most commonly affects school-age children. Following a nonspecific febrile illness, affected children experience frequent repetitive multifocal seizures that are notoriously refractory to anti-seizure medications and often require anesthetic infusion to induce variable degrees of background suppression. cEEG monitoring is essential to detect and treat subclinical seizures. Outcomes in these children are most often poor, although some can achieve a relatively good outcome [1, 2], particularly when the need for prolonged anesthesia can be avoided [3].

Key Neuromonitoring Findings

During the first hour of cEEG, multifocal repetitive seizures arose independently over both hemispheres in the context of a continuous background and bilateral independent periodic discharges (Figure C28.1) sometimes with concurrent contralateral seizures (Figure C28.2). As a high-dose midazolam infusion was increased, generalized periodic discharges (GPDs) and a burst suppression pattern emerged, yet seizures continued to break through (Figure C28.3). A barbiturate coma extended the inter-burst interval (at times exceeding 5 minutes) and led to improved seizure control. However, the patient remained on the ictal-interictal continuum [4] for the next 6 weeks of monitoring, fluctuating between GPD burst suppression (varying inter-burst intervals), continuous and rhythmic GPDs, and definite electrographic seizures (Figure C28.3). Stimulus-induced periodic discharges and seizures are common in this clinical scenario (Figure C28.4) [5].

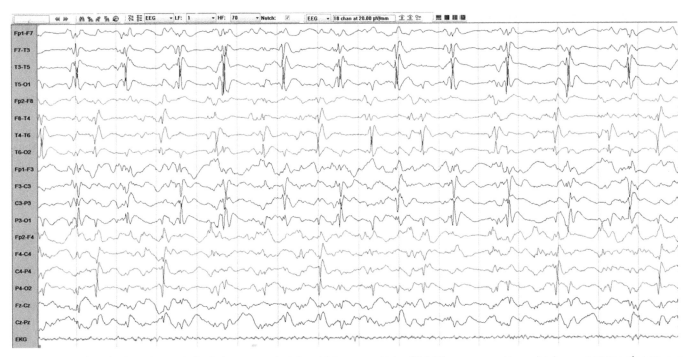

Figure C28.1 Bilateral independent periodic discharges over the left and right temporal lobes (T5 & T6) were apparent immediately upon initiation of continuous EEG monitoring.

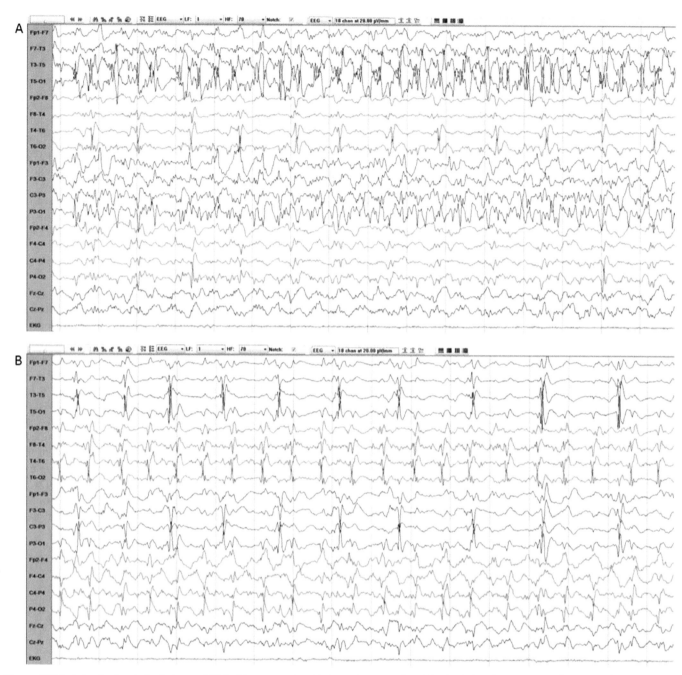

Figure C28.2 Lateralized periodic discharges (LPDs) with concurrent and independent contralateral focal subclinical seizures. (A) Left temporal focal subclinical seizure (maximal at T5) with spread to the left hemisphere and concurrent independent right temporal LPDs (maximal at T6). (B) Right hemisphere subclinical seizure and concurrent independent left temporal LPDs (maximal at T5).

References

1. Kramer U, Chi CS, Lin KL, et al. Febrile infection-related epilepsy syndrome (FIRES): pathogenesis, treatment, and outcome: a multicenter study on 77 children. *Epilepsia*. 2011;**52** (11):1956–65.

2. Kenney-Jung DL, Vezzani A, Kahoud RJ, et al. Febrile infection-related epilepsy

syndrome treated with anakinra. *Ann Neurol*. 2016;**80**(6):939–45.

3. Kramer U, Chi CS, Lin KL, et al. Febrile infection-related epilepsy syndrome (FIRES): does duration of anesthesia affect outcome? *Epilepsia*. 2011; **52** (Suppl 8):28–30.

4. Chong DJ, Hirsch LJ. Which EEG patterns warrant treatment in the critically ill? Reviewing the evidence

for treatment of periodic epileptiform discharges and related patterns. *J Clin Neurophysiol*. 2005;**22** (2):79–91.

5. Hirsch LJ, Claassen J, Mayer SA, Emerson RG. Stimulus-induced rhythmic, periodic, or ictal discharges (SIRPIDs): a common EEG phenomenon in the critically ill. *Epilepsia*. 2004;**45**(2):109–23.

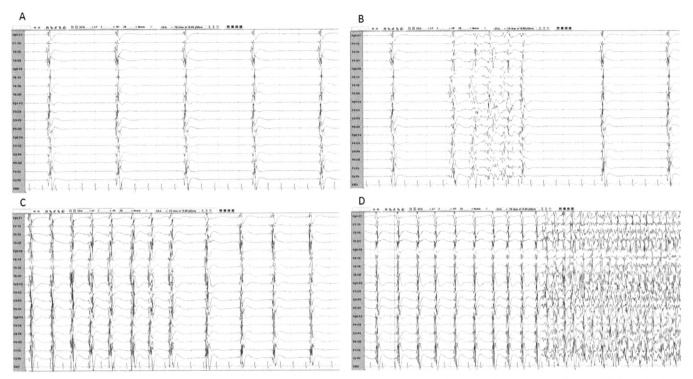

Figure C28.3 Ictal-interictal continuum during ongoing barbiturate (high-dose phenobarbital) coma for super-refractory status epilepticus. (A) Generalized periodic discharges (GPDs), <1 Hz, variable frequency over time. (B) GPDs intermixed with a brief (3-second) subclinical bi-hemispheric "ictal-like" discharge. (C) Rhythmic and continuous GPDs, 1–2 Hz, lacking clear electrographic evolution and any clinical correlate. (D) Rhythmic GPDs evolve to produce a sustained subclinical bi-hemispheric seizure.

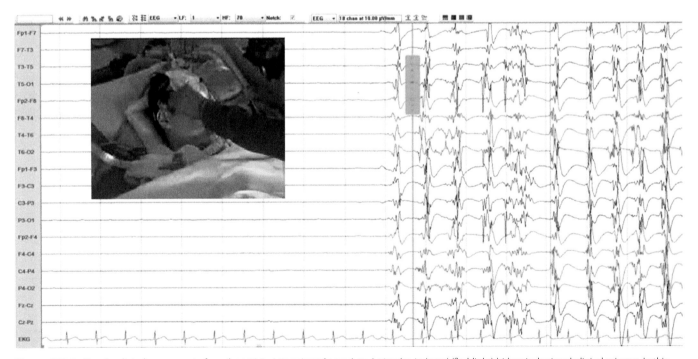

Figure C28.4 Regular clinical assessment of pupil reactivity intermittently produced stimulus-induced (flashlight) bi-hemispheric subclinical seizures. In this instance, a GPD had just fired prior to flashlight stimulation, triggering the seizure.

Baclofen Intoxication

Chusak Limotai, Iris Noyman, and Cecil D. Hahn

Clinical Presentation

A previously healthy 14-year-old girl was found by her parents unconscious in bed in a pool of vomit. She was last observed to be normal 6 hours earlier. Paramedics were called, and she was intubated on the scene and rushed to hospital. Upon arrival she was normotensive, bradycardic, and made no respiratory effort. She had a Glasgow Coma Scale score of 3 and absent brainstem and deep tendon reflexes. Blood gases, serum glucose, electrolytes, liver enzymes, a complete blood count, and toxicology screens of urine and blood were normal. No improvement was seen following administration of glucose or naloxone. She subsequently developed hypotension requiring a dopamine infusion. Brain CT was normal. She was admitted to the intensive care unit, where upon reexamination her pupils remained fixed at 4 mm bilaterally, but corneal and oculocephalic reflexes were present and she demonstrated a weak cough. Her tone was flaccid, deep tendon reflexes were absent, there were no spontaneous movements, and there was no response to deep painful stimuli. Brain MRI, MRA, and MRV were normal. CSF examination was normal. Continuous EEG

monitoring was commenced after return from MRI (Figures C29.1–C29.4). She regained consciousness 35 hours after coma onset. Upon further questioning, it became clear that she had deliberately overdosed on her grandmother's "back pain medication," oral baclofen.

Discussion

Baclofen, a derivative of gamma-aminobutyric acid (GABA), is an agonist at presynaptic $GABA_B$ receptors in the spinal cord and also has central nervous system depressant effects. Baclofen is primarily used to treat spasticity. Toxicity may result from oral or intrathecal overdose. Signs and symptoms of baclofen toxicity include nausea, ataxia, and agitation, followed by profound coma, flaccid areflexia, respiratory depression, absent brainstem reflexes including pupillary responses, hypotension, bradycardia or tachycardia, hypersalivation, hypothermia, myoclonus, and seizures. There is no antidote, so treatment is limited to supportive care. Complete recovery is common, but deaths have been reported due to rhabdomyolysis and multisystem organ failure.

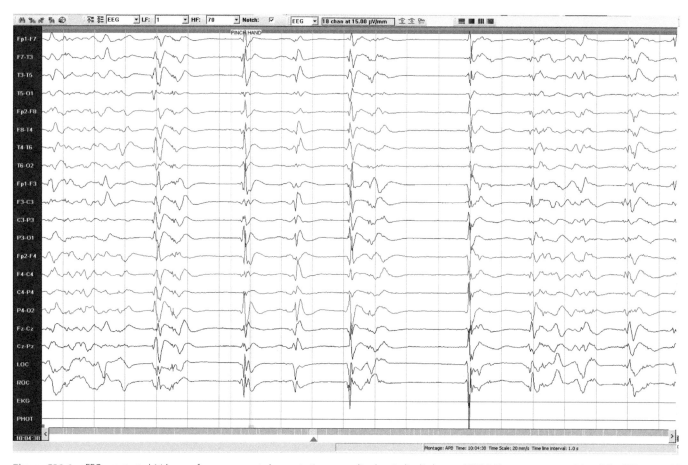

Figure C29.1 cEEG was started 14 hours after coma onset, demonstrating generalized periodic discharges (GPDs). There was no reactivity of the EEG to painful stimulation (see annotation).

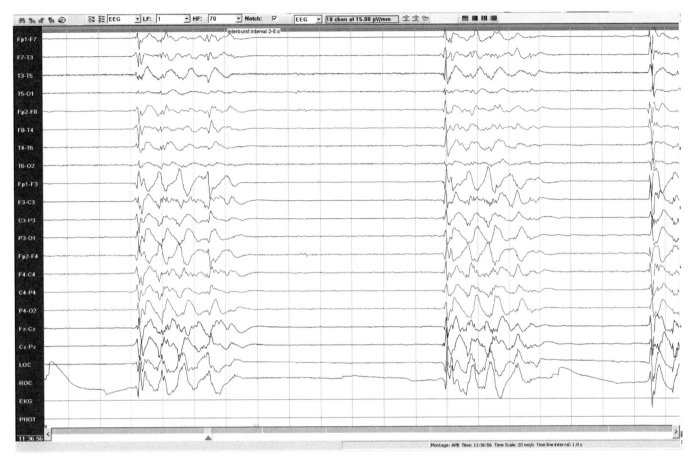

Figure C29.2 Ninety minutes later, GPDs began to alternate with periods of generalized background suppression lasting 2–8 seconds.

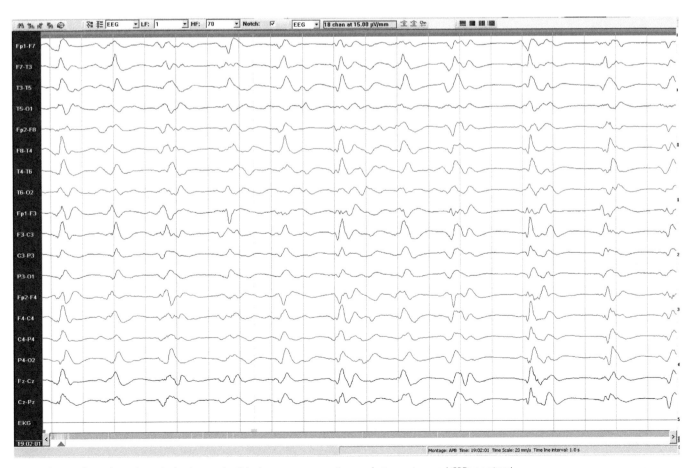

Figure C29.3 Seven hours later, the background activity became more continuous, but superimposed GPDs persisted.

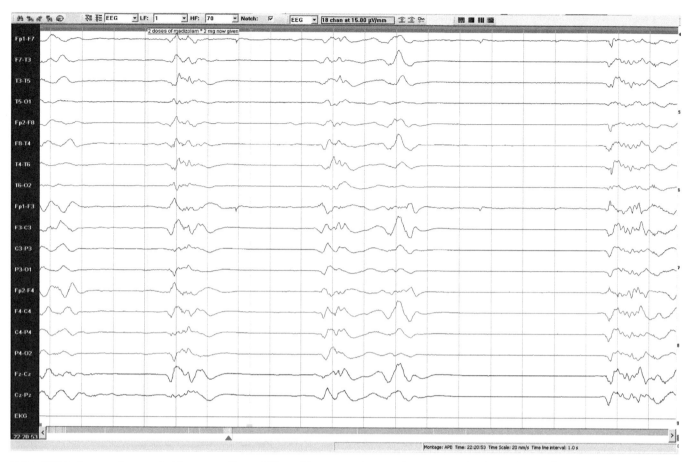

Figure C29.4 Because of concern that the near-continuous GPDs could represent seizures, an intravenous midazolam trial was performed (2 doses of 2 mg), which resulted in greater background discontinuity but no clinical change.

Key Neuromonitoring Findings

Reported EEG findings of baclofen intoxication include a burst suppression background, generalized polymorphic or monomorphic delta activity, and generalized periodic discharges, which may have triphasic morphology and may be stimulus induced. In this case, the discordance between the severe clinical presentation and EEG suppression, and the normal MRI including absence of diffusion restriction, raised suspicion of intoxication. Without a history of baclofen exposure, the diagnosis would have been difficult because the drug is not detected by routine toxicology screening and serum levels are not readily obtainable.

References

1. Darbari FP, Melvin JJ, Piatt JH, Jr., Adirim TA, Kothare SV. Intrathecal baclofen overdose followed by withdrawal: clinical and EEG features. *Pediatr Neurol.* 2005;**33**(5):373–7.

2. Kumar G, Sahaya K, Goyal MK, Sivaraman M, Sahota PK. Electroencephalographic abnormalities in baclofen-induced encephalopathy. *J Clin Neurosci.* 2010;**17**(12): 1594–6.

3. Skjei KL, Kessler SK, Abend NS. Stimulus-induced rhythmic, periodic, or ictal discharges in a 13-year-old girl after an overdose and respiratory arrest. *Pediatr Neurol.* 2011; **45**(5):350–1.

Intraventricular Tumor

Adam Wallace and Eric T. Payne

Clinical Presentation

A 2-week-old, ex–35 week gestation girl presented to hospital with persistent vomiting and a bulging anterior fontanelle. Neuroimaging demonstrated a large intraventricular tumor causing obstructive hydrocephalus (Figure C30.1A). Pathology confirmed a grade IV embryonal tumor. Despite chemotherapy, the tumor continued to grow. At age 3 months, resection with a right frontal transcallosal approach was performed. Only partial resection was possible due to difficulty with excessive bleeding. On post-operative day 2, during sedation wean, paroxysmal events of left lower extremity clonic activity and sustained gaze deviation to the left were observed. Continuous video-EEG monitoring confirmed clinical and subclinical seizures emanating from the right frontocentral region (Figure C30.2). Anticonvulsant medications were promptly administered, and seizures abated. Repeat neuroimaging demonstrated residual blood products and expected post-operative changes along the surgical tract but no evidence of ischemia (Figure C30.1B).

Discussion

Neurosurgical manipulation can be complicated by post-operative seizures. The transcallosal and transcortical approaches for accessing ventricular tumors are associated with a particularly increased risk for post-operative seizures [1]. Furthermore, since patients often remain sedated following neurosurgical intervention, seizures are often subclinical. Following neurosurgical intervention, careful clinical observation and a low threshold for continuous EEG monitoring are necessary for accurate seizure detection. In this instance, EEG-confirmed seizures were found to originate over cortex adjacent to the surgical tract.

Key Neuromonitoring Findings

Continuous EEG monitoring revealed a background activity that was continuous, of moderate amplitude, and reactive to stimulation. Excessive negative sharp transients were present, consistent with a mild degree of encephalopathy of nonspecific etiology. Prior to any seizures being observed, focal repetitive negative sharp transients occurred over the right frontocentral and central midline regions, suggesting a propensity toward focal onset seizures. A quantitative EEG trend panel clearly demonstrated four brief focal right hemisphere seizures (Figure C30.2A). These seizures were subclinical. Full EEG confirmed a focal seizure arising over the right frontocentral region (Figure C30.2B,C).

Reference

1. Milligan B, Meyer F. Morbidity of transcallosal and transcortical approaches to lesions in and around the lateral and third ventricles: a single-institution experience. *Neurosurgery*. 2010;67(6):1483.

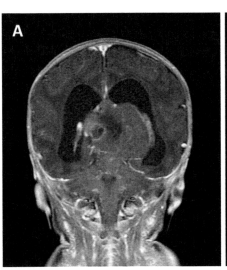
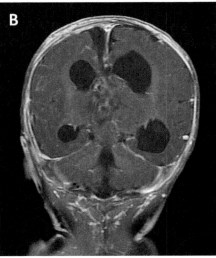

Figure C30.1 Brain MRI pre- and post-transcallosal tumor debulking. (A) Pre-operative coronal T1 with gadolinium demonstrates a large heterogeneous non-enhancing cystic third ventricular mass that extends into the lateral ventricles and posterior fossa causing obstructive hydrocephalus. (B) Post-operative coronal T1 with gadolinium demonstrates post-operative changes in the right frontal and interhemispheric regions.

A

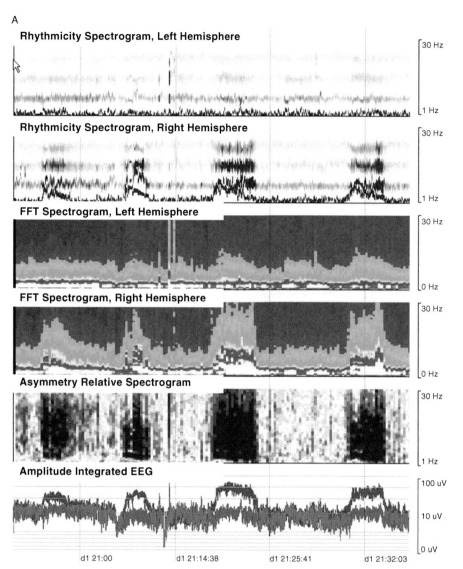

Rhythmicity Spectrogram, Left Hemisphere

Rhythmicity Spectrogram, Right Hemisphere

FFT Spectrogram, Left Hemisphere

FFT Spectrogram, Right Hemisphere

Asymmetry Relative Spectrogram

Amplitude Integrated EEG

Figure C30.2 Continuous EEG monitoring began 52 hours post-surgery to characterize clinical paroxysms suspicious for seizures. (A) A 30-minute epoch of quantitative EEG clearly identifies four electrographic seizures arising over the right hemisphere (right rhythmicity spectrogram, right FFT [power] spectrogram, right asymmetry spectrogram, and elevated lower and upper margins on amplitude-integrated EEG). (B & C) Focal electrographic seizure arises over the right central area and rapidly spreads to the right frontal and midline frontal areas.

B

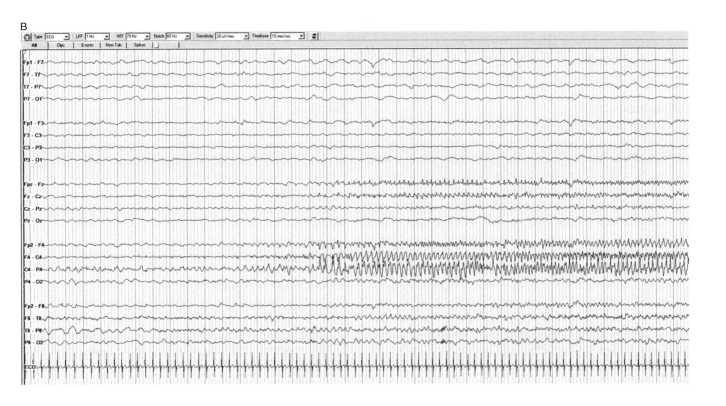

C

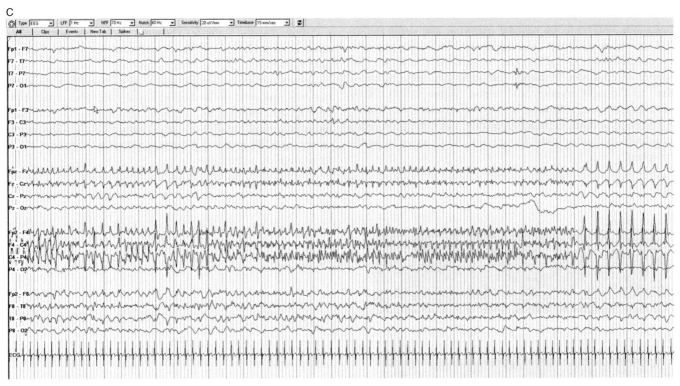

Figure C30.2 (cont.)

Multimodality Monitoring of Acute Stroke

Shefali Aggarwal and Brian Appavu

Clinical Presentation

A 6-year-old female with congenital heart disease (atrioventricular septal defect, pulmonary atresia with fenestrated Fontan repair) was admitted for worsening heart failure. Her course was complicated by line-related non-occlusive upper extremity deep vein thromboses, treated with enoxaparin. One week into her hospital course, she developed sudden loss of bladder and bowel control with progressively altered mental status and gait instability. Stat CT head scan was unremarkable. The following morning, her mental status remained altered, and she developed a new right-sided hemiplegia and facial droop with concern for acute middle cerebral artery (MCA) stroke. Her last known well time was 12–16 hours prior to presentation. Bedside transcranial Doppler (TCD) ultrasound showed asymmetric MCA mean flow velocities (MFVs), with normal right MCA MFVs at 46 cm/sec and decreased left MCA MFVs at 24 cm/sec with dampened waveform morphology (thrombolysis in brain ischemia [TIBI] classification III) (Figures C31.1 & C31.2). MRI brain showed complete left MCA occlusion (proximal M1 segment) with infarction in the left basal ganglia and external capsule (Figure C31.3A, B). An urgent cerebral angiogram with mechanical thrombectomy was performed. Two clots were successfully removed. Postoperatively, she was placed on neurological monitoring including continuous EEG, cerebral regional oximetry, and daily TCDs. EEG showed polymorphic delta slowing over the left hemisphere and quantitative EEG (QEEG) analysis revealed a decreased left anterior spectral edge frequency and alpha-delta ratio as compared to the right anterior head region (Figure C31.4). TCD velocities improved following her revascularization procedure. She received post-stroke standard of care, was started on anticoagulation and anti-platelet therapy, and later received a heart transplant.

Discussion

This case highlights the utility of advanced neuromonitoring techniques in a child with an acute arterial ischemic stroke. Although initial CT head was negative despite acute clinical changes in mental status and gait, additional neuromonitoring techniques supported the diagnosis of an acute stroke secondary to a large vessel occlusion. TCD can assess cerebral blood flow through assessment of MFVs and waveform analysis and grading [1]. TCD demonstrated asymmetry in cerebral blood flow between the MCAs in real time, which was then confirmed to be a left MCA occlusion on MRI/MRA. QEEG can assess differences in cerebral perfusion after pediatric stroke, with decreased spectral edge frequency and alpha and beta power often observed in injured regions [2, 3]. The concurrent use of TCDs, cerebral regional oximetry and continuous EEG with QEEG provides noninvasive measures of cerebral hemodynamics after mechanical thrombectomy.

Key Neuromonitoring Findings

Acute reduction in cerebral regional oximetry along with asymmetric MCA MFVs and waveforms on TCD were the key findings suggestive of a left MCA occlusion (Figures C31.1 & C31.2). Daily TCDs were performed to monitor changes in MCA MFVs as a surrogate for vessel patency post-thrombectomy, which improved markedly and remained symmetric. Although continuous EEG monitoring was initiated following revascularization, asymmetric hemispheric slowing (left > right) also supported the diagnosis of a large vessel occlusion (Figure C31.4). The asymmetry on EEG eventually normalized with improved blood flow after thrombectomy.

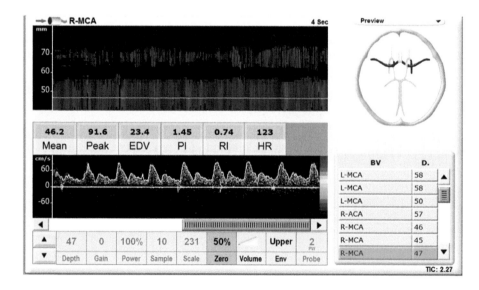

Figure C31.1 Right middle cerebral artery (MCA) mean flow velocity (46.2 cm/sec) is within the normal range with mildly elevated (1.45) pulsatility index (PI).

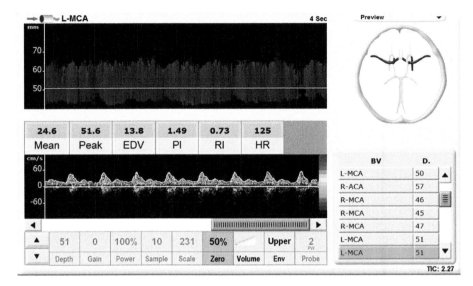

Figure C31.2 Left middle cerebral artery (MCA) mean flow velocity (24 cm/sec) is below the normal range and decreased compared to the right MCA. The pulsatility index (PI) for the left MCA is also mildly elevated (1.49). Given a sharp systolic upstroke with MFVs decreased by 47%, the left MCA waveform is concerning for dampened morphology (grade III) by the TIBI grading scale [1].

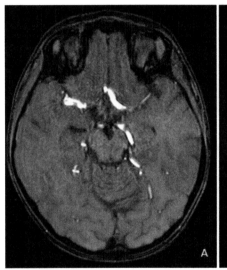
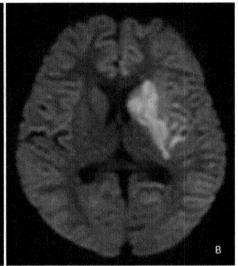

Figures C31.3 Panel A: Magnetic resonance angiography (MRA) shows complete occlusion of the left middle cerebral artery (MCA). Panel B: Diffusion-weighted imaging (DWI) demonstrates infarction in the left MCA distribution, primarily affecting the left basal ganglia and external capsule.

References

1. Demchuk AM, Burgin WS, Christou I, et al. Thrombolysis in brain ischemia (TIBI) transcranial Doppler flow grades predict clinical severity, early recovery, and mortality in patients treated with intravenous tissue plasminogen activator. *Stroke*. 2001 Jan;**32**(1):89–93.

2. Appavu BL, Temkit MH, Foldes ST, et al. Quantitative electroencephalography after pediatric anterior circulation stroke. *J Clin Neurophysiol*. 2020 Dec 29; Online ahead of print.

3. Foreman B, Claassen J. Quantitative EEG for the detection of brain ischemia. *Crit Care*. 2012 Dec 12;**16**(2):216.

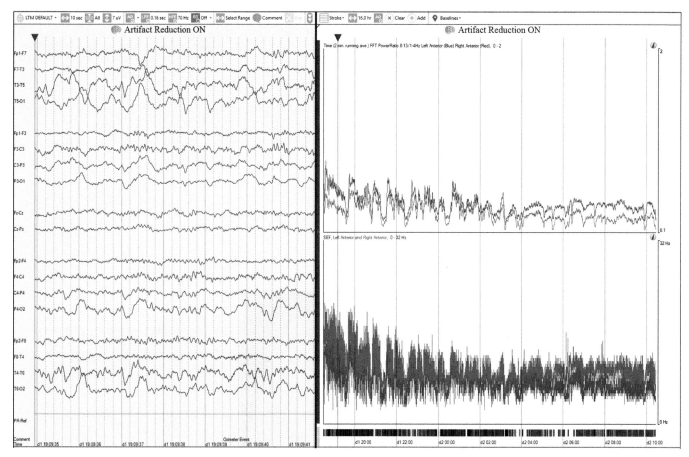

Figure C31.4 Continuous EEG demonstrates left hemispheric slowing on the raw EEG tracing and QEEG shows reduced alpha–delta ratio (upper right trend) and spectral edge frequency (lower right trend) over the left anterior head region (the left anterior head region is displayed in blue trends and the right anterior head region is displayed in red trends).

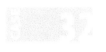

Multimodal Neurological Monitoring: Ventilation and Cerebral Perfusion

Rudolph Wong and Brian Appavu

Clinical Presentation

A 12-year-old boy collapsed while running outside. He had a temperature of 40.4°C and was unresponsive but hemodynamically stable. He was intubated due to a Glasgow Coma Score of 4 and treated for dehydration and heat stroke. He demonstrated a severe systemic inflammatory response with renal and hepatic failure. He was also found to have multifocal cerebral infarctions (Figure C32.1). Due to worsening hepatic encephalopathy and concerns for cerebral edema, mild hyperventilation was induced. Later, ventilation needs were reassessed in consideration of optimizing cerebral blood flow (CBF) and ventilation targets returned to normal. The effects of changes in ventilation on CBF were analyzed with continuous transcranial Doppler ultrasound (TCD) in conjunction with multimodal monitoring (MMM) incorporating continuous measurements of end-tidal CO_2 (EtCO$_2$), mean arterial blood pressure (mABP), and cerebral oximetry. He was treated with immunomodulation for severe inflammatory response and had a near full neurological recovery.

Discussion

Hepatic encephalopathy is a serious neurological condition that can lead to cerebral edema, severe intracranial hypertension (ICH) and death [1, 2]. ICH can be associated with systemic hypertension, and moderate hyperventilation is often used as a treatment strategy [3]. While ICH is a worrisome secondary insult, clinicians need to be mindful of the physiological parameters that drive CBF, particularly when limited to noninvasive monitoring.

Increases in arterial carbon dioxide content (Paco$_2$) cause cerebral vasodilation resulting in increased CBF, whereas decreases in Paco$_2$ cause cerebral vasoconstriction resulting in decreased CBF. Arterial carbon dioxide content (Paco$_2$) is primarily determined by minute ventilation, a product of respiratory rate and tidal volume, and can be approximated noninvasively by measuring EtCO$_2$. In the presence of ICH, hyperventilation can be used to reduce Paco$_2$, thereby causing vasoconstriction and reducing CBF, which can mitigate intracranial pressure elevations. However, in the absence of ICH from malignant cerebral edema, hyperventilation may actually be deleterious. In this patient, initial TCD findings were not suggestive of ICH from malignant cerebral edema as evidenced by Pulsatility Indices (PIs) < 1.1 [4]. With a decrease in ventilation, TCD left middle cerebral artery (MCA) mean flow velocities (MFVs) and cerebral oximetry increased, affirming that this change led to increased CBF and cerebral oxygenation. Furthermore, improved CBF led to a decrease in mABP as a result of normal cerebral autoregulation mechanisms.

Multimodal monitoring in this clinical scenario enabled a targeted ventilation strategy to optimize CBF and was able to demonstrate in real time the anticipated physiological effects.

Key Neuromonitoring Findings

On continuous EEG monitoring, the patient was noted to have generalized periodic discharges with triphasic morphology indicative of hepatic encephalopathy (Figure C32.2). Hyperventilation induced through a respiratory rate of 16–20 breaths per minute (bpm) resulted in an EtCO$_2$ level approximating 27 mmHg. Mean arterial blood pressure remained elevated, between 120 and 130 mmHg. Cerebral oximetry, assessed using near-infrared spectroscopy (NIRS), approximated 63%–68%. Transcranial Doppler ultrasound was performed with insonation of the left MCA. Initial left MCA MFVs approximated 43 cm/sec with a PI between 0.6 and 0.7 (Figure C32.3). The respiratory rate was then reduced from 16 to 10 bpm. Over the subsequent 30 minutes, EtCO$_2$ increased to 37 mmHg, left MCA MFVs increased from 43 to 50 cm/sec and cerebral oximetry increased from 63% to 72% (Figure C32.4). Mean arterial blood pressure decreased from 126 mmHg to 110–115 mmHg.

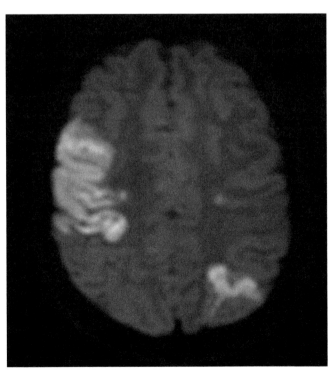

Figure C32.1 MRI brain scan reveals multifocal cerebral infarctions as evident on diffusion weighted imaging.

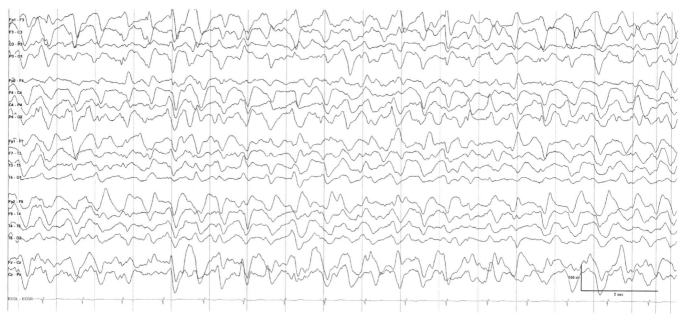

Figure C32.2 After worsening hepatic function, continuous EEG reveals generalized periodic discharges with triphasic morphology.

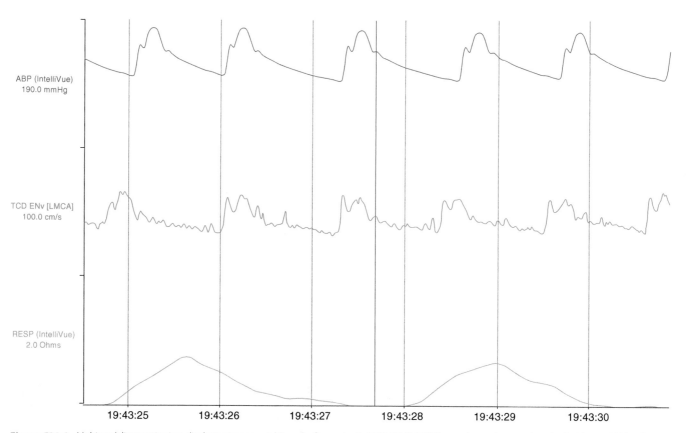

Figure C32.3 Multimodality monitoring, displaying transcranial Doppler flow velocity (TCD ENV [LMCA]) waveforms time synchronized with arterial blood pressure (ABP) and respirations (RESP).

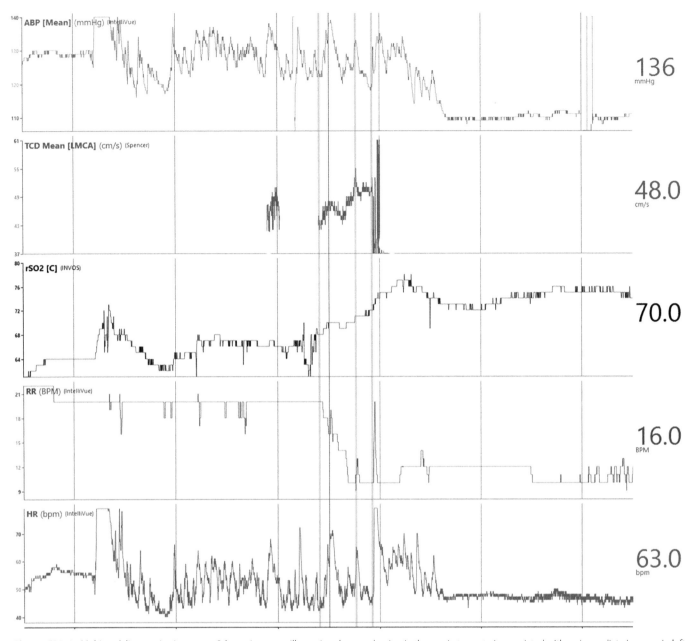

Figure C32.4 Multimodality monitoring over a 3-hour timespan, illustrating that a reduction in the respiratory rate is associated with an immediate increase in left transcranial Doppler mean flow velocities (TCD Mean [LMCA]) and cerebral regional oximetry (rSO$_2$ [C]), suggestive of increased blood flow. In the subsequent hour, mean arterial blood pressure (ABP [Mean]) decreases.

References

1. Reynolds AS, Brush B, Schiano T, Reilly K, Dangayach NS. Neurological monitoring in acute liver failure. *Hepatology*. 2019 Nov;**70**(5):1830–5.

2. Rashke RA, Curry SC, Rempe S, et al. Results of a protocol for management of patients with fulminant liver failure. *Crit Care Med*. 2008;**36**:2244–8.

3. Rangel-Castillo L, Gopinath S, Robertson CS. Management of intracranial hypertension. *Neurol Clin*. 2008 May;**26**(2):521–41.

4. O'Brien NF, Maa T, Reuter-Rice K. Noninvasive screening for intracranial hypertension in children with acute, severe traumatic brain injury. *J Neurosurg Pediatr*. 2015 Oct;**16**(4):420–5.

Index

abusive head trauma, 152, 275–6, 277, 278. *See also* non-accidental injury
ACNS. *See* American Clinical Neurophysiology Society
ACP. *See* antegrade cerebral perfusion
activation procedures, 24
  hyperventilation, 25
  photic stimulation, 25
activité moyenne, 60–1, 62
activity band, 49–50, 51
acute bilirubin encephalopathy, 227, 228, 229
acute brain injury, seizures risk with, 150
acute ischemic stroke, 116–17, 118
  cEEG monitoring of, 160–1, 300, 301, 302
  seizure risk with, 152
aEEG monitoring. *See* amplitude-integrated EEG monitoring
allopurinol, 171–3
alpha–delta power ratio, ischemia monitoring with, 159–60
American Academy of Pediatrics, clinical practice guidelines for use of therapeutic hypothermia in neonatal encephalopathy, 12
American Clinical Neurophysiology Society (ACNS)
  clinical practice guidelines and consensus statements
    cEEG monitoring in children, 12
    cEEG monitoring in neonates, 11–12, 173
  electrode placement recommendations, 19, 20
  patient selection guidelines, 30
  standard montages, 21
amplitude
  abnormal, 77–8
  artifactual asymmetry in, 67
  normal, 50–2, 57–9

amplitude grading system, for aEEG, 105–6, 107, 110
amplitude trends, 27
amplitude-integrated EEG (aEEG) monitoring
  abnormal patterns on, 43, 44, 90–3, 94, 95, 97
  artifacts on, 69, 206–7
  background continuity on, 49–50, 51
  bedside, 35–6
  documentation of, 45–6
  of electrographic seizures in critically ill children, 14–15
  of electrographic seizures in critically ill neonates, 13–15
  in neonatal encephalopathy, 103–4
    findings in HIE, 105–7, 110
    outcome prediction using, 112–14
    sedation and other neuroprotective agent effects on, 108–9
  of neonatal onset epilepsy, 129–31
  of newborn heart surgery, 175–6
  normal amplitudes in, 50, 51, 57–9
  normal patterns on, 40, 41
    overview of preterm and full-term newborns, 56–9
    at 24–27 weeks conceptional age, 59
    at 28–31 weeks conceptional age, 59–60
    at 32–35 weeks conceptional age, 60
    at 36–37 weeks conceptional age, 60
    at 38–42 weeks conceptional age, 61
  post-cardiac arrest, 191–5, 196–7
  seizure detection with, 91–3, 95, 97, 138–9
  technical aspects of, 25, 26
anesthetic therapies
  EEG effects of, 160

  for refractory status epilepticus, 144–5
antegrade cerebral perfusion (ACP), 167, 176
anti-seizure medications (ASMs)
  diazepam, 140, 142–3
  EEG/aEEG effects of, 108–9
  levetiracetam, 140–1, 142–3, 176
  lidocaine, 176
  lorazepam, 140, 142–3
  in neonatal epilepsies, 131
  observational studies of neonatal outcomes with, 9–10
  pentobarbital, 142–3, 144
  phenobarbital, 108–9, 140–1, 142–3, 144–5, 176
  phenytoin, 140–1, 142–3, 176
  for post-operative seizure after newborn heart surgery, 176
  propofol, 142–3, 144–5, 160
  for status epilepticus
    benzodiazepines, 140, 142–3, 144
    continuous infusions of, 144–5
    non-benzodiazepines, 140–1, 142–3
  thiopental, 142–3, 144
  topiramate, 176
  valproate, 140–1, 142–3
artifact reduction, 27
artifacts, 48, 66
  during ECMO, 182–7
  EEG filters for, 22
    high frequency, 23
    low frequency, 23
    notch, 23, 24
  extracerebral channels in detection of, 23–4
  neonatal, 106
  physiological, 66–7, 68, 69, 70, 71, 72, 73
  on QEEG, 69, 206–7
  review for, 43–4
  technical and environmental, 67–8, 74, 75
ARX mutations, 132

ASMs. *See* anti-seizure medications
asymmetry
  artifactual, 67
  background, 52, 53
  recognition of, 43
attenuated featureless background, 79–80, 82
autoimmune encephalitis, 145, 152, 289–90
average reference, 21

background, EEG
  abnormal patterns on, 43, 76, 93
    in infants and children, 79–80, 81, 82, 83
    in neonates, 76–9, 80
    seizure risk with, 151
  age-related specific activity in, 54
  asymmetry in, 52, 53
  continuity of, 48–50, 51
  global analysis of, 48–53
  in neonatal epilepsies, 128, 129
  in newborn heart surgery, 167–9, 170
  normal patterns on, 40, 41, 42
  post-cardiac arrest, 196–7
  prognostication using, 4–5, 77–80, 81, 82, 83
  variability and reactivity of, 52–3
baclofen intoxication, 294–6
bacterial meningoencephalitis, 119, 152, 279–81
bedside neuromonitoring
  monitors used for, 35–6
  nurse roles in, 35, 36, 46, 47
    abnormal pattern reporting, 43–5
    clinical event marking, 40
    documentation in patient records, 45–6
    education and training in brain monitoring, 46
    equipment selection, 36
    interprofessional communication facilitation, 45
    maintenance of brain monitoring, 37–40